RECLAIM YOUR HEALTH

Learn how to overcome the most common chronic illnesses

STEM CELLS

The Future of Regenerative Medicine

By Award Winning Author

Dr. Harris Phillip

BSc, MSc, MBBS, FRCOG, FACOG, LLM

Death is the result of degeneration of the body. Let's stop the degeneration and begin the regenerative process. Stem cells, with functional guard rails, the future of Regenerative Medicine.

Table of Contents

Foreword

By Professor Ali Nakash

While continuing with his 30+ years of experience in clinical practice, Harris has decided to sum up much of what he has gained from seeing and treating thousands, maybe millions, of patients with many medical problems over the years. In his summary, compiled into a series of twelve chunk-sized books, the reader is provided with usable tools presented in a simple, readily digestible format to allow everyone to benefit. From the least medically inclined among us to the nursing student, the pharmacy student, the nurse, the pharmacist, the midwifery student, the midwife, the medical student, and the trained doctor, whether junior or senior. In essence, there are useful nuggets of easy-to-follow guidance for all. In the first book in the series, he starts with a disease we all dread. Many, including my wife, call it that disease.... You certainly know the disease to which I refer; it is cancer. Reading through the pages of the first book in this series, I was immediately impressed with the presentation. Such a complex condition was condensed into such simple and easy-to-follow guidance. Not only has he addressed cancer from its cellular level, but he has also extended the discussion to allow you, the reader, to appreciate plausible causative agents for this condition once it is initiated. He gives some Reclaim Your Health-Cancer, he gives some insight into how the disease process flourishes, and towards the end of the book, he addresses how we can make ourselves cancer-proof. Making ourselves cancer-proof, I find, is particularly interesting since it allows both medical and non-medical personnel to explore avenues through which they can empower both themselves and their patients as together we fight this dreaded disease. In the other books of this series, which are being completed, the approach is the same, whether it is addressing Alzheimer's disease, cardiovascular disease, diabetes, or the other chronic health challenges of our time. I am particularly impressed with the presentation, the relative simplicity, and the inherent usefulness of this series, which doubtlessly will empower and serve as a useful companion handbook on our journey to reclaiming our health. Mr Phillip is an award-winning author for his book STOP! It's Not Too Late: Adding Years to Your Life and Life to Your Years Using the BMS Model, a book which I call an encyclopaedic guide to healthy living. But in this book series, I think he has outdone himself as he seeks to provide the tools that we all need to reclaim our health. He has most definitely put his years of training and experience in capsule form through the various books in this series. Mr Phillip is a trained senior consultant obstetrician and gynaecologist. He has displayed his abundance of knowledge through the ease with which he addresses the various chronic health challenges of our times. This series, for me, represents an interesting and empowering piece of medical science which has been presented in a digestible format for even the non-medical personnel among us. I am therefore moved to make this bold prediction that once you start reading these books, you will find it difficult to stop because of the timeliness and appropriateness of their contents.

A Note from the author

In a world where healthcare often feels impersonal, reactive, and fragmented, Reclaim Your Health offers a bold and compassionate alternative. This twelve-book series was born from a simple yet powerful conviction: that patients deserve not only access to care, but ownership of it. As a clinician, innovator, and educator, I have witnessed first-hand the transformative impact of knowledge—when patients understand their bodies, their conditions, and their options, they become active participants in their healing. This series is designed to bridge the gap between clinical expertise and everyday experience, translating complex medical concepts into clear, actionable guidance. Nine volumes have already been published, each tackling a vital dimension of conservative care—with clarity, empathy, and scientific rigor. The remaining three volumes are in advanced stages of preparation, and I will complete the series in the coming year. Reclaim Your Health is more than a collection of books. It is a movement toward autonomy, dignity, and informed decision-making. It complements our broader mission—through medical device innovation and workforce development—to reshape healthcare from the ground up. Whether you are a patient seeking answers, a clinician striving to educate, or a policymaker looking to support sustainable care models, this series is for you. May it inspire confidence, spark dialogue, and above all, help you reclaim what matters most: your health.

Harris Phillip Founder,

Philburn Academy

Healthcare Entrepreneur & Innovator United Kingdom

Introduction

Several years ago, I was employed as a teacher, which incidentally was my first professional job. While entering the classroom to deliver a biology lecture to a group of students at Saint Andrews High School, who were preparing to write the General Certificate of Education examination (GCE or GCSE as referred to in the UK), a young man who claimed he had no interest in biology collected his books and was leaving the classroom to go to the library. The lecture was designed to highlight the characteristics of living things and to help distinguish the living from the dead. I commenced the lecture with the statement, 'Once one starts living, he/she starts dying'. Inherent in that statement is that both living and dying are processes. Even deeper is the realisation that what we refer to as life is simply a grant. You see, we are given two dates and a dash. The dash is our life, the period between our date of birth and our date of death. Upon hearing this introduction, the young man made an about-turn and asked permission to attend my lecture. I did not convert him into a biologist, but he left the class much better informed. Today, this young man is a politician. The dash is the focus of this book: how can we extend the dash to delay our date of death? I prefer to look at the whole scenario as a rubber band that can be stretched between two points, the two points being the date of birth and the date of death. We can do nothing about our date of birth; that date is beyond our control, but if my analogy of a rubber band is fully understood and since our date of birth cannot be seriously influenced by our action or inaction, the rubber band concept to hold, it means that the dash can be extended and thus we can delay our date of death. My paternal grandmother, for instance, lived to a ripe old age of 115. She lived a fully independent life, still being able to cook and care for herself in her 115th year. This is not widespread, I hear you say, and my response is: why not? Do we have any skills, knowledge, or abilities in the current era to approach this lifespan and make it more of the expected norm as opposed to an occasional event? It is with this burning desire that I have used my medical knowledge gleaned in the field, as well as my extensive research, the skills of which I learned as a university student in organic and biochemistry at a top 10 USA university, as I pursued a PhD degree in Biochemistry. This training not only provided me with the skills and tools which I needed to pursue the more inquisitive aspect of my person but also alerted me to the value of research. Thus, when faced with a challenging question, I revert to research to help me determine the answer. In observing the lifestyle of my paternal grandmother, my 30+ years of medical practice, drawing on the knowledge gleaned through my research and from my study in organic chemistry, leading to my master's degree and my sojourn through the biochemistry classroom, I believe that we have an opportunity to delay the second date, the date of death, by stretching in rubber band style the duration of the dash. This is the purpose of this book series: providing tools, suggestions, and basic information that will hopefully allow you to prolong your dash and live a more dynamic and healthier lifestyle, thus adding years to your life and life to your years. I will aim to provide books on each of the nine chronic ailments, suggesting how best one can delay the insult on our bodies, hence allowing us to live a more complete, fun-filled life, a guide to which has been developed in one of my earlier books, using the BMS approach, an award-winning book. In this book series, we will look at cancer, Alzheimer's, dementia and diseases of the brain, heart disease and strokes, diabetes, arthritis, obesity, chronic lung disease, and chronic kidney diseases, hoping that this serves as a useful handbook – guide, if you will – in understanding and defeating the most common chronic ailments affecting human beings on planet earth. I know that you may be stunned: why have a trained obstetrician and gynaecologist got involved in the writing of books addressing various aspects of health, some of which may be remote from obstetrics (care of pregnant ladies during their pregnancy and childbirth) and gynaecology (the branch of medicine which deals with the functions and diseases specific to women and girls, specifically those related to the reproductive system)? This discipline is the only medical discipline which allows one to practise all the facets of medicine. It, therefore, means that any good obstetrician or gynaecologist, because of the demands on his scope of practice, needs to be above average in his knowledge of internal medicine, surgery, paediatrics, social and preventive medicine, care of the elderly, and neonatology. Hence, my familiarity with these various disciplines and the related physiology has empowered me in the provision of this book series, which I am hopeful will be an empowering tool to help many understand elements of their health while simultaneously allowing them to know when things are wrong and therefore the need to seek medical advice. Hopefully, the message is that the earlier a disease process is found, the more options will be available for management, and the more likely a full cure will be realised.

Chapter 1
Introduction to Stem Cell Biology

Overview of Stem Cell Types

Stem cells are classified into various types, each with distinct properties and potential applications in medicine. The two primary categories are embryonic stem cells (ESCs) and adult stem cells (ASCs). ESCs, derived from early-stage embryos, possess the unique ability to differentiate into any cell type in the body, making them incredibly versatile for research and therapeutic purposes. In contrast, ASCs, which are found in various tissues throughout the body, have a more limited differentiation potential but are crucial for tissue maintenance and repair.

The therapeutic applications of ESCs and ASCs differ significantly. ESCs have shown promise in regenerative medicine due to their pluripotency, allowing for the generation of specific cell types needed for repairing damaged tissues. Clinical trials have explored the use of ESCs in treating conditions such as spinal cord injuries and degenerative diseases. Conversely, ASCs have been successfully employed in therapies for conditions like blood disorders and certain cancers, showcasing their role in established treatment protocols.

When evaluating the efficacy of stem cell sources, the differentiation potential of ESCs often gives them an edge in experimental settings. However, ASCs are generally less controversial and may elicit a lower immune response, making them preferable for certain patient populations. This immune compatibility is particularly relevant in the context of allogeneic therapies, where the stem cells are sourced from a donor rather than the patient.

Long-term outcomes of treatments derived from various stem cell types remain a critical area of research. Preliminary findings suggest that while ESC-based therapies may offer greater initial benefits due to their versatility, ASCs might provide more sustainable outcomes with fewer complications over time. Additionally, the cost-effectiveness of these therapies is a growing concern, as the production and application of ESCs can be more resource-intensive compared to ASCs, which can often be harvested from the patient and used in a more straightforward manner.

The role of stem cell niches in tissue engineering and repair is another vital aspect of understanding stem cell functionality. These niches provide the necessary microenvironment for stem cells to thrive and differentiate effectively. Investigating how these niches contribute to the regeneration process can enhance the development of targeted therapies. As research evolves, the comparison of ESCs and ASCs will continue to shape clinical applications and ethical considerations in the field of regenerative medicine.

Historical Context of Stem Cell Research

The historical context of stem cell research is deeply intertwined with advancements in medical science and ethical debates that have shaped its trajectory over the decades. The discovery of stem cells dates to the early 20th century, when scientists first identified the unique properties of these cells that allow them to differentiate into various cell types. This foundational work laid the groundwork for understanding both embryonic and adult stem cells, and their potential applications in regenerative medicine and therapeutic interventions.

In the 1970s and 1980s, significant milestones were achieved, particularly in the isolation and culture of hematopoietic stem cells, which are responsible for blood formation. This period marked the beginning of clinical applications that utilised adult stem cells for treating conditions such as leukaemia through bone marrow transplants. As researchers gained insights into the differentiation potential of these cells, interest in embryonic stem cells surged, especially following their successful isolation in the late 1990s. This breakthrough ignited a fervent debate regarding the ethical implications of using human embryos in research.

The ethical discussions surrounding embryonic stem cell research have predominantly revolved around the moral status of the human embryo and the implications of potential life. These debates have led to varying regulatory frameworks across countries, influencing funding, research directions, and clinical applications. Notably, the United States experienced significant political fluctuations in stem cell policy, impacting both public and private funding for research. Conversely, countries such as the UK established more permissive guidelines that allowed for extensive research and clinical trials involving embryonic stem cells.

As the field matured, the comparative efficacy of embryonic versus adult stem cells became a focal point for researchers and clinicians alike. Numerous clinical trials have been initiated to evaluate the long-term outcomes of therapies derived from both sources. These studies aim to elucidate the advantages and limitations inherent in each type of stem cell, particularly concerning their immune response, differentiation potential, and overall effectiveness in treating diverse conditions. The results of these trials are pivotal in determining the future direction of stem cell therapies in clinical practice.

In contemporary research, the emphasis has shifted towards harnessing the advantages of both embryonic and adult stem cells while also exploring novel approaches such as induced pluripotent stem cells (iPSCs). These advancements highlight the ongoing dialogue between scientific innovation and ethical considerations, as the medical community seeks to balance efficacy with moral responsibilities. Understanding the historical context of stem cell research is essential for medical personnel, researchers, and ethicists as they navigate the complexities of therapeutic applications and regulatory frameworks in their pursuit of regenerative medicine.

Ethical Considerations in Stem Cell Research

The ethical considerations surrounding stem cell research are multifaceted and deeply significant, particularly in the context of embryonic and adult stem cells. Ethical dilemmas often arise from the source of the stem cells, as embryonic stem cells are derived from human embryos, leading to debates about the moral status of the embryo. Medical personnel and ethicists must navigate these complex discussions, balancing the potential for groundbreaking therapies against the respect for human life and the implications of embryo destruction. This tension highlights the need for clear ethical guidelines that can inform research practices while considering societal values.

In comparison, adult stem cells, which can be sourced from tissues such as bone marrow and adipose tissue, present a different ethical landscape. The use of adult stem cells raises fewer moral objections, as their extraction typically does not involve the destruction of embryos. This aspect makes adult stem cells a more palatable option for many stakeholders, including oversight bodies and the public. However, the limitations in differentiation potential and the efficacy of adult stem cells in certain therapeutic applications must be carefully considered, prompting discussions on the balance between ethical acceptability and clinical effectiveness.

The efficacy of stem cell sources is crucial for advancing regenerative medicine. Clinical trials comparing the outcomes of therapies using embryonic versus adult stem cells reveal varying degrees of success, with embryonic stem cells often demonstrating superior differentiation potential. It is essential for biomedical research scientists to assess the long-term outcomes of treatments involving different stem cell types, as these findings directly impact clinical decision-making and patient care. Understanding the complexities of these outcomes helps in shaping future research directions and therapeutic strategies.

Furthermore, the immune response to stem cell therapies is an important consideration that intersects with ethical discussions. While embryonic stem cells may provoke less of an immune response due to their pluripotent nature, adult stem cells often require careful matching to the recipient to avoid rejection. This aspect not only influences the effectiveness of treatments but also raises ethical questions regarding patient consent, risk, and the potential for unforeseen complications in therapy. Addressing these issues is vital for ensuring that stem cell research adheres to the highest ethical standards.

Lastly, the cost-effectiveness of embryonic and adult stem cell therapies must be evaluated within the broader context of healthcare resources. As healthcare systems worldwide grapple with budget constraints, the economic implications of stem cell interventions play a significant role in their adoption. Stakeholders must consider not only the financial aspects but also the societal benefits of improved health outcomes. In this light, a comprehensive approach to ethical considerations in stem cell research will support informed decision-making that respects both scientific advancement and ethical integrity.

Embryonic Stem Cells

Characteristics of Embryonic Stem Cells

Embryonic stem cells (ESCs) are unique in their ability to differentiate into virtually any cell type in the human body, a characteristic known as pluripotency. This remarkable potential arises from their origin in the early stages of embryonic development, where they exist as a clump of cells prior to the formation of specific tissues. The inherent plasticity of ESCs makes them a focal point in regenerative medicine, offering the possibility of treating a wide range of conditions, from neurodegenerative diseases to spinal cord injuries.

One of the defining characteristics of ESCs is their self-renewal capability, allowing them to divide indefinitely while maintaining their undifferentiated state. This property is crucial for both research and therapeutic applications, as it enables the production of large quantities of stem cells for use in clinical settings. Unlike adult stem cells, which are often limited in their ability to proliferate and differentiate, ESCs provide a more versatile platform for developing novel treatments that require extensive cell populations.

The immune response to ESC therapies is another critical aspect to consider when evaluating their clinical applications. Since ESCs are derived from embryos, their introduction into a patient's body can elicit an immune reaction, depending on the genetic compatibility between the donor and recipient. This potential for rejection contrasts with adult stem cells, which are typically harvested from the patient, thereby reducing the risk of immunogenicity and making them a more favourable option in some cases.

In terms of long-term outcomes, studies have shown that therapies using ESCs can lead to significant improvements in tissue repair and regeneration. However, concerns remain regarding the ethical implications of using embryonic sources, as well as the potential for tumour formation due to the uncontrolled growth of pluripotent cells. Hence, a careful evaluation of the risks and benefits is essential when considering ESCs in therapeutic applications, especially in comparison to adult stem cell alternatives.

Finally, the cost-effectiveness of employing ESCs versus adult stem cells in clinical settings often comes under scrutiny. While ESCs may offer superior differentiation potential and self-renewal capabilities, the overall costs associated with their use, including sourcing, culturing, and regulatory compliance, can be substantial. Therefore, ongoing clinical trials comparing the efficacy of these two stem cell types are vital in establishing a clearer understanding of their respective roles in therapeutic contexts and determining the most economically viable options for patient care.

Sources of Embryonic Stem Cells

Embryonic stem cells (ESCs) are derived from the inner cell mass of blastocysts, typically harvested from in vitro fertilisation (IVF) clinics. These cells possess unique properties, including the ability to self-renew indefinitely and differentiate into any cell type in the human body. This pluripotency makes them exceptionally valuable for regenerative medicine, as they can potentially be used to generate tissues and organs for transplantation, addressing a wide range of degenerative diseases and injuries. The ethical considerations surrounding the use of ESCs primarily stem from the destruction of embryos, which necessitates stringent oversight and guidelines from regulatory bodies.

In contrast, adult stem cells (ASCs) are found in various tissues throughout the body, such as bone marrow, fat, and blood. Unlike ESCs, ASCs are multipotent, meaning they can only differentiate into a limited range of cell types relevant to their tissue of origin. While ASCs have been used successfully in therapies, such as hematopoietic stem cell transplantation for blood disorders, their differentiation potential is often considered less robust compared to ESCs.

This limitation raises questions regarding the efficacy of ASCs in complex tissue regeneration compared to their embryonic counterparts.

The therapeutic applications of ESCs extend beyond mere differentiation, as they hold potential for drug testing and disease modelling. By generating specific cell types from ESCs, researchers can create in vitro models that closely mimic human diseases, allowing for the screening of new drugs and the understanding of disease mechanisms. This application underscores the importance of ESCs in biomedical research, providing insights that could lead to novel therapeutic strategies. The comparative analysis of ESCs and ASCs in clinical trials further elucidates their respective advantages and limitations in therapeutic contexts.

One significant aspect of stem cell therapies is the immune response elicited by the host. ESCs, being derived from embryos, may possess antigens that can provoke an immune reaction when transplanted into an adult recipient. Conversely, ASCs, particularly those harvested from the same individual (autologous sources), tend to be less immunogenic, reducing the risk of rejection. Understanding these immune dynamics is crucial for developing effective stem cell therapies and ensuring long-term success in clinical applications.

Lastly, the cost-effectiveness of stem cell therapies remains a pivotal consideration for healthcare systems. While ESC therapies may offer greater differentiation potential and broader applications, the ethical, regulatory, and procedural costs associated with their procurement can be substantial. In contrast, ASCs, often more accessible and less controversial, can provide immediate therapeutic benefits with potentially lower costs. The ongoing debate about the efficacy and application of both stem cell types necessitates a thorough examination of clinical outcomes, patient safety, and economic viability in the field of regenerative medicine.

Differentiation Potential and Applications

The differentiation potential of stem cells is a crucial aspect that determines their applicability in therapeutic contexts. Embryonic stem cells (ESCs) possess an unparalleled ability to differentiate into any cell type within the human body, making them a prime candidate for regenerative medicine. In contrast, adult stem cells (ASCs), while capable of differentiating into a limited range of cell types specific to their tissue of origin, offer a unique advantage in terms of ethical considerations and lower immunogenicity. Understanding these differences is vital for medical personnel and researchers exploring the most effective treatment pathways for various conditions.

In terms of therapeutic applications, ESCs have shown promise in treating complex conditions such as spinal cord injuries and neurodegenerative diseases due to their pluripotent nature. However, the use of ESCs raises ethical concerns due to the destruction of embryos during their procurement. Adult stem cells, sourced from tissues such as bone marrow or adipose tissue, have demonstrated efficacy in treating blood disorders and certain musculoskeletal injuries, presenting a more ethically acceptable alternative. This juxtaposition highlights the need for a balanced evaluation of both sources in clinical practice.

The efficacy of stem cell sources in regenerative medicine is further influenced by their ability to integrate into existing tissues and engender functional recovery.

Clinical trials have begun to provide comparative data on the outcomes of treatments using ESCs versus ASCs, revealing that while ESCs may offer superior differentiation potential, ASCs often lead to more favourable long-term outcomes due to their compatibility with the recipient's immune system. This aspect is particularly relevant in the context of immune response, as ASC therapies tend to elicit a lower incidence of rejection than their embryonic counterparts.

Cost-effectiveness is another critical factor when considering the application of stem cell therapies. While ESCs may initially appear more expensive due to the complexities involved in their use, the long-term benefits they offer in terms of regenerative capabilities could justify the investment. Conversely, ASCs are often more readily available and less costly to obtain in clinical settings, making them an attractive option for many healthcare providers. This economic analysis is essential for oversight bodies when evaluating which therapies to endorse and support in clinical practice.

Lastly, the role of stem cell niches in tissue engineering and repair cannot be overlooked. Both ESCs and ASCs require specific microenvironments to thrive and differentiate effectively. Research into these niches has revealed that manipulating the local cellular environment can enhance the therapeutic potential of stem cells, thereby improving outcomes in regenerative applications. Future studies aimed at elucidating these interactions will be pivotal in advancing stem cell therapies and ensuring their successful integration into standard medical practice.

Adult Stem Cells

Characteristics of Adult Stem Cells

Adult stem cells are a unique population of undifferentiated cells found in various tissues throughout the body. Unlike embryonic stem cells, which are pluripotent and can differentiate into any cell type, adult stem cells are typically multipotent, meaning they are limited to differentiating into a narrower range of cell types. This characteristic makes them particularly valuable in regenerative medicine, where they can contribute to the repair and maintenance of specific tissues. For instance, haematopoietic stem cells in the bone marrow give rise to various blood cells, illustrating their critical role in blood regeneration and immune function.

In terms of therapeutic applications, adult stem cells have demonstrated significant efficacy in treating a variety of conditions. For example, they are commonly used in bone marrow transplants for patients with leukaemia and other blood disorders. Clinical trials have shown that these stem cells can improve patient outcomes and reduce recovery times. The ability of adult stem cells to be harvested from the patient's own body also reduces the risk of immune rejection, a significant advantage over embryonic stem cells that may provoke an immune response.

The differentiation potential of adult stem cells, while more limited compared to embryonic counterparts, is nonetheless impressive. Research has shown that certain adult stem cells can exhibit plasticity, allowing them to differentiate into cell types outside their typical lineage under specific conditions. This adaptability opens new avenues for tissue engineering and the development of therapies for various degenerative diseases. However, the mechanisms governing this plasticity remain an area of active investigation, as understanding these processes could enhance the utility of adult stem cells in clinical settings.

Another critical aspect to consider is the long-term outcomes associated with different stem cell types. Studies have indicated that therapies using adult stem cells often lead to more stable and durable results, potentially due to their role in tissue maintenance and repair. In contrast, while embryonic stem cells may provide initial advantages in differentiation, issues related to tumorigenesis and long-term integration into host tissues pose challenges. This distinction is crucial for medical personnel and researchers when evaluating the best stem cell sources for specific therapeutic applications.

Cost-effectiveness is also a significant factor in the ongoing debate between embryonic and adult stem cell therapies. Adult stem cell procedures, such as bone marrow transplants, have established protocols and a history of successful outcomes, making them more readily accessible and financially viable in many healthcare settings. In contrast, embryonic stem cell therapies are often still in experimental stages, which can lead to higher costs and uncertainties in their clinical application. Understanding these economic implications is essential for oversight bodies and ethicists as they consider the future of stem cell research and therapy.

Sources of Adult Stem Cells

Adult stem cells, also known as somatic or tissue stem cells, are found throughout the human body and play a crucial role in tissue repair and regeneration. Unlike embryonic stem cells, which have the potential to differentiate into any cell type, adult stem cells are typically limited to differentiating into the cell types of their tissue of origin. This unique characteristic makes them particularly valuable in regenerative medicine, as they are already adapted to specific environments and functions within the body.

The primary sources of adult stem cells include bone marrow, adipose tissue, and peripheral blood. Bone marrow is the most extensively studied source and contains hematopoietic stem cells, which are responsible for producing blood cells. Adipose tissue, often discarded during surgical procedures, contains mesenchymal stem cells that can differentiate into a variety of cell types, including osteoblasts, chondrocytes, and adipocytes. Peripheral blood is another source, where mobilised stem cells can be harvested, particularly in the context of certain diseases or after chemotherapy.

In addition to these sources, umbilical cord blood has emerged as an important reservoir of hematopoietic stem cells, offering a less invasive option for stem cell collection. The use of umbilical cord blood stem cells presents ethical advantages over embryonic stem cells, as the collection process does not involve harm to the donor. This has led to an increase in cord blood banking and its application in various therapeutic contexts, including blood disorders and transplantation.

The immunological properties of adult stem cells also warrant discussion, as they generally exhibit reduced immunogenicity compared to embryonic stem cells. This characteristic makes adult stem cells less likely to provoke an immune response when transplanted into a host, thereby improving their utility in clinical settings. However, the effectiveness of adult stem cells can vary based on the source, age of the donor, and the specific therapeutic application being targeted.

In conclusion, while adult stem cells may not possess the same extensive differentiation potential as embryonic stem cells, their readily available sources and lower ethical concerns make them a vital component of contemporary therapeutic strategies. Continued research into the various sources and applications of adult stem cells is essential for enhancing their efficacy in regenerative medicine and improving long-term outcomes for patients.

Differentiation Potential and Applications

Differentiation potential is a fundamental characteristic that distinguishes embryonic stem cells (ESCs) from adult stem cells (ASCs). ESCs possess the unique ability to differentiate into any cell type in the body, which is attributed to their pluripotent nature. This capacity allows for extensive applications in regenerative medicine, where the goal is to repair or replace damaged tissues and organs. In contrast, ASCs are multipotent and can only differentiate into a limited range of cell types related to their tissue of origin, which can restrict their therapeutic applications. Understanding these differences is crucial for clinicians and researchers when considering the best approaches for patient treatment and tissue engineering.

The therapeutic applications of stem cells have gained considerable attention in recent years, with both ESCs and ASCs showing promise in various clinical trials. ESCs have been explored for their potential in treating conditions such as spinal cord injuries, neurodegenerative disorders, and heart diseases. These applications leverage their ability to generate diverse cell types that can integrate into damaged tissues. Conversely, ASCs have been successfully employed in therapies for certain blood disorders, orthopaedic injuries, and skin regeneration, showcasing their effectiveness in specific contexts. The ongoing research into the comparative efficacy of these two stem cell sources continues to yield insights that could guide future clinical practices.

Regenerative medicine relies heavily on the differentiation potential of stem cells, making the understanding of their source paramount. ESCs, due to their pluripotency, can be cultured to produce large quantities of specific cell types needed for therapeutic purposes. This trait makes them highly desirable for developing tissue-engineered products. On the other hand, ASCs are often more readily available and ethically accepted, although their differentiation potential may limit the range of applications. Nevertheless, researchers are investigating innovative techniques to enhance the efficacy of ASCs, such as reprogramming them to exhibit pluripotent characteristics, thereby expanding their therapeutic potential.

The immune response to stem cell therapies is another critical consideration in the field. ESCs, being derived from embryos, may provoke an immune reaction in patients due to their foreign nature. In contrast, ASCs, which are derived from the patients themselves or closely related donors, often present a lower risk of immune rejection. This aspect significantly influences the long-term outcomes of treatments using different stem cell types, as minimising immune response can lead to improved patient outcomes. Ongoing clinical trials are essential to elucidate these dynamics further and inform best practices in stem cell therapy.

Finally, the cost-effectiveness of embryonic and adult stem cell therapies remains a topic of significant interest. While ESCs may offer broader therapeutic possibilities, the costs associated with their procurement, ethical considerations, and regulatory hurdles can be substantial. In contrast, ASCs are generally less expensive to harvest and utilise, making them more accessible in many clinical settings. Evaluating the financial implications alongside the clinical efficacy of these therapies is vital for healthcare providers and oversight bodies as they navigate the complexities of stem cell applications in modern medicine.

Comparative Efficacy of Stem Cell Sources

Mechanisms of Action

The mechanisms of action of stem cells, particularly in the context of embryonic and adult sources, represent a pivotal area of inquiry in regenerative medicine. Embryonic stem cells (ESCs) possess an inherent ability to differentiate into any cell type within the body, which is attributed to their pluripotent nature. This distinguishes them from adult stem cells (ASCs), which are generally multipotent and limited to differentiating into a narrower range of cell types. Understanding these fundamental differences in differentiation potential is essential for evaluating the efficacy of stem cell therapies across various clinical applications.

In regenerative medicine, the therapeutic applications of ESCs and ASCs showcase diverse capabilities. ESCs have shown promise in treating conditions such as spinal cord injuries and neurodegenerative diseases due to their extensive differentiation potential. Conversely, ASCs, derived from tissues like bone marrow or adipose tissue, are often employed in the repair of specific organs, such as the heart and liver, due to their ability to regenerate tissue within their native niches. This functional disparity highlights the importance of selecting an appropriate stem cell source based on the intended therapeutic outcome.

The immune response to stem cell therapies is another critical mechanism of action that influences treatment efficacy and safety. ESCs are often associated with a higher risk of immune rejection due to their foreign nature, especially when derived from donors. In contrast, ASCs, being autologous in many cases, tend to elicit a more favourable immune response, thus reducing the likelihood of complications. This aspect not only affects patient outcomes but also underscores the need for rigorous assessment of immunogenicity in clinical trials comparing different stem cell sources.

Long-term outcomes of treatments using various stem cell types further elucidate the mechanisms of action involved in regenerative therapies. Studies have shown that while ESC-based treatments may initially provide robust improvements, the longevity of these effects can vary significantly. ASCs, on the other hand, often demonstrate more sustainable outcomes in certain contexts, primarily due to their inherent role in tissue homeostasis and repair. Evaluating these long-term effects is vital for understanding the overall effectiveness and safety profile of stem cell therapies.

Finally, the cost-effectiveness of embryonic and adult stem cell therapies plays a crucial role in their clinical application. ESCs may entail higher initial research and development costs due to ethical and regulatory hurdles, while ASCs are often more readily available and less expensive to procure. Balancing these economic considerations with the potential benefits of each stem cell type is essential for healthcare providers, ethicists, and oversight bodies as they navigate the complex landscape of stem cell research and application in medicine.

Efficacy in Regenerative Medicine

The efficacy of regenerative medicine largely relies on the source and characteristics of stem cells employed in clinical applications. Embryonic stem cells (ESCs) are renowned for their pluripotency, enabling them to differentiate into any cell type, thus presenting a broader therapeutic potential compared to adult stem cells (ASCs). However, ethical considerations surrounding the use of embryonic cells often overshadow their scientific advantages, leading to a complex landscape where the efficacy of both cell types must be critically assessed in relation to their clinical applications.

When comparing the therapeutic applications of ESCs and ASCs, one must consider the specific conditions being treated. ESCs have shown promising results in preclinical studies for conditions such as spinal cord injuries and neurodegenerative diseases due to their ability to generate a wider variety of cell types. Conversely, ASCs, derived from adult tissues, have demonstrated efficacy in treatments such as cardiac repair and bone regeneration, where the niche environment plays a crucial role in their functionality and integration into existing tissues.

The differentiation potential of stem cells is a key factor influencing their efficacy in regenerative medicine. While ESCs can easily transform into various cell lineages, the differentiation of ASCs is often limited to their tissue of origin, which can restrict their therapeutic applications. Nonetheless, the unique properties of ASCs, such as their ability to modulate immune responses and promote tissue repair, make them valuable candidates for specific therapeutic contexts, particularly where minimising immunogenicity is essential.

Long-term outcomes of treatments using different stem cell types also reveal contrasting efficacy profiles. Clinical trials have demonstrated that while ESC-based therapies may offer robust initial responses, concerns regarding teratoma formation and long-term stability remain. In contrast, ASC therapies have generally shown more predictable outcomes and fewer adverse effects, making them a safer option in many cases. This aspect is crucial for patients and healthcare providers when considering the viability of stem cell therapies over extended periods.

Finally, the cost-effectiveness of stem cell therapies is an increasingly important consideration for healthcare systems. ESC therapies, often associated with higher research and development costs, may not always translate to better outcomes compared to ASC therapies, which can be sourced more readily and are often less expensive. The role of stem cell niches in tissue engineering and repair further complicates this landscape, as understanding these environments can enhance the efficacy of both ESCs and ASCs in clinical settings, ultimately leading to improved patient outcomes and more sustainable treatment options.

Case Studies: Success and Limitations

Case studies of stem cell therapies provide invaluable insights into both the successes and limitations of embryonic and adult stem cells. In regenerative medicine, several clinical trials have demonstrated the remarkable efficacy of embryonic stem cells in treating conditions such as spinal cord injuries and certain neurodegenerative diseases. These studies highlight the unique differentiation potential of embryonic stem cells, which can give rise to virtually any cell type, thereby offering a broader scope for therapeutic applications. However, the challenges associated with ethical considerations and immune rejection remain significant hurdles in the widespread adoption of these therapies.

Conversely, adult stem cells, particularly those derived from sources like bone marrow and adipose tissue, have shown promising results in various clinical settings. Case studies reveal that these cells can effectively promote tissue repair and regeneration while exhibiting a lower risk of immune rejection compared to embryonic stem cells. Adult stem cells are already utilised in established therapies, such as haematopoietic stem cell transplantation for blood disorders, showcasing their practical applications and relative safety in patients. Nevertheless, the limited differentiation potential of adult stem cells compared to their embryonic counterparts poses challenges for treating a wider range of diseases.

The immune response to stem cell therapies is another critical area highlighted in case studies. While embryonic stem cells may provoke a more robust immune response due to their foreign nature, adult stem cells tend to be more immunologically compatible, particularly when sourced from the same individual. This aspect is crucial for patient outcomes, as minimising immune rejection can significantly enhance the long-term viability of the treatment. Studies focusing on the immune dynamics during stem cell therapy have underscored the need for personalised approaches, especially in cases where immunogenicity could impact the success of the therapy.

Long-term outcomes of treatments involving different stem cell types also reveal a nuanced picture. While embryonic stem cell therapies may offer immediate benefits, some case studies indicate concerns regarding tumorigenesis and other adverse effects that may arise in the long term. In contrast, adult stem cell therapies, despite their limited scope, often demonstrate more stable long-term outcomes, with fewer complications reported over time. These findings necessitate a careful consideration of the risk-benefit ratio when selecting the appropriate stem cell source for clinical applications.

Lastly, the cost-effectiveness of stem cell therapies remains a pivotal concern in the healthcare landscape. Case studies comparing the economic implications of both embryonic and adult stem cell therapies indicate that while embryonic stem cell treatments may carry higher initial costs due to extensive research and development, the potential for broader applications and improved patient outcomes could justify the investment. Adult stem cell therapies, being more established, often present lower costs but may not offer the same level of regenerative capacity. As the field evolves, ongoing assessments of these factors will be essential for guiding future research and clinical practices in stem cell therapy.

Therapeutic Applications

Applications of Embryonic Stem Cells

Embryonic stem cells (ESCs) hold significant promise in the field of regenerative medicine due to their unique properties, including pluripotency and the ability to differentiate into any cell type. These characteristics make ESCs particularly valuable in therapeutic applications, as they can potentially regenerate damaged tissues and organs. In comparison to adult stem cells, which have limited differentiation potential, ESCs offer a broader range of applications in treating various diseases and injuries, thereby positioning them at the forefront of experimental and clinical research.

The therapeutic applications of embryonic stem cells extend across various medical disciplines, including neurology, cardiology, and orthopaedics. For instance, ESCs have shown potential in treating neurodegenerative diseases such as Parkinson's and Alzheimer's by facilitating the regeneration of neuronal cells. Additionally, their application in cardiac repair after myocardial infarctions has been explored, showing promising results in improving heart function and reducing scar tissue formation. This versatility highlights the efficacy of ESCs in addressing complex medical conditions that traditional therapies struggle to manage.

In terms of differentiation potential, embryonic stem cells exhibit a distinct advantage over adult stem cells. ESCs can be directed to differentiate into a wide variety of cell types, which is crucial for developing targeted treatments. Conversely, adult stem cells are often limited to their tissue of origin, which can restrict their therapeutic use. This difference in differentiation capacity is a critical factor in evaluating the long-term outcomes of treatments derived from either stem cell type, as it directly impacts the effectiveness and applicability of regenerative strategies.

Another important consideration is the immune response to stem cell therapies. ESCs, due to their embryonic origin, may pose a risk of immune rejection when transplanted into a non-matching host. However, advancements in techniques such as induced pluripotent stem cells (iPSCs) are being researched to mitigate this issue. In contrast, adult stem cells often exhibit a more favourable immune profile, as they are less likely to provoke an adverse response. Understanding these immunological aspects is paramount for clinical applications and developing safe, effective therapies using either stem cell type.

Finally, the cost-effectiveness of employing embryonic stem cells compared to adult stem cells is a vital aspect for healthcare systems. While the initial research and development costs associated with ESC therapies can be higher, their potential to provide comprehensive treatments for a range of conditions may lead to significant long-term savings in healthcare expenditures. Clinical trials are ongoing to compare the efficacy and cost-effectiveness of these stem cell sources, with promising preliminary results favouring the use of embryonic stem cells in certain contexts. This ongoing research is crucial for establishing best practices and guidelines for stem cell therapies in clinical settings.

Applications of Adult Stem Cells

Adult stem cells have emerged as pivotal players in the realm of regenerative medicine, offering promising avenues for therapeutic interventions. Unlike their embryonic counterparts, adult stem cells possess the unique capacity to differentiate into various cell types relevant to specific tissues, such as haematopoietic stem cells in the bone marrow that generate blood cells. This intrinsic ability not only facilitates tissue repair but also reduces the ethical concerns often associated with embryonic stem cell research. Furthermore, adult stem cells can be harvested from various tissues, including adipose tissue, bone marrow, and umbilical cord blood, making them a more readily accessible resource for clinical applications.

In clinical settings, the applications of adult stem cells span a wide array of conditions, particularly in the treatment of degenerative diseases and injuries. For instance, mesenchymal stem cells derived from bone marrow have shown efficacy in treating osteoarthritis and myocardial infarctions, where they promote tissue regeneration and reduce inflammation. Additionally, ongoing clinical trials are investigating the potential of adult stem cells in treating neurological disorders such as multiple sclerosis and spinal cord injuries, highlighting their versatility and therapeutic potential. These applications underscore the significance of adult stem cells in addressing various medical challenges, often with fewer complications compared to embryonic stem cells.

A critical consideration in the utilisation of stem cells is the immune response elicited by these therapies. Adult stem cells, particularly those derived from the patient's own tissues, exhibit reduced immunogenicity, leading to a lower risk of rejection compared to embryonic stem cells. This characteristic not only enhances the safety profile of adult stem cell therapies but also extends the range of potential applications in personalised medicine. As research progresses, understanding the nuances of immune response will be paramount in optimising treatment protocols and ensuring successful long-term outcomes for patients receiving stem cell therapies.

The cost-effectiveness of adult stem cell therapies presents another compelling argument for their adoption in clinical practice. While the initial investment in research and development is significant, the potential for fewer side effects, reduced hospital stays, and improved patient outcomes translates into substantial economic benefits over time. Additionally, as the field of regenerative medicine advances, the scalability of adult stem cell applications promises to enhance accessibility and affordability, making these therapies more viable for widespread use in healthcare settings.

In summary, the applications of adult stem cells in therapeutic contexts are diverse and expanding. Their unique properties, coupled with a favourable safety profile and cost-effectiveness, position them as a critical component in the future of regenerative medicine. As ongoing research continues to elucidate the full potential of adult stem cells, it is imperative for medical personnel, researchers, and ethicists to collaborate closely in navigating the complexities of stem cell therapies, ensuring that patients receive the most effective and ethically responsible treatments available.

Comparative Outcomes in Clinical Settings

In the realm of regenerative medicine, the comparative outcomes of embryonic and adult stem cells have been a focal point for clinical research and application. Embryonic stem cells, known for their pluripotency, exhibit a remarkable ability to differentiate into various cell types, making them highly attractive for therapeutic applications. In contrast, adult stem cells, while limited in their differentiation potential, have shown promising efficacy in treating specific conditions, particularly within the same tissue type from which they are derived. This distinction raises critical questions about the optimal use of each stem cell type in clinical settings.

Clinical trials have provided valuable insights into the therapeutic applications of both embryonic and adult stem cells. For instance, studies have demonstrated the efficacy of embryonic stem cells in the treatment of degenerative diseases such as Parkinson's and spinal cord injuries. Conversely, adult stem cells have been successfully utilised in the treatment of blood disorders and certain forms of cancer. The outcomes from these trials highlight not only the effectiveness of each stem cell type but also their respective roles in targeted therapies, where the nature of the disease may dictate the choice of stem cell source.

An important aspect of stem cell therapies is the immune response they elicit. Embryonic stem cells are often associated with a higher risk of immune rejection due to their foreign origin, necessitating immunosuppressive therapies. On the other hand, adult stem cells, being derived from the patient's own tissues, generally exhibit a lower risk of rejection, thus reducing the need for additional immunosuppression. This difference can significantly influence long-term outcomes, as therapies with lower rejection rates tend to result in more sustained and successful results.

Cost-effectiveness also plays a crucial role in the decision-making process for the implementation of stem cell therapies. While the initial investment for embryonic stem cell research and application may be higher due to the complexity of sourcing and handling, adult stem cell therapies often prove to be more cost-effective in the long run due to their lower complication rates and reduced need for follow-up treatments. Evaluating these financial implications alongside clinical efficacy is essential for medical personnel and oversight bodies when considering the broader adoption of these therapies in clinical practice.

Lastly, the role of stem cell niches in tissue engineering and repair cannot be overlooked. The microenvironment surrounding stem cells influences their behaviour and differentiation potential. Understanding how to manipulate these niches can enhance the efficacy of both embryonic and adult stem cells in clinical applications. Continued research into these areas will provide further clarity on how best to utilise each stem cell type, ultimately leading to improved patient outcomes in regenerative medicine.

Stem Cell Differentiation Potential

Factors Influencing Differentiation

Differentiation of stem cells is influenced by a multitude of factors that are crucial for understanding their therapeutic potential. Environmental cues, including the presence of specific growth factors and extracellular matrix components, play a significant role in guiding stem cell fate. In the context of embryonic versus adult stem cells, the inherent properties of these cells also dictate their differentiation capabilities. For instance, embryonic stem cells are pluripotent and possess a greater ability to differentiate into various cell types compared to their adult counterparts, which are usually multipotent and limited in their differentiation potential.

The niche in which stem cells reside is another critical factor influencing differentiation. Stem cell niches provide the necessary microenvironment that supports stem cell maintenance and regulates their activity. In regenerative medicine, understanding these niches can lead to innovations in tissue engineering and repair. For both embryonic and adult stem cells, the interaction with their niche can enhance or inhibit differentiation, making it essential to consider these factors when designing therapeutic strategies.

The immune response to stem cell therapies is also a significant consideration in differentiation. Adult stem cells, being more immunologically compatible with the recipient, often elicit a lower immune response compared to embryonic stem cells. This difference can affect the long-term outcomes of treatments, as a robust immune reaction may lead to rejection of the transplanted cells, thereby compromising the efficacy of the therapy. Consequently, the choice between embryonic and adult stem cells must account for the immunological context and its impact on differentiation and integration into host tissues.

Cost-effectiveness is another factor that cannot be overlooked when evaluating the use of embryonic versus adult stem cells in clinical applications. The financial implications of sourcing, processing, and implementing stem cell therapies vary significantly between these two types. Adult stem cell therapies often have lower associated costs due to their availability and the complexity involved in handling embryonic cells. Therefore, when considering differentiation potential and therapeutic applications, a comprehensive analysis of cost-effectiveness is essential for healthcare providers and oversight bodies.

Finally, ongoing clinical trials comparing the efficacy of different stem cell sources are vital for advancing our understanding of differentiation. These trials provide critical data on the long-term outcomes of treatments, informing best practices in regenerative medicine. As research progresses, the insights gained from these studies will clarify the roles of embryonic and adult stem cells in clinical settings, ultimately guiding decisions that impact patient care and treatment efficacy.

Comparative Analysis of Differentiation

The comparative analysis of differentiation between embryonic and adult stem cells is a pivotal aspect in understanding their therapeutic potential. Embryonic stem cells, derived from the early stages of development, possess a unique ability to differentiate into any cell type within the human body, offering unprecedented opportunities for regenerative medicine. In contrast, adult stem cells, which are found in specific tissues, exhibit a more limited differentiation capacity, typically restricted to their tissue of origin. This fundamental difference in differentiation potential plays a crucial role in determining the efficacy of stem cell therapies across various clinical applications.

When examining the therapeutic applications of these two stem cell sources, the versatility of embryonic stem cells becomes evident. They have shown promise in treating a range of conditions, including neurodegenerative diseases and spinal cord injuries, due to their capacity to generate diverse cell types. On the other hand, adult stem cells have been successfully utilised in treating diseases such as leukaemia and other blood disorders, primarily through haematopoietic stem cell transplantation. The ongoing research efforts aim to bridge the gap between these two sources, exploring ways to enhance the differentiation and therapeutic efficacy of adult stem cells, thereby expanding their applicability in clinical settings.

The immune response to stem cell therapies is another critical factor in the comparative analysis of differentiation. Embryonic stem cells, while offering greater differentiation potential, can provoke significant immunogenic responses when transplanted into an immunologically mismatched host. Conversely, adult stem cells derived from the patient's own tissues tend to elicit a more favourable immune response, reducing the risk of rejection and complications. This aspect is particularly important for long-term outcomes of treatments, as a less aggressive immune response can contribute to sustained therapeutic benefits and improved patient quality of life.

Cost-effectiveness is also a vital consideration in the comparative analysis of embryonic and adult stem cell therapies. While embryonic stem cell research has the potential to yield innovative treatments, the associated ethical concerns and regulatory hurdles often lead to increased costs and prolonged timelines for clinical applications. Adult stem cell therapies, although sometimes offering less versatility, have established protocols and a clearer regulatory pathway, making them more accessible and often more cost-effective for widespread clinical use. This economic aspect influences the decision-making processes of healthcare providers and oversight bodies, impacting the availability of specific therapies for patients.

Finally, the role of stem cell niches in tissue engineering and repair cannot be overlooked. Understanding how different stem cell sources interact with their microenvironment is essential for optimising their differentiation and therapeutic outcomes. Embryonic stem cells can be influenced by various signalling pathways within engineered niches, potentially enhancing their regenerative capabilities. Meanwhile, adult stem cells thrive within their natural niches, which support their maintenance and functionality. Further research into these interactions will be key to advancing the field of regenerative medicine and ensuring that both embryonic and adult stem cell therapies reach their full potential in clinical applications.

Therapeutic Implications of Differentiation Potential

The differentiation potential of stem cells has profound therapeutic implications, particularly when comparing embryonic and adult stem cells. Embryonic stem cells are pluripotent, meaning they can differentiate into any cell type, providing a vast array of possibilities for regenerative medicine. This capability allows for the potential treatment of various degenerative diseases and injuries, positioning embryonic stem cells as a powerful tool in clinical applications. In contrast, adult stem cells are multipotent, with a more limited differentiation potential, mainly restricted to the tissue from which they are derived. Understanding these differences is crucial for medical professionals and researchers when considering treatment options.

Recent clinical trials have revealed significant variances in efficacy between embryonic and adult stem cells in therapeutic applications. Embryonic stem cells have shown promising results in early-phase trials for conditions such as spinal cord injuries and certain types of cancer. These findings are pivotal as they provide insights into the advantages of embryonic stem cells in potentially regenerating complex tissues. Conversely, adult stem cells have been successfully employed in treatments for conditions like blood disorders and certain cardiac diseases, demonstrating their importance in current therapeutic strategies.

The immune response to stem cell therapies is another critical factor influencing the choice between embryonic and adult stem cells. Embryonic stem cells, being foreign to the recipient, often elicit a stronger immune response, which can complicate long-term outcomes. In contrast, adult stem cells, derived from the patient's own tissue, typically have a lower risk of rejection. This aspect is particularly relevant in the context of personalised medicine, where minimising immune complications is essential for successful therapy.

Moreover, the role of stem cell niches in tissue engineering and repair cannot be overlooked. Embryonic stem cells, due to their high differentiation potential, can be integrated into engineered tissues more effectively, potentially leading to better functional outcomes. Adult stem cells, however, thrive in specific microenvironments that support their survival and differentiation, making the understanding of these niches vital for enhancing their therapeutic applications. The interplay between stem cell sources and their niches is fundamental in developing effective regenerative therapies.

Lastly, the cost-effectiveness of embryonic versus adult stem cell therapies remains a significant consideration for healthcare systems. While embryonic stem cell therapies may offer broader therapeutic potential, they often come with higher research and development costs, alongside ethical concerns. Adult stem cell therapies, being more established, might present a more immediate return on investment. Balancing these factors is essential for oversight bodies and healthcare policymakers as they navigate the complex landscape of stem cell research and its clinical applications.

Immune Response to Stem Cell Therapies

Immune Rejection Mechanisms

Immune rejection mechanisms play a critical role in the success of stem cell therapies, particularly when considering the differences between embryonic and adult stem cells. The immune system's response to transplanted cells can lead to significant complications, including graft rejection. This is particularly relevant in cases where embryonic stem cells are used, as they possess a different immunological profile compared to adult stem cells, which are more likely to be accepted by the host due to their origin from the same individual.

Embryonic stem cells are often perceived as more immunogenic than adult stem cells because they express a unique set of antigens. This difference can provoke a robust immune response, potentially resulting in acute rejection of the transplanted cells. Conversely, adult stem cells, which can be derived from the patient's own tissues, typically exhibit lower immunogenicity, allowing for more seamless integration and function within the host environment. Understanding these mechanisms is vital for optimising therapeutic applications and ensuring better patient outcomes.

The therapeutic applications of stem cells are heavily influenced by their immune properties. In regenerative medicine, the ability of adult stem cells to evade immune detection can lead to more effective treatments with fewer adverse effects. This aspect is crucial when considering long-term outcomes of therapies, as patients receiving adult stem cell transplants often report a reduced incidence of complications related to immune rejection compared to those treated with embryonic stem cells.

Moreover, the differentiation potential of stem cells is closely linked to their immune responses. Embryonic stem cells have a higher capacity for differentiation into various cell types, which can be advantageous in treating a range of diseases. However, this potential comes at the risk of immunogenic rejection. Adult stem cells, while perhaps less versatile in differentiation, offer a more stable and lower-risk alternative that can be tailored to the patient's immune profile, enhancing their therapeutic efficacy.

Lastly, the cost-effectiveness of stem cell therapies cannot be overlooked. While embryonic stem cell treatments may promise broader applications, the costs associated with managing immune rejection and its complications can outweigh the initial benefits. In contrast, adult stem cell therapies may provide a more sustainable and economically viable approach in clinical settings. As research continues, understanding the complex interplay of immune rejection mechanisms will be essential for advancing stem cell therapies and improving patient care across diverse medical fields.

Strategies to Enhance Acceptance

Enhancing acceptance of stem cell therapies, particularly in the context of embryonic versus adult stem cells, requires a multifaceted approach that addresses both scientific and ethical dimensions. Medical personnel and researchers play a crucial role in educating patients and the public about the potential benefits and risks associated with various stem cell sources. By providing clear, evidence-based information, they can help to demystify stem cell research and alleviate concerns regarding moral implications, thereby fostering a more informed dialogue within the community.

One effective strategy is to promote transparency in clinical trials comparing the efficacy of embryonic and adult stem cells. Oversight bodies should ensure that trial results are disseminated promptly and comprehensively, highlighting both successes and failures. This openness not only builds trust among stakeholders but also encourages more extensive participation in research studies. In doing so, it is vital to communicate the long-term outcomes of treatments, as understanding these results can significantly influence public perception and acceptance of stem cell therapies.

Another strategy involves engaging ethicists and public opinion leaders in discussions about the potential of regenerative medicine. Workshops and forums can be organised to address ethical considerations surrounding stem cell use, particularly focusing on the differentiation potential of embryonic versus adult cells. By involving diverse perspectives, these discussions can help create a more balanced understanding of the ethical landscape, which is essential in guiding policy and regulatory frameworks.

Additionally, cost-effectiveness analyses of embryonic and adult stem cell therapies should be made accessible to healthcare providers and policymakers. By demonstrating the economic implications of different stem cell sources, stakeholders can make informed decisions that align with both clinical efficacy and fiscal responsibility. This approach not only aids in resource allocation but also enhances the overall acceptance of therapies that may have higher upfront costs but offer substantial long-term benefits.

Lastly, fostering collaborations between biomedical scientists, clinicians, and industry stakeholders can lead to innovative solutions that enhance acceptance. By working together, these groups can develop targeted educational campaigns that address specific concerns related to immune responses and the role of stem cell niches in tissue engineering. Such initiatives can help bridge the gap between scientific advancements and public understanding, ultimately leading to improved patient outcomes and greater acceptance of stem cell therapies in clinical practice.

Clinical Implications of Immune Response

The clinical implications of immune response in stem cell therapies are profound, influencing treatment outcomes across various conditions. When considering the use of embryonic versus adult stem cells, it is crucial to understand how the immune system reacts to these different cell types. Embryonic stem cells, being pluripotent, can provoke a stronger immune response due to their foreign nature when introduced into a host. In contrast, adult stem cells, which are often derived from the patient's own tissues, generally elicit a more favourable immune response, reducing the risk of rejection and complications associated with transplantation.

In regenerative medicine, the efficacy of stem cell sources is heavily tied to their differentiation potential and the immune environment of the recipient. Embryonic stem cells have a greater capacity for differentiation into various cell types, offering promising therapeutic avenues. However, the challenge remains in managing the immune response to prevent potential rejection. Adult stem cells, while more limited in differentiation capabilities, often lead to more stable long-term outcomes due to their compatibility with the host's immune system. This compatibility can be particularly advantageous in chronic conditions where continuous therapy is necessary.

Clinical trials comparing the efficacy of embryonic and adult stem cell sources have highlighted the importance of immune factors in treatment success. Studies have shown that while embryonic stem cells may offer superior initial results in certain applications, the long-term persistence of treatment effects tends to favour adult stem cells. This trend underscores the necessity of considering not just the short-term benefits but also the long-term viability and safety of stem cell therapies, particularly in patients with compromised immune systems.

Additionally, the cost-effectiveness of these therapies cannot be overlooked. Embryonic stem cell therapies often require extensive immunosuppressive regimens, which can increase the overall treatment costs. Adult stem cell therapies, in contrast, may offer a more economically viable option by reducing the need for long-term immunosuppression. This financial aspect is essential for healthcare providers and policymakers when determining the best approaches to stem cell-based treatments.

Lastly, the role of stem cell niches in tissue engineering and repair plays a significant part in understanding immune responses. Each stem cell type interacts differently with its microenvironment, influencing not only differentiation but also immune modulation. Research continues to unravel these complex interactions, paving the way for innovative therapies that harness the immune system's potential to enhance the efficacy of stem cell treatments. Overall, recognising the clinical implications of immune response is vital for optimising therapeutic strategies in stem cell medicine.

Long-term Outcomes of Stem Cell Treatments

Tracking Efficacy Over Time

The efficacy of stem cell therapies is a critical aspect to consider in both clinical and research settings. Over time, tracking the outcomes of treatments that utilise embryonic versus adult stem cells provides invaluable insights into their respective therapeutic potentials. As medical personnel and researchers evaluate the effectiveness of these therapies, long-term follow-up studies become essential to ascertain the durability of the benefits conferred by these interventions. Understanding the nuances of stem cell differentiation potential, as well as the immune response elicited by these different sources, is paramount in assessing their efficacy.

Clinical trials serve as a cornerstone in the comparison of efficacy between embryonic and adult stem cell sources. These trials not only provide data on short-term outcomes but also illuminate the long-term effects associated with various treatments. The role of preclinical studies, particularly those that investigate the regenerative capabilities of different stem cell types, cannot be overstated. Such investigations allow for a deeper understanding of how these cells perform in vivo, particularly in the context of tissue engineering and repair.

Monitoring the immune response to stem cell therapies is critical, as it can significantly impact the success of treatment protocols. Different sources of stem cells may provoke varying immune reactions, influencing both the immediate effectiveness and the long-term sustainability of the therapy. This is particularly relevant in regenerative medicine, where the goal is to restore function while minimising adverse effects. The interplay between the stem cell niche and the host environment plays a vital role in determining the outcome of these therapies.

Cost-effectiveness is another vital factor to consider in the assessment of stem cell sources. As the field of regenerative medicine evolves, understanding the economic implications of using embryonic versus adult stem cells becomes increasingly important. Health care systems and oversight bodies must evaluate not only the clinical outcomes but also the financial burdens associated with each treatment type. This evaluation will aid in making informed decisions about resource allocation and treatment options.

In summary, tracking the efficacy of stem cell therapies over time presents a multifaceted challenge that encompasses clinical outcomes, immune responses, and economic considerations. As research continues to advance, a comprehensive approach that includes long-term monitoring and comparative studies will be essential in determining the best practices for utilising embryonic and adult stem cells in clinical applications. Ultimately, the goal is to optimise therapeutic outcomes while ensuring patient safety and resource efficiency.

Complications and Side Effects

The utilisation of stem cells in clinical applications presents a range of potential complications and side effects that warrant careful consideration. Both embryonic and adult stem cells can lead to adverse outcomes, which can significantly impact patient health and the overall efficacy of therapies. One major concern is the risk of tumour formation, particularly associated with embryonic stem cells, which possess a high differentiation potential. This uncontrolled growth can result in teratomas or other malignancies, necessitating rigorous monitoring and management strategies in clinical settings.

Additionally, the immune response elicited by stem cell therapies can pose challenges, particularly when using allogeneic (donor-derived) cells. Adult stem cells, while generally inducing a milder immune reaction, may still provoke graft-versus-host disease (GVHD) if not properly matched to the recipient. Conversely, embryonic stem cells are less likely to be rejected due to their pluripotent nature, yet their use raises ethical questions and potential for immune-related complications. Understanding the immunological aspects of both stem cell types is essential for optimising patient outcomes and minimising adverse effects.

Long-term outcomes of treatments involving different stem cell sources are also a critical consideration. While some studies indicate promising results with adult stem cells in regenerative medicine, there is a need for extensive follow-up to ascertain the durability of therapeutic benefits and any late-onset complications. In contrast, the long-term effects of embryonic stem cell therapies remain less well-defined, necessitating vigilance in ongoing clinical trials. The comparison of efficacy between these two sources must take into account not only immediate therapeutic success but also the potential for chronic complications.

Cost-effectiveness is another important factor when evaluating stem cell therapies. Adult stem cell treatments may often be less expensive due to the streamlined processes involved in their extraction and application. However, the initial high costs associated with embryonic stem cell research and therapies can be justified if the long-term benefits outweigh the financial investments. A thorough economic evaluation, alongside a comparative analysis of treatment outcomes, is crucial for informing policy and funding decisions in the field of regenerative medicine.

Finally, the role of stem cell niches in tissue engineering and repair cannot be overlooked. The microenvironments surrounding stem cells play a pivotal role in their behaviour and differentiation potential. Understanding how these niches influence the efficacy of embryonic versus adult stem cells could lead to innovative approaches that enhance therapeutic outcomes while minimising risks. As research progresses, continuous assessment of complications and side effects will be essential for refining clinical applications and ensuring patient safety in stem cell therapies.

Patient Quality of Life Post-Treatment

The quality of life for patients following stem cell treatment is a critical area of investigation, particularly when comparing the efficacy of embryonic versus adult stem cells. Post-treatment outcomes can vary significantly based on the source of stem cells used, reflecting their distinct properties and therapeutic potentials. For instance, patients receiving treatments derived from embryonic stem cells may experience different recovery trajectories and quality of life improvements compared to those treated with adult stem cells, which are often more restricted in their differentiation potential.

Regenerative medicine relies heavily on the ability of stem cells to differentiate into various cell types, impacting patient outcomes profoundly. Embryonic stem cells possess a broader differentiation capacity, potentially leading to more effective restoration of damaged tissues. However, adult stem cells, while limited in differentiation, have been shown to elicit a more favourable immune response in some cases, reducing the risk of complications that can adversely affect quality of life.

Long-term outcomes are integral to evaluating the success of any therapeutic intervention, and stem cell therapies are no exception. Studies have shown that patients who undergo stem cell treatments often report improvements in mobility, pain reduction, and overall well-being. Such enhancements are crucial for the elderly and those with chronic conditions, where the aim is to not only prolong life but also improve its quality significantly.

Cost-effectiveness is another vital consideration in assessing patient quality of life post-treatment. While embryonic stem cell therapies may offer superior efficacy in certain applications, the financial implications for patients and healthcare systems must be weighed against the outcomes achieved with adult stem cell treatments. This economic evaluation plays a significant role in determining accessibility and affordability for patients, ultimately influencing their quality of life.

Finally, ongoing clinical trials comparing the efficacy of stem cell sources are essential for providing robust data on long-term patient outcomes. Understanding how different stem cell types interact with the body's systems will inform future treatments and enhance patient care. By focusing on these comparisons, medical personnel can better guide patients through their treatment options, ensuring informed decisions that prioritise quality of life.

Cost-effectiveness of Stem Cell Therapies

Economic Considerations in Treatment Choices

The economic considerations surrounding treatment choices in stem cell therapies are increasingly relevant as the medical community seeks to balance efficacy with affordability. In the context of embryonic versus adult stem cells, the costs associated with sourcing, processing, and administering these treatments can vary significantly. Embryonic stem cell therapies often involve complex ethical and regulatory frameworks, which can lead to increased costs in clinical trials and product development. In contrast, adult stem cells are generally more accessible, potentially reducing the financial burden on healthcare systems and patients alike.

Cost-effectiveness analysis plays a crucial role in determining the viability of different stem cell treatments. Understanding the long-term outcomes associated with each type of stem cell is essential for making informed economic decisions. For instance, while embryonic stem cells may offer superior differentiation potential and regenerative capabilities, the costs involved in managing complications or adverse immune responses can offset these benefits. Comparatively, adult stem cells, although sometimes perceived as less versatile, may lead to better overall cost savings due to their lower incidence of complications and shorter treatment timelines.

Clinical trials comparing the efficacy of embryonic and adult stem cell therapies provide valuable data that can inform economic considerations. These trials often assess not only the clinical outcomes but also the associated costs of treatment protocols, including hospital stay durations, follow-up care, and the need for additional interventions. By understanding the comprehensive economic impact of each stem cell type, stakeholders can better allocate resources and develop strategies that enhance patient access to effective therapies.

Moreover, the role of stem cell niches in tissue engineering and repair can influence economic decisions regarding treatment options. The ability of a stem cell type to integrate effectively into its target tissue not only affects clinical outcomes but also the long-term costs associated with treatment failures or the need for repeat procedures. As research continues to advance our understanding of these niches, it may lead to the identification of more cost-effective applications for both embryonic and adult stem cells.

In conclusion, economic considerations in treatment choices for stem cell therapies should encompass a comprehensive analysis of efficacy, long-term outcomes, and cost-effectiveness. As the field evolves, it is essential for medical personnel, biomedical researchers, ethicists, and oversight bodies to collaborate in evaluating the financial implications of these therapies. Ultimately, informed economic decisions can enhance patient care and ensure that advancements in stem cell research translate into accessible clinical applications.

Cost Analysis of Embryonic vs Adult Therapies

The cost analysis of embryonic versus adult stem cell therapies plays a crucial role in determining their viability within clinical applications. Embryonic stem cells, derived from early-stage embryos, often involve significant ethical considerations and regulatory hurdles, which can escalate costs associated with research and development. On the other hand, adult stem cell therapies, which utilise cells sourced from fully developed tissues, typically face fewer ethical issues and may be more readily accepted in the clinical setting. However, this does not inherently mean that adult stem cell therapies are less expensive, as the complexity of treatment protocols and the required technologies can vary significantly.

When evaluating the cost-effectiveness of these therapies, it is essential to consider not only the immediate financial implications but also the long-term outcomes associated with each type of stem cell. Embryonic stem cells have shown higher differentiation potential in preclinical studies, which could translate into better therapeutic results, potentially reducing the need for multiple treatments. Conversely, adult stem cells may provide more predictable outcomes due to their established roles in tissue repair and regeneration, but their efficacy can be limited by their differentiation capacity.

Clinical trials comparing the efficacy of embryonic and adult stem cell therapies further inform cost analysis by providing data on the success rates and potential complications associated with each treatment. Trials often reveal that the initial costs of embryonic therapies may be offset by superior long-term benefits for certain conditions, suggesting that a broader perspective on cost should be adopted. This highlights the necessity for a comprehensive evaluation of both direct and indirect costs, including the overall quality of life improvements for patients.

The immune response to stem cell therapies is another critical factor influencing cost analysis. Adult stem cell therapies are typically associated with a lower risk of immune rejection, which can lead to reduced costs in managing post-treatment complications. In contrast, embryonic stem cell therapies may require immunosuppressive protocols that increase overall treatment expenses. Understanding these dynamics is vital for stakeholders when making informed decisions about resource allocation in regenerative medicine.

Ultimately, the cost analysis of embryonic versus adult stem cell therapies should encompass a multidimensional approach, integrating financial, ethical, and clinical considerations. As the field of regenerative medicine continues to evolve, ongoing research and comparative studies will be essential in shaping guidelines that optimise both the use of resources and patient outcomes. The balance between ethical implications, treatment efficacy, and cost will be pivotal in steering future clinical practices in stem cell therapies.

Implications for Healthcare Systems

The implications for healthcare systems with regard to the use of embryonic versus adult stem cells are vast and multifaceted. As medical personnel and researchers delve deeper into the therapeutic applications of these stem cells, they must consider not only the efficacy of each type but also the broader systemic impacts. This includes the potential for regulatory changes, shifts in funding priorities, and the necessity for updated training programmes for healthcare providers to ensure they are equipped to implement these advanced therapies in clinical settings.

Cost-effectiveness is another critical consideration for healthcare systems when evaluating stem cell therapies. While embryonic stem cells may offer greater differentiation potential, the financial implications of their usage cannot be overlooked. Adult stem cells, often derived from less controversial sources, may present a more economically viable option in certain contexts. Healthcare administrators must weigh these factors alongside clinical efficacy and patient outcomes to make informed decisions about resource allocation and investment in stem cell research.

The immune response to stem cell therapies also poses significant implications for healthcare. Understanding how different stem cell types interact with the immune system is essential for minimising adverse effects and maximising therapeutic efficacy. This knowledge impacts not only patient management strategies but also the design of clinical trials aimed at comparing the effectiveness of embryonic and adult stem cell treatments. A robust framework for evaluating these interactions will be necessary to establish safe and effective guidelines for practice.

Long-term outcomes of treatments using various stem cell sources are crucial for assessing their viability within healthcare systems. Continuous monitoring and evaluation of patient outcomes will inform best practices and enhance the overall quality of care. The integration of long-term data into healthcare decision-making processes will also support the development of evidence-based policies that govern the use of stem cells in regenerative medicine, ultimately benefiting patient populations.

Finally, the role of stem cell niches in tissue engineering and repair must not be underestimated. Understanding how these niches contribute to the success of stem cell therapies can provide valuable insights into optimising treatment protocols. As healthcare systems adapt to incorporate these innovative therapies, a focus on the biological context in which stem cells operate will help to improve therapeutic outcomes and foster advancements in regenerative medicine. The collaboration between medical personnel, researchers, and oversight bodies will be critical in navigating these complex implications effectively.

Clinical Trials and Research

Overview of Key Clinical Trials

The exploration of key clinical trials involving embryonic and adult stem cells reveals significant insights into their respective therapeutic potentials. Clinical trials serve as the backbone of evidence-based medicine, providing data that helps delineate the efficacy and safety of various stem cell therapies. Notably, trials focusing on regenerative medicine have showcased how embryonic stem cells exhibit a higher differentiation potential compared to their adult counterparts. This characteristic is crucial for applications in conditions requiring extensive tissue repair and regeneration, such as spinal cord injuries and degenerative diseases.

In the context of therapeutic applications, several clinical trials have compared the outcomes of treatments using embryonic stem cells with those derived from adult sources. For example, trials investigating the use of embryonic stem cells in treating Parkinson's disease have demonstrated promising results in restoring function. In contrast, while adult stem cells have shown efficacy in treating certain conditions, their limited differentiation potential often requires more complex strategies to achieve similar outcomes. This comparison not only highlights the benefits of each stem cell type but also informs future research directions in regenerative medicine.

The immune response to stem cell therapies is another critical aspect observed in clinical trials. Trials have indicated that while embryonic stem cells may elicit a more robust immune response due to their foreign nature, adult stem cells tend to have an immunomodulatory effect that can mitigate rejection. Understanding these immune dynamics is essential for developing long-term treatment strategies and ensuring patient safety. Moreover, the long-term outcomes of treatments involving different stem cell types are vital for assessing the durability and effectiveness of therapies, guiding clinicians in making informed decisions.

Cost-effectiveness is an increasingly important consideration in the development and implementation of stem cell therapies. Clinical trials evaluating the economic aspects of embryonic versus adult stem cell treatments indicate that despite the initial high costs associated with embryonic stem cell research, the potential for lasting therapeutic benefits could justify the investment. Furthermore, the integration of stem cell niches in tissue engineering and repair plays a pivotal role in enhancing the efficacy of these therapies, as observed in several innovative clinical studies.

In summary, the overview of key clinical trials elucidates the complexities surrounding the use of embryonic and adult stem cells in clinical applications. As the body of research expands, it will be crucial for medical personnel, biomedical researchers, and ethicists to evaluate the findings critically. This collective understanding will pave the way for more effective, safe, and ethically sound stem cell therapies that can significantly improve patient outcomes across various medical disciplines.

Comparative Studies of Efficacy

Comparative studies of the efficacy of embryonic versus adult stem cells are crucial for understanding their potential in clinical applications. Embryonic stem cells, known for their pluripotency, can differentiate into any cell type, offering a wide range of therapeutic possibilities. In contrast, adult stem cells, while more limited in their differentiation potential, have shown promise in specific regenerative medicine applications, particularly in tissue repair and regeneration. These differences highlight the need for thorough comparative analyses to establish the most effective stem cell sources for various treatments.

Therapeutic applications of both embryonic and adult stem cells have been explored extensively in recent years. Clinical trials have demonstrated that embryonic stem cells can lead to significant advancements in treating conditions such as Parkinson's disease and spinal cord injuries. However, adult stem cells have also made remarkable contributions in areas like cardiovascular disease and orthopaedics, where they are often favoured due to their lower immunogenicity and ethical considerations. Understanding the unique advantages of each stem cell type is essential for developing tailored therapies.

The efficacy of stem cell sources in regenerative medicine is also influenced by their differentiation potential. Embryonic stem cells possess a higher capacity for differentiation, which allows for the generation of a diverse range of specialised cell types. Adult stem cells, while limited, can still differentiate effectively within their specific niches, such as haematopoietic stem cells in blood regeneration. This aspect is vital for clinicians and researchers as they navigate the complexities of tissue engineering and repair.

Moreover, the immune response to stem cell therapies varies significantly between embryonic and adult stem cells. The immunogenic profile of embryonic stem cells can lead to complications, necessitating careful consideration of immunosuppressive strategies in clinical settings. In contrast, adult stem cells generally elicit a milder immune response, making them more suitable for autologous transplants. Understanding these immune dynamics is critical for improving patient outcomes and minimising adverse effects in stem cell therapy.

Finally, long-term outcomes of treatments using different stem cell types warrant careful evaluation. While embryonic stem cell therapies show great promise, the potential for teratoma formation poses significant risks. Adult stem cells, on the other hand, often demonstrate more predictable and safer long-term results. Additionally, the cost-effectiveness of these therapies is an important factor for healthcare systems, as the economic implications of stem cell treatments continue to evolve. A comprehensive understanding of these factors is essential for medical personnel and oversight bodies as they formulate guidelines and policies for stem cell research and application.

Future Directions in Stem Cell Research

The future of stem cell research holds immense promise, particularly in the realm of regenerative medicine. As researchers continue to investigate the differences between embryonic and adult stem cells, the potential therapeutic applications are becoming clearer. While embryonic stem cells are renowned for their pluripotency, adult stem cells, with their more limited differentiation capacity, have proven effective in various clinical applications. The ongoing comparative studies on the efficacy of these stem cell sources will play a crucial role in shaping future therapies and treatment protocols.

One significant avenue for future research is the differentiation potential of both embryonic and adult stem cells. Understanding the mechanisms that govern this differentiation can lead to enhanced regenerative therapies tailored for specific conditions. For instance, researchers are exploring how to maximise the differentiation of adult stem cells to achieve outcomes previously attributed to embryonic sources. This exploration not only addresses efficacy but also the ethical concerns surrounding the use of embryonic stem cells, thereby influencing public and institutional support for different research paths.

The immune response to stem cell therapies is another critical aspect that warrants further investigation. As clinical trials progress, understanding how the immune system interacts with transplanted stem cells will be essential. Findings could lead to strategies that minimise rejection and enhance the long-term success of stem cell therapies. Additionally, the cost-effectiveness of these treatments remains a pressing issue. Future studies should focus on the economic implications of utilising embryonic versus adult stem cells, providing vital information for health care providers and policymakers.

Long-term outcomes from various stem cell treatments will also shape future research directions. Monitoring the durability of treatment effects and potential complications over extended periods will inform best practices in clinical settings. Moreover, the role of stem cell niches in tissue engineering and repair is emerging as a significant area of study. Understanding how to manipulate these niches could maximise the regenerative potential of stem cells, paving the way for innovative therapies that harness the body's natural healing processes.

In conclusion, the future directions in stem cell research will likely focus on the comparative efficacy of embryonic and adult stem cells, their therapeutic applications, and the underlying biological mechanisms governing their behaviours. As the field evolves, interdisciplinary collaboration among medical personnel, researchers, ethicists, and oversight bodies will be vital in navigating the complexities of stem cell therapies. This collaborative approach will ensure that advancements in stem cell applications are both scientifically sound and ethically responsible, ultimately benefiting patient care and outcomes.

Role of Stem Cell Niches in Tissue Engineering

Understanding Stem Cell Niches

Stem cell niches play a crucial role in the maintenance and regulation of stem cells, influencing their behaviour and fate. These microenvironments provide the necessary signals and support for stem cell survival, proliferation, and differentiation. Understanding the specific characteristics of stem cell niches is essential for improving therapeutic outcomes, particularly when comparing the efficacy of embryonic and adult stem cells in clinical applications. The intricate interactions between stem cells and their niches can significantly affect regenerative processes and the overall success of stem cell therapies.

In the context of regenerative medicine, the efficacy of different stem cell sources hinges on their ability to differentiate into desired cell types and integrate into host tissues. Embryonic stem cells (ESCs) possess a broader differentiation potential compared to adult stem cells (ASCs), which are typically limited to specific lineages. This inherent property of ESCs allows for greater versatility in therapeutic applications, although ethical considerations surrounding their use remain contentious. Conversely, ASCs, while limited in differentiation, are often more readily accepted by the immune system, reducing the risk of rejection and complications in transplantation settings.

The immune response to stem cell therapies is another critical factor influenced by the niche environment. ESCs, derived from early embryos, may provoke a stronger immune response due to their foreign origin, whereas ASCs, which are often harvested from the same individual, tend to elicit a more favourable immunological profile. Consequently, the choice between using embryonic or adult stem cells not only hinges on their differentiation capabilities but also on the anticipated immune interactions within the therapeutic context. This aspect underscores the importance of niche characteristics in determining the long-term outcomes of stem cell-based treatments.

Cost-effectiveness is a significant consideration when evaluating different stem cell therapies. While ESCs may offer superior differentiation potential, the costs associated with their procurement, ethical oversight, and potential complications can be substantial. In contrast, ASCs, often more straightforward to obtain and ethically less contentious, may present a more economically viable option despite their limitations. Clinical trials comparing the efficacy of various stem cell sources often highlight these factors, providing valuable insights into the practical implications of niche-dependent outcomes on treatment costs and accessibility.

Finally, the role of stem cell niches in tissue engineering and repair cannot be overstated. By mimicking the natural microenvironments that support stem cells, researchers can enhance the efficacy of both ESCs and ASCs in regenerative applications. This approach holds promise for developing advanced therapies that leverage the unique properties of both stem cell types, ultimately leading to innovative solutions in treating a variety of degenerative conditions. As research progresses, a deeper understanding of stem cell niches will be pivotal in harnessing the full therapeutic potential of stem cells in clinical practice.

Implications for Tissue Repair and Engineering

The exploration of tissue repair and engineering through stem cell therapies presents significant implications for medical practice and research. Embryonic stem cells (ESCs) exhibit pluripotency, allowing for differentiation into various cell types, which is crucial for regenerating damaged tissues. In contrast, adult stem cells (ASCs), while more limited in their differentiation potential, are often more readily accepted by the immune system, thereby reducing the risk of rejection in therapeutic applications. This fundamental difference shapes the ongoing debate about the most effective sources for tissue engineering in clinical settings.

Clinical applications of ESCs have shown promising results in regenerative medicine, particularly in fields such as cardiology and neurology. However, ethical considerations surrounding the use of embryonic tissues continue to provoke intense discussions among ethicists and oversight bodies. The balance between potential therapeutic benefits and ethical implications necessitates careful examination of both ESCs and ASCs in clinical trials. This scrutiny is vital in ensuring that the advancements in regenerative medicine uphold ethical standards while maximising patient benefits.

The immune response to stem cell therapies also plays a crucial role in their efficacy. While ASCs typically elicit a more favourable immune profile, ESCs can provoke immune responses that complicate their use. Understanding these immune interactions is essential for developing effective protocols that enhance the success rates of stem cell therapies. As research progresses, it is becoming increasingly clear that tailoring approaches based on the source of stem cells can significantly influence long-term treatment outcomes.

The cost-effectiveness of ESC versus ASC therapies is another key consideration for healthcare providers and policymakers. While ESCs may offer superior differentiation capabilities, the associated costs, including those from potential complications due to immune rejection, can be prohibitive. Conversely, ASCs, being more established in clinical practice, may present a more economical option, albeit with limitations in their regenerative capacity. This economic analysis must be factored into decision-making processes regarding the adoption of stem cell therapies in clinical settings.

In conclusion, the role of stem cell niches in tissue engineering and repair underscores the complex interplay between different stem cell types and their therapeutic applications. The microenvironment surrounding stem cells significantly impacts their behaviour and differentiation potential, which is critical for successful tissue regeneration. Ongoing research into these niches will illuminate new avenues for enhancing the efficacy of both ESCs and ASCs, driving forward the field of regenerative medicine and improving patient outcomes.

Future Perspectives on Niche Development

As we look to the future of stem cell research and its applications in medicine, the comparative efficacy of embryonic versus adult stem cells remains a pivotal topic. Evidence suggests that while embryonic stem cells possess greater differentiation potential, adult stem cells have shown remarkable efficacy in various therapeutic applications. This dichotomy invites ongoing investigation, particularly in the context of regenerative medicine, where the choice of stem cell source can significantly influence treatment outcomes. The need for rigorous clinical trials that evaluate not only efficacy but also safety and long-term impacts of these therapies is paramount.

The therapeutic applications of embryonic and adult stem cells differ significantly, with each type offering unique advantages and challenges. Embryonic stem cells, with their pluripotent nature, provide opportunities for generating a wide range of cell types for tissue repair. In contrast, adult stem cells are already integrated within specific tissues, which may enhance their ability to promote repair and regeneration in a more natural environment. As we advance our understanding of these cells, it becomes crucial to explore their respective roles in various therapeutic contexts, particularly in diseases where tissue degeneration is prominent.

Regenerative medicine stands at the forefront of this exploration, as the effectiveness of stem cell sources directly correlates with patient outcomes. Recent studies have underscored the importance of understanding the immune response to different stem cell therapies. The interaction between the host immune system and transplanted stem cells can significantly influence the success of treatments, making it essential to consider immunological factors when designing future therapies. Ongoing research must focus on how to mitigate adverse immune responses while maximising therapeutic benefits.

The long-term outcomes of treatments using various stem cell types are another critical area of investigation. Understanding the durability of treatment effects and the potential for adverse events over time will be vital for the acceptance of stem cell therapies in clinical practice. Moreover, the cost-effectiveness of embryonic and adult stem cell therapies will play a crucial role in their integration into healthcare systems, necessitating comprehensive economic evaluations alongside clinical efficacy studies.

Finally, the role of stem cell niches in tissue engineering and repair cannot be overlooked. These microenvironments are crucial for supporting stem cell function and differentiation, influencing their therapeutic potential. Future research should aim to elucidate the mechanisms underlying niche interactions and how they can be harnessed to enhance stem cell therapies. As we navigate these complex landscapes, collaborative efforts among medical personnel, researchers, ethicists, and oversight bodies will be essential to ensure that advancements in stem cell science translate into meaningful clinical benefits.

Conclusion and Future Directions

Summary of Key Findings

The comparison between embryonic and adult stem cells has unveiled critical insights into their respective efficacy and therapeutic applications. Embryonic stem cells, characterised by their pluripotency, exhibit a greater differentiation potential compared to adult stem cells, which are typically multipotent. This inherent capability allows embryonic stem cells to develop into various cell types, presenting a promising avenue for regenerative medicine. In contrast, adult stem cells are more limited in their differentiation pathways, which has implications for their use in treating complex diseases and injuries.

Therapeutic applications of both stem cell types have been explored through numerous clinical trials, revealing a spectrum of outcomes. Embryonic stem cells have shown significant promise in the treatment of conditions such as spinal cord injuries and degenerative diseases, while adult stem cells have been successfully employed in haematopoietic stem cell transplants and tissue repair. However, the immune response elicited by these therapies varies, with adult stem cells generally exhibiting a lower risk of rejection due to their autologous sources, whereas embryonic stem cells can provoke stronger immune reactions, necessitating immunosuppressive therapies.

Long-term outcomes of treatments using different stem cell types are another critical factor in evaluating their efficacy. Studies indicate that while embryonic stem cell therapies may offer immediate benefits, concerns regarding teratoma formation and long-term safety remain. Adult stem cell therapies, on the other hand, have demonstrated more stable long-term results with fewer adverse events. This dichotomy presents a challenging decision-making landscape for medical personnel and oversight bodies when considering treatment options for patients.

Cost-effectiveness is a pivotal consideration in the deployment of stem cell therapies. The initial investment in research and development for embryonic stem cell therapies can be substantial, yet the potential for groundbreaking treatments may justify these costs. Conversely, adult stem cell therapies often have lower upfront costs and established protocols, making them more accessible for clinical practice. Evaluating the economic implications alongside the clinical benefits is essential for informed decision-making in healthcare settings.

Finally, the role of stem cell niches in tissue engineering and repair cannot be overlooked. Understanding the microenvironments that support stem cell function is vital for enhancing therapeutic outcomes. Both embryonic and adult stem cells rely on their niches for optimal differentiation and integration into host tissues. Future research should focus on harnessing these niches to improve the efficacy of stem cell therapies, ultimately bridging the gap between laboratory findings and clinical applications.

Ethical and Clinical Considerations Moving Forward

As the field of regenerative medicine continues to evolve, ethical and clinical considerations surrounding the use of embryonic and adult stem cells remain paramount. Medical personnel and biomedical researchers must navigate a landscape where the promise of innovative therapies is often tempered by moral questions. The efficacy of embryonic versus adult stem cells is a central theme in these discussions, particularly in light of recent clinical trials that have revealed significant differences in their therapeutic applications. Understanding these distinctions is crucial for informed decision-making in clinical practice and research.

One of the key ethical considerations is the source of stem cells. While embryonic stem cells are derived from pre-implantation embryos, adult stem cells can be harvested from various tissues, including bone marrow and adipose tissue. This fundamental difference has implications not only for the potential differentiation capacity of these cells but also for the ethical acceptability of their use. Oversight bodies play a vital role in establishing guidelines that balance scientific advancement with respect for human life and dignity, ensuring that all stem cell therapies are subject to rigorous ethical scrutiny.

The immune response to stem cell therapies is another critical factor that healthcare providers must consider. Adult stem cells tend to provoke a less intense immune reaction, making them more suitable for autologous treatments.

In contrast, embryonic stem cells, due to their allogenic nature, may elicit stronger immune responses, complicating their clinical application. Understanding these immune dynamics is essential for optimising treatment protocols and improving long-term outcomes for patients undergoing stem cell therapies.

Cost-effectiveness also plays a significant role in the ongoing debate over stem cell sources. Adult stem cell therapies are often more accessible and less expensive due to lower regulatory hurdles and a more straightforward harvesting process. In contrast, the development of embryonic stem cell therapies can be prohibitively costly, both financially and ethically. As healthcare systems grapple with budgeting for innovative treatments, the cost-benefit analysis of these therapies will significantly influence their integration into clinical practice.

Finally, the role of stem cell niches in tissue engineering and repair is an emerging area of interest. Both embryonic and adult stem cells exhibit unique interactions with their microenvironments, which can impact their differentiation potential and therapeutic efficacy. Understanding these relationships is vital for advancing regenerative medicine and developing strategies that harness the full potential of stem cells. As we move forward, interdisciplinary collaboration among medical personnel, ethicists, and researchers will be essential to address these complexities and optimise patient outcomes in the evolving landscape of stem cell therapies.

The Future of Stem Cell Research and Applications

The future of stem cell research is poised for remarkable advancements, particularly in the comparative efficacy between embryonic and adult stem cells.

As research progresses, the understanding of how these cells can be harnessed for therapeutic applications continues to expand. The potential for regenerative medicine, utilising both embryonic and adult sources, raises important questions about not only the efficacy of these treatments but also their ethical implications and societal acceptance. With ongoing clinical trials, the landscape is shifting, offering promising avenues for treatment that could redefine medical practices in the years to come.

One of the most exciting areas of exploration is stem cell differentiation potential. Embryonic stem cells are known for their pluripotency, allowing them to develop into any cell type, whereas adult stem cells are typically multipotent, limited to specific lineages. Understanding these differences is crucial, as they directly influence the therapeutic applications of these stem cells in diseases such as Parkinson's, diabetes, and spinal cord injuries. As researchers continue to delve into the mechanisms of differentiation, the possibilities for innovative treatments grow, highlighting the need for meticulous oversight and ethical considerations in the field.

The immune response to stem cell therapies is another critical factor that will shape their future applications. Autologous adult stem cells generally elicit a lower immune response, making them a favourable choice for patients. In contrast, the use of embryonic stem cells can provoke immune rejection, necessitating advancements in immunosuppression techniques or the development of universal donor cells. Addressing these immunological challenges is essential for the successful integration of stem cell therapies into mainstream medicine, particularly as the demand for personalised medicine increases.

Long-term outcomes of treatments using different stem cell types will be pivotal in informing clinical practices and patient choices. As long-term data becomes available from ongoing clinical trials, comparisons of the efficacy and safety profiles of embryonic versus adult stem cells will help establish best practices for different conditions. Furthermore, the cost-effectiveness of these therapies will play a significant role in their adoption within healthcare systems, as stakeholders seek to balance innovation with economic viability in patient care.

Finally, the role of stem cell niches in tissue engineering and repair cannot be understated. The microenvironment surrounding stem cells is influential in determining their function and efficacy. Future research must focus on how to manipulate these niches effectively to enhance stem cell therapies. By understanding and utilising these biological frameworks, researchers can develop more effective strategies to repair and regenerate damaged tissues, thereby enhancing the overall impact of stem cell research on health care and medicine.

Pause for Thought

- Two primary types of stem cells based on their source. The primary categories are embryonic stem cells (ESC) and adult stem cells (ASC). The ESCs are derived from early-stage embryo's, they possess the unique ability to differentiate into any cell type in the body making them very versatile for research and therapeutic purposes. ASCs found in various tissues through-out the body have a more limited differentiation potential but are crucial for tissue maintenance and repair.

- ESCs have shown promise in regenerative medicine due to their pluripotency, allowing for the generation of specific cell types needed for repairing damaged tissues. ASCs have been successfully employed in therapies for conditions like blood disorders and certain cancers showcasing their role in established treatment protocols.

- Long term outcomes of treatments derived from various stem cell types remain an area for much research. Preliminary findings suggest that while ESC – based therapies may offer greater initial benefits due to their versatility, ASCs might provide more sustainable outcomes and fewer complications over time. The cost effectiveness is also a factor for concern. ESCs being more resource intensive, ASCs can often be sourced from the patient and used in a straighter forward manner.

- The role of stem cell niches in tissue engineering and repair is a vital aspect of understanding stem cell functionality. Those niches provide the necessary microenvironment for stem cells to thrive and differentiate effectively. Understanding how these niches contribute to the regeneration process can enhance the development of targeted therapies.

- The discovery of stem cells date to the early 20th century, when scientist first identified the unique properties of these cells. In the 1970's and '80'shaemopoetic stem cells were isolated and cultured. Embryonic stem cells were successfully isolated in the late 1990's

- ESC's have a self-renewal capability, which allows them to divide indefinitely while maintaining their undifferentiated state. This property makes them ideal for research and therapeutic applications as it enables the production of large quantities of stem cells for use in clinical settings. ESCs thus provide a versatile platform for developing novel treatments that require extensive cell populations.

- ASCs, since they are typically harvested from the patient, reduces the risk of immunogenicity making them a more favourable option in some cases, but unfortunately do not share as wide a utility as ESCs.

- The cost effectiveness of stem cell therapies remains a pivotal consideration for health care systems. ESC therapies may offer greater differentiation potential and broader applications, the ethical, regulatory, and procedural cost associated with their procurement can be substantial. ASCs are often more accessible and less controversial; they can provide immediate therapeutic benefits at potentially lower cost.

- Adult stem cells are typically multipotent, meaning they are limited to differentiating into a narrower range of cell types. This makes them valuable in regenerative medicine since with that capacity, they can contribute to the repair and maintenance of specific tissues.

- ASC's have demonstrated significant efficacy in treating a variety of conditions for example, they are commonly used in bone marrow transplants for patients with leukaemia and other blood disorders. Clinical trials have shown that these stem cells can improve patient outcomes and reduce recovery times.

Take Home Nuggets

- *ASC also referred to as somatic, or tissue stem cells are found through-out the human body and play a crucial role in tissue repair and regeneration. These are typically limited to differentiating into the cell types of their tissue of origin which makes them valuable in regenerative medicine.*

- The primary sources of ASCs include bone marrow, adipose tissue, and peripheral blood. Umbilical cord blood has emerged as an important reservoir of haemopoietic stem cells and so offers a less invasive option for stem cell collection. Additionally, the effectiveness of adult stem cells can vary based on the source, age of the donor and specific therapeutic applications being targeted.

- The unique properties of ASCs such as their ability to modulate immune responses and promote tissue repair, make them valuable candidates for specific therapeutic contexts, particularly where minimising immunogenicity is essential.

- Teratoma formation is an ongoing concern as a plausible long-term feature associated with ESC treatment, despite its initial robust response

- Therapeutic applications of stem cells are heavily influenced by their immune properties. In regenerative medicine, the ability of ASC to evade immune detection can lead to more effective treatments with fewer adverse effects. Patients receiving ASC transplants often report a reduced incidence of complications related to immune rejections compared to those treated with ESCs.

- Among various strategies for enhancing stem cell use is that of transparency in clinical trials comparing the efficacy of ESC and ASC. Oversight bodies should ensure that trial results are disseminated promptly and comprehensively. Involving ethicist and public opinion leaders in discussions about the potential of regenerative medicine, workshops and forums can be organised to address ethical considerations surrounding stem cell use.

- Tracking the outcomes of treatment that utilise embryonic versus adult stem cells provides invaluable insights their respective therapeutic potentials. Long-term follow-up studies become essential to ascertain the durability of the benefits conferred by these interventions.

- The utilisation of stem cells in clinical applications present a range of potential complications and side effects that warrant careful considerations. Both ESC and ASC can lead to adverse outcomes, which can significantly impact patient health and the overall efficacy of therapies. One major concern is the risk of tumour formation particularly associated with ESC because of their high differentiation potential. There is the lingering view that this uncontrolled growth can result in teratomas or other malignancies thus necessitating rigorous monitoring and management strategies in clinical settings. The immune response is also a cause for concern.

- The quality of life for patients following stem cell treatment is a critical area of investigation. Post treatment outcomes can vary significantly based on the source of stem cells used reflecting their distinct properties and therapeutic potentials. Patients receiving treatments derived from ESC may experience different recovery trajectories and quality of life improvement compared to those treated with ASC.

- The economic considerations surrounding treatment choices in stem cell therapies are increasingly relevant as the medical community seeks to balance efficacy and affordability.

Chapter 2
Stem Cells: The Beginnings

Embryonic Stem Cells

Embryonic stem cells (ESCs) are unique in their ability to differentiate into any cell type in the body, making them a focal point in stem cell research. Derived from early-stage embryos, these cells hold immense potential for understanding developmental processes and the mechanisms underlying various diseases. Their pluripotent nature allows them to generate virtually any cell type, which is crucial for advancements in regenerative medicine. The exploration of ESCs not only sheds light on developmental biology but also opens avenues for innovative therapies aimed at degenerative diseases.

Ethical considerations surrounding the use of embryonic stem cells are significant and often contentious. The extraction of these cells typically involves the destruction of the embryo, which raises moral and ethical dilemmas. Health care professionals and researchers must navigate these complex issues while advocating for the potential benefits that ESCs may offer in treating conditions such as Parkinson's disease, spinal cord injuries, and heart disease. Engaging in informed discussions about these ethical implications is essential for fostering a responsible approach to stem cell research.

The role of embryonic stem cells in regenerative medicine is particularly promising, as they could lead to breakthroughs in tissue engineering and organ replacement. Scientists are investigating ways to harness the regenerative capabilities of ESCs to repair damaged tissues and to develop therapies that can restore function in degenerative diseases. The ability to create specific cell types from ESCs could revolutionise the treatment landscape, offering hope to patients with previously untreatable conditions.

Advances in stem cell technology have propelled the field forward, with innovative techniques enhancing our understanding of ESC biology. Techniques such as CRISPR gene editing and advanced cell culture methods have enabled researchers to manipulate ESCs more effectively, facilitating the study of genetic disorders and the development of personalised medicine. These advancements not only improve the efficiency of stem cell research but also expand the possibilities for therapeutic applications, paving the way for tailored treatments based on individual genetic profiles.

Public perception and misconceptions surrounding embryonic stem cell research also play a critical role in the progress of this field. Misinformation can hinder funding and support for research initiatives, making it crucial for health care professionals to communicate the facts clearly. Educating the public about the scientific basis and potential benefits of ESC research can foster a more informed discourse, ultimately leading to broader acceptance and support for stem cell applications in both human and veterinary medicine.

Adult Stem Cells

Adult stem cells, also known as somatic stem cells, are undifferentiated cells found throughout the body after development. They play a crucial role in tissue homeostasis and repair by providing a reservoir of cells that can replenish damaged or lost tissues. Unlike embryonic stem cells, adult stem cells are limited in their ability to differentiate into various cell types, typically giving rise to the cell types of their tissue of origin. This intrinsic limitation does not diminish their significance; rather, it highlights their role in maintaining the functionality of adult organs.

Ethical considerations surrounding the use of adult stem cells have generated much discussion in both scientific and public domains. Since adult stem cells can be harvested from tissues such as bone marrow, adipose tissue, and blood, their collection often involves less ethical controversy compared to embryonic stem cells. This aspect has made adult stem cells a more acceptable option in research and therapy, helping to alleviate some concerns regarding the moral implications of stem cell use.

The potential of adult stem cells in regenerative medicine is vast, particularly in treating degenerative diseases such as Parkinson's disease, diabetes, and various forms of arthritis. Researchers are exploring the utilisation of these cells to replace damaged cells in affected tissues, thereby restoring function and improving patient outcomes. Clinical trials are ongoing to assess the efficacy and safety of therapies derived from adult stem cells, showcasing their promise in the field of regenerative medicine.

Recent advances in stem cell technology have further expanded the capabilities of adult stem cells. Techniques such as induced pluripotent stem (iPS) cell technology allow for the reprogramming of adult cells to regain pluripotency, enabling them to differentiate into any cell type. This innovation holds significant implications for personalised medicine, as it allows for the development of patient-specific therapies tailored to individual genetic backgrounds, potentially minimising the risk of rejection and enhancing treatment efficacy.

Public perception of adult stem cell research remains mixed, with misconceptions often stemming from a lack of understanding. Education and transparent communication about the science behind adult stem cells and their applications are vital in shaping an informed public opinion. As advancements continue and more successful therapies emerge, it is crucial for health care professionals to engage with the community, addressing concerns and promoting awareness of the transformative potential of adult stem cells in medicine.

Induced Pluripotent Stem Cells

Induced pluripotent stem cells (iPSCs) represent a remarkable advancement in the field of regenerative medicine, providing a means to generate pluripotent stem cells from somatic cells. This innovative technique, developed by Shinya Yamanaka and his team in 2006, allows for the reprogramming of differentiated cells back to a pluripotent state, effectively creating cells that have the potential to develop into any cell type in the body. iPSCs hold significant promise for understanding developmental biology and disease pathology, as well as for developing personalised therapies that are tailored to individual patients' needs.

One of the most compelling aspects of iPSCs is their potential application in personalised medicine. By obtaining a patient's somatic cells and reprogramming them into iPSCs, researchers can create patient-specific cell lines that can be used for drug screening, disease modelling, and even cell replacement therapies.

This approach not only enhances the efficacy of medical treatments but also reduces the risk of immune rejection, a critical concern in traditional stem cell therapies derived from embryonic sources.

Despite the tremendous promise of iPSCs, ethical considerations remain paramount in the discourse surrounding stem cell research. Since iPSCs can be derived from readily available tissues without the ethical dilemmas associated with embryonic stem cells, they provide a more ethically acceptable alternative. However, the potential for misuse and the need for stringent regulatory frameworks to govern their use in research and therapy must be continuously addressed to ensure responsible scientific advancement.

The advances in iPSC technology have also accelerated research into genetic disorders, offering new avenues for understanding the molecular mechanisms underlying these conditions. By generating iPSCs from patients with specific genetic mutations, scientists can study disease progression in a controlled environment, paving the way for innovative therapeutic strategies. Additionally, iPSCs can serve as a valuable tool in the discovery of novel drugs and treatment protocols, significantly impacting the future of medicine.

Finally, the application of iPSCs is not limited to human medicine; veterinary applications are also emerging, demonstrating their versatility. iPSCs are being explored for use in treating degenerative diseases in animals, which could lead to improved health outcomes and longevity for pets and livestock alike. As public perception evolves and misconceptions about stem cell research are addressed, the potential of iPSCs to revolutionise both human and veterinary medicine becomes increasingly evident.

Ethical Considerations in Stem Cell Research

Ethical Frameworks and Guidelines

The ethical frameworks and guidelines surrounding stem cell research are crucial for guiding health care professionals and biomedical scientists in their work. This area of research, while promising, raises various ethical considerations, especially when it involves human embryos or foetal tissues. Establishing a robust ethical framework ensures that the potential benefits of stem cell therapies for degenerative diseases are realised without compromising moral standards or human dignity. Moreover, these guidelines help navigate the complex landscape of regenerative medicine, where interventions may significantly impact patients' lives.

Health care professionals must understand the importance of informed consent in stem cell research. This process not only respects the autonomy of donors but also fosters trust in the research community. Clear communication regarding the purpose and potential outcomes of research is vital, as it allows donors to make knowledgeable decisions. In addition, ethical frameworks advocate for transparency in research practices, which is essential for maintaining public confidence in stem cell applications and their implications for personalised medicine.

The role of regulatory bodies in overseeing stem cell research cannot be overstated. These organisations establish protocols that researchers must follow to ensure ethical compliance and safety in stem cell applications. By providing guidelines on issues such as stem cell banking and its implications, regulatory bodies help mitigate risks associated with stem cell therapies. This oversight is particularly important in addressing public perception and misconceptions surrounding stem cell research, as misinformation can hinder progress and innovation in this field.

As advances in stem cell technology and techniques continue to evolve, so too must the ethical considerations that accompany them. New methodologies may present unforeseen ethical dilemmas, necessitating ongoing dialogue among researchers, ethicists, and health care professionals. By remaining engaged in this conversation, the scientific community can adapt and refine ethical frameworks to address emerging challenges in stem cell research, ensuring that the advancements benefit society while upholding ethical integrity.

In conclusion, the ethical frameworks and guidelines that govern stem cell research are essential for balancing scientific innovation with moral responsibility. For health care professionals and biomedical scientists, understanding these frameworks is crucial for navigating the complexities of stem cell therapies and their applications. By adhering to established ethical guidelines, the potential of stem cells in treating degenerative diseases and advancing regenerative medicine can be harnessed responsibly, paving the way for future breakthroughs in personalised medicine and beyond.

Public and Religious Perspectives

The exploration of stem cells has prompted a wide array of public and religious perspectives, significantly influencing the discourse surrounding their research and application. Many religious groups maintain traditional stances regarding the sanctity of life, which often leads to opposing views on the use of embryonic stem cells. These perspectives are rooted in deep philosophical beliefs about the beginning of life, prompting a complex dialogue between scientific advancement and ethical considerations. Health care professionals must navigate these discussions with sensitivity, recognising the diverse beliefs that inform public opinion.

Public perception of stem cell research is also shaped by a myriad of factors, including media representation and personal experiences with degenerative diseases. Misconceptions about the potential of stem cells often persist, leading to unrealistic expectations among patients and their families. It is crucial for biomedical scientists and medical personnel to engage in transparent communication, educating the public about the realistic applications and limitations of stem cell therapies. This not only aids in dispelling myths but also fosters a more informed and supportive environment for ongoing research.

The ethical considerations surrounding stem cell research are further complicated by the potential for personalised medicine. As scientists explore the capabilities of stem cells to tailor treatments based on individual genetic profiles, ethical dilemmas regarding access and equity arise. This presents a challenge for health care professionals who must advocate for fair practices while considering the diverse socio-economic backgrounds of patients. Engaging with these ethical questions is essential for advancing research in a manner that respects both scientific integrity and human dignity.

Moreover, the impact of stem cells extends beyond human medicine; their applications in veterinary medicine also raise public interest and ethical questions. As veterinary science increasingly incorporates stem cell therapies for animal health, parallels can be drawn with human applications, prompting discussions about the moral implications of such treatments. This intersection calls for a broader consideration of the role of stem cells in both human and animal health, urging professionals to think critically about the ethical frameworks that guide their practices.

In conclusion, the public and religious perspectives on stem cell research present both challenges and opportunities for health care professionals and biomedical scientists. By fostering open dialogue and addressing misconceptions, the scientific community can work towards a more informed public understanding of stem cells. This approach not only enhances the credibility of the research but also strengthens the collaborative efforts needed to navigate the ethical landscape of emerging stem cell technologies.

Controversies and Debates

Stem cell research has been at the forefront of scientific innovation and medical advancement, yet it is also fraught with controversies and debates. The ethical considerations surrounding stem cell research are among the most contentious issues in the field. Questions about the moral status of embryos, the consent of donors, and the potential for exploitation have led to significant public and governmental scrutiny. Health care professionals must navigate these ethical waters carefully, ensuring that their practices align with both scientific integrity and societal values.

The application of stem cells in therapies for degenerative diseases raises additional debates regarding efficacy and safety. While preliminary studies show promise in treating conditions such as Parkinson's disease and spinal cord injuries, concerns about the long-term effects and potential complications remain. Biomedical scientists and medical personnel in training must be equipped to evaluate these risks critically, balancing the potential benefits of new treatments against the uncertainties that accompany them.

Advances in stem cell technology and techniques have also sparked discussions about the implications of personalised medicine. The ability to tailor treatments based on an individual's genetic profile presents exciting possibilities, yet it also raises questions about access and equity. The potential for stem cell therapies to be available primarily to wealthier patients could exacerbate existing health disparities, making it essential for health care professionals to advocate for equitable access to these innovations.

Moreover, public perception and misconceptions about stem cell research significantly influence its progress and funding. Misunderstandings regarding the science behind stem cells can lead to fear and hesitance to support research initiatives. Health care professionals have a critical role in educating the public, dispelling myths, and fostering informed discussions about the real potential and limitations of stem cell therapies.

Lastly, the implications of stem cell banking present further ethical and practical considerations. The idea of storing stem cells for future use raises questions about consent, ownership, and the long-term viability of stored cells. As stem cell applications expand into areas such as veterinary medicine, the debates surrounding these issues are likely to intensify. Health care professionals must stay informed and engaged in these conversations, contributing their expertise to shape the future of stem cell research responsibly.

Stem Cell Therapies for Degenerative Diseases

Mechanisms of Action

The mechanisms of action of stem cells are fundamental to understanding their potential applications in medicine. Stem cells possess unique properties, such as self-renewal and the ability to differentiate into various cell types. These characteristics enable them to play crucial roles in tissue repair and regeneration. By understanding the underlying biological processes, healthcare professionals can better appreciate how stem cells can be harnessed for therapeutic purposes.

One of the primary mechanisms of action is the ability of stem cells to secrete a range of bioactive factors. These factors can modulate the immune response, promote cell survival, and stimulate the repair of damaged tissues. This paracrine effect is essential in regenerative medicine, as it allows stem cells to influence their microenvironment and facilitate healing without necessarily differentiating into specific cell types.

Moreover, the process of differentiation is another critical mechanism of action. When exposed to specific stimuli, stem cells can differentiate into specialised cells, such as neurons, cardiomyocytes, or insulin-producing cells. This differentiation is influenced by intrinsic factors, such as genetic programming, and extrinsic factors, including the presence of growth factors and extracellular matrix components. Understanding this process is vital for developing targeted stem cell therapies for degenerative diseases.

Ethical considerations also play a significant role in shaping the landscape of stem cell research. The mechanisms of action must be understood not only from a scientific perspective but also through the lens of ethical implications. This includes the source of stem cells, particularly embryonic versus adult stem cells, and the potential for creating personalised medicine solutions while respecting moral boundaries.

Lastly, advancements in stem cell technology have led to innovative techniques that enhance the efficiency of stem cell therapies. Techniques such as gene editing and the use of biomaterials can improve the survival and integration of stem cells in host tissues. As these technologies evolve, the mechanisms of action will continue to be refined, leading to more effective treatments for a variety of conditions while addressing public misconceptions about stem cell research.

Case Studies: Parkinson's Disease

Parkinson's disease (PD) is a progressive neurodegenerative disorder characterised by the degeneration of dopaminergic neurons in the substantia nigra, leading to motor symptoms such as tremors, rigidity, and bradykinesia. Recent advances in stem cell research have opened new avenues for potential therapies aimed at repairing or replacing the damaged neurons in patients suffering from this debilitating condition. Understanding the mechanisms of PD and the role of stem cells in its treatment is crucial for healthcare professionals and biomedical scientists alike, as it paves the way for innovative strategies in regenerative medicine.

Case studies have highlighted various approaches to utilising stem cells for Parkinson's disease. One notable example is the transplantation of induced pluripotent stem cells (iPSCs) derived from patients' skin cells. These iPSCs can differentiate into dopaminergic neurons, offering a personalised medicine approach that reduces the risk of immune rejection. Clinical trials have begun to show promising results, with patients exhibiting improvements in motor functions and overall quality of life after receiving these stem cell therapies.

Ethical considerations remain a significant aspect of stem cell research in Parkinson's disease. The use of embryonic stem cells has raised concerns regarding the moral implications of sourcing these cells. However, the development of iPSCs has alleviated some of these ethical dilemmas, as they can be generated from adult cells without the need for embryos. This shift not only enhances the acceptance of stem cell research within the public sphere but also encourages further investment and exploration of stem cell applications in treating degenerative diseases.

Moreover, the impact of stem cell banking on Parkinson's disease cannot be overlooked. By storing stem cells for future use, researchers can ensure a readily available supply for developing therapies tailored to individual patients. This practice not only enhances the prospects of personalised medicine but also contributes to a better understanding of the disease's progression and response to various treatments, ultimately leading to improved outcomes for patients.

In conclusion, the case studies surrounding Parkinson's disease and stem cell research illustrate the immense potential of these technologies in regenerative medicine. As advancements continue, it is essential for healthcare professionals and medical personnel in training to stay informed about the latest developments, benefits, and ethical considerations in stem cell therapies. The future of treating Parkinson's disease may very well lie in the harnessing of stem cells, offering hope to millions affected by this condition.

Case Studies: Alzheimer's Disease

Alzheimer's disease, a progressive neurodegenerative disorder, poses significant challenges for healthcare professionals and biomedical researchers alike. Recent case studies have highlighted the potential of stem cell therapies in addressing the complexities of this condition. By understanding the pathological mechanisms of Alzheimer's, researchers can explore how stem cells may offer rejuvenation to damaged neural tissues and restore cognitive functions in affected individuals.

One prominent case study involved the use of induced pluripotent stem cells (iPSCs) derived from patients with familial Alzheimer's disease. These iPSCs were differentiated into neurons to model the disease in vitro. The findings revealed toxic protein accumulations, which provided insights into disease progression and potential therapeutic targets. Such studies underscore the importance of patient-specific stem cell lines in developing personalised medicine strategies for Alzheimer's treatment.

Ethical considerations remain paramount in stem cell research, particularly concerning the sourcing of stem cells and the implications for patient consent. In the context of Alzheimer's, the need for ethical frameworks is amplified due to the involvement of vulnerable populations. Case studies that address these ethical dilemmas contribute to a more nuanced understanding of how to advance stem cell research while respecting the rights and dignity of participants.

Another notable case study examined the application of mesenchymal stem cells (MSCs) in animal models of Alzheimer's disease. Results indicated that MSCs could improve cognitive function and reduce neuroinflammation, shedding light on their regenerative potential. Such findings not only pave the way for clinical trials in humans but also stimulate discussions around the efficacy and safety of stem cell therapies in neurodegenerative diseases.

As advancements in stem cell technology continue to progress, the integration of findings from case studies into clinical practice becomes essential. The ongoing research into Alzheimer's disease serves as a testament to the transformative potential of stem cells in regenerative medicine. Through collaborative efforts among health care professionals and scientists, there is hope for developing effective strategies to combat this debilitating condition, ultimately improving quality of life for patients and their families.

0zqasThe Role of Stem Cells in Regenerative Medicine

Tissue Engineering

Tissue engineering represents a pioneering frontier in the realm of regenerative medicine, intertwining principles of biology and engineering to create functional tissues that can restore or replace damaged biological structures. By harnessing the unique properties of stem cells, researchers are exploring innovative ways to fabricate tissues that not only mimic the natural architecture of human organs but also integrate seamlessly with the host's biological systems. This approach has profound implications for treating degenerative diseases, where traditional therapies often fall short.

The ethical considerations surrounding stem cell research remain a pivotal concern, particularly in the context of tissue engineering. The sourcing of stem cells, especially embryonic stem cells, raises significant moral and ethical dilemmas that healthcare professionals must navigate. It is essential to engage with these ethical discussions to ensure that advancements in tissue engineering are pursued responsibly, balancing scientific progress with respect for human dignity and rights.

Advancements in stem cell technology and techniques have catalysed significant progress in tissue engineering. Techniques such as 3D bioprinting and scaffolding technologies are paving the way for the creation of complex tissue structures that can be used in both research and clinical applications. These innovations not only enhance the functional capabilities of engineered tissues but also improve their viability and integration within the host organism, offering new hope for patients with conditions that currently lack effective treatment options.

As the field of personalised medicine continues to evolve, the role of stem cells in tailoring therapies to individual patients becomes increasingly prominent. Tissue engineered products can be designed using a patient's own stem cells, minimising the risk of rejection and maximising therapeutic efficacy. This personalised approach not only enhances treatment outcomes but also aligns with the growing demand for patient-centric healthcare solutions.

Finally, the public perception and misconceptions surrounding stem cell research and tissue engineering play a crucial role in shaping policy and funding for these innovative therapies. Educating both the public and healthcare professionals about the scientific realities of stem cell applications is vital for fostering a supportive environment for research. Addressing misconceptions and highlighting the tangible benefits of tissue engineering can help garner public trust and facilitate the advancement of regenerative medicine in society.

Stem Cell Transplantation

Stem cell transplantation represents a significant advancement in modern medicine, offering hope for patients with various degenerative diseases. This procedure involves the transfer of stem cells into a patient's body to replace damaged or diseased cells. The origins of these stem cells can vary, including embryonic stem cells, adult stem cells, and induced pluripotent stem cells, each with its unique potential and ethical considerations. Understanding the different types of stem cells and their origins is crucial for healthcare professionals who are involved in this field.

Ethical considerations surrounding stem cell research have been a topic of intense debate. The use of embryonic stem cells raises moral questions regarding the beginning of life and the rights of embryos. Healthcare professionals must navigate these ethical dilemmas while staying informed about regulatory guidelines and public sentiment. Ongoing discussions about the moral implications of stem cell sourcing are essential for fostering responsible research and application in clinical settings.

Stem cell therapies have shown promise in treating degenerative diseases such as Parkinson's and Alzheimer's, where traditional treatments may fall short. By replenishing damaged cells, stem cell transplantation can potentially restore function and improve quality of life for affected individuals. Medical personnel in training should be educated about the latest advancements in these therapies, including ongoing clinical trials and emerging techniques that enhance the effectiveness of stem cell treatments.

In the realm of regenerative medicine, stem cells play a pivotal role in repairing and regenerating damaged tissues. This field is rapidly evolving, with innovations in technology allowing for more targeted and effective interventions. The potential of stem cells in personalised medicine is particularly compelling, as it opens avenues for tailored therapies that consider the unique genetic makeup of each patient, increasing the likelihood of successful outcomes.

Lastly, the impact of stem cells extends beyond human medicine, with applications in veterinary medicine also being explored. Stem cell banking has emerged as a significant aspect of this research, allowing for the preservation of stem cells for future use. Public perception and misconceptions surrounding stem cell research can greatly influence funding and support for ongoing studies, making it essential for healthcare professionals to engage with the community and disseminate accurate information about the benefits and limitations of stem cell transplantation.

Clinical Applications

The clinical applications of stem cells have garnered significant attention in recent years, reflecting their potential to revolutionise medicine. These applications range from treating degenerative diseases to advancing regenerative medicine. Health care professionals and biomedical scientists are increasingly exploring how these remarkable cells can be utilised to repair damaged tissues, restore function, and improve the quality of life for patients suffering from various ailments.

One of the most promising areas of stem cell therapy is in the treatment of degenerative diseases such as Parkinson's disease, Alzheimer's, and spinal cord injuries. Clinical trials are underway to determine how stem cells can replace lost or damaged neurons, aiming to restore cognitive and motor functions. This research not only highlights the therapeutic potential of stem cells but also underscores the importance of ethical considerations in their application, as the source and manipulation of these cells must be conducted responsibly.

Regenerative medicine stands at the forefront of clinical applications, where stem cells are employed to regenerate damaged organs and tissues. This approach offers hope for patients with conditions previously deemed irreversible. Advances in techniques such as 3D bioprinting and gene editing further enhance the capabilities of stem cells in creating personalised treatment plans, which cater to the unique genetic makeup of patients, thereby improving outcomes.

The impact of stem cells extends beyond human medicine, finding applications in veterinary medicine as well. Stem cell therapies are being developed to treat a variety of conditions in animals, including osteoarthritis and tendon injuries. This not only benefits animal health but also informs clinical practices in human health, as parallels can be drawn between veterinary and human applications of stem cell technology.

Public perception and misconceptions about stem cell research remain significant barriers to the advancement of clinical applications. Educating health care professionals and the wider community about the potential benefits and ethical considerations is crucial. As knowledge increases, so too does the potential for stem cells to become a cornerstone of modern medicine, paving the way for innovative therapies and improved patient care.

Advances in Stem Cell Technology and Techniques

CRISPR and Gene Editing

CRISPR technology has revolutionised the field of gene editing, offering unprecedented precision and efficiency in modifying genetic material. This innovative approach allows scientists to target specific sequences in DNA, effectively enabling the manipulation of genes associated with various diseases. For healthcare professionals and biomedical scientists, understanding CRISPR's mechanisms is essential, as it provides the tools necessary for advancing stem cell therapies and regenerative medicine practices.

Three-Dimensional Cell Cultures

Three-dimensional (3D) cell cultures represent a significant advancement in the field of biomedical research, particularly in stem cell studies. Unlike traditional two-dimensional (2D) cultures, which can lead to artificial behaviour of cells, 3D cultures provide a more physiologically relevant environment. This innovation allows for better mimicry of in vivo conditions, enabling researchers to observe how stem cells interact within a more natural context. As a result, 3D cultures are increasingly being utilised to study the differentiation and functionality of stem cells.

The application of 3D cell cultures in stem cell research has profound implications for regenerative medicine. By cultivating stem cells in a 3D matrix, scientists can create organoids that closely resemble real organs. These organoids offer a unique platform for investigating various degenerative diseases, providing insights into disease mechanisms and potential therapeutic targets. Moreover, this method enhances the potential for personalised medicine, as patient-specific stem cells can be used to generate organoids for tailored treatments.

Ethical considerations remain a critical aspect of stem cell research. The shift to 3D cultures does not eliminate ethical dilemmas but rather shifts the focus towards how stem cells are sourced and their applications in therapy. Ensuring that stem cells are ethically obtained and used in research is fundamental for maintaining public trust and advancing scientific inquiry. Furthermore, the development of 3D cultures may lead to reduced reliance on animal models, addressing some ethical concerns associated with traditional research practices.

In addition to their applications in human medicine, 3D cell cultures also play a role in veterinary medicine. The ability to study stem cells in a 3D environment can lead to breakthroughs in treating genetic disorders and degenerative diseases in animals. This cross-disciplinary approach highlights the versatility of stem cell research, showcasing its potential benefits not only for human health but also for animal welfare and veterinary practices.

As the field of stem cell technology advances, the integration of 3D cell cultures is poised to revolutionise our understanding of cell behaviour and therapeutic efficacy. Ongoing research and development in this area promise to enhance the effectiveness of stem cell therapies, paving the way for innovative treatments. As healthcare professionals and biomedical scientists continue to explore these technologies, the future of regenerative medicine looks increasingly promising, with 3D cultures at the forefront of this progress.

Bioprinting of Tissues

Bioprinting of tissues represents a revolutionary advancement in the field of regenerative medicine, offering the potential to create functional living tissues that can be used for transplantation and drug testing. This technique utilises bioinks, which are materials that can support cell growth and mimic the natural extracellular matrix. By precisely depositing these bioinks layer by layer, researchers can engineer tissues that closely resemble their natural counterparts, thereby addressing the critical shortage of organ donors and the ethical dilemmas associated with organ transplantation.

One of the most significant advantages of bioprinting is its ability to customise tissues for individual patients. This personalised approach is particularly beneficial in treating degenerative diseases, where tailored solutions can enhance treatment efficacy. By using a patient's own cells to create bioprinted tissues, the risks of rejection and complications associated with immunosuppressive therapies can be significantly reduced. This innovation aligns with the growing trend towards personalised medicine, which seeks to provide more effective and targeted therapies for patients.

However, the bioprinting of tissues does not come without ethical considerations. The process raises questions about the source of stem cells used for bioprinting, particularly when derived from embryonic sources. Ethical frameworks must be established to ensure that research is conducted responsibly and that the rights of donors are protected. Moreover, as bioprinting technology advances, there is a need to consider the implications of creating complex tissues and organs, including the moral status of these engineered constructs and their potential uses in society.

Advancements in bioprinting techniques are rapidly evolving, with researchers continuously exploring new methods to improve the resolution and functionality of printed tissues. Innovations such as 3D printing combined with stem cell technology are paving the way for creating more sophisticated tissue structures that can better mimic the physiological properties of human tissues. These advancements have the potential to revolutionise not only regenerative medicine but also pharmacological testing, enabling more accurate assessments of drug efficacy and safety.

In conclusion, bioprinting of tissues stands at the forefront of stem cell research and regenerative medicine. As this technology continues to develop, it holds the promise of transforming the landscape of medical treatments, providing solutions to previously unsolvable problems in tissue and organ transplantation. Healthcare professionals and biomedical scientists must remain informed about these advancements to harness their potential effectively and navigate the ethical landscape that accompanies such innovations.

Stem Cells and Their Potential in Personalised Medicine

Customised Treatments

Customised treatments represent a revolutionary approach in modern medicine, particularly in the realm of stem cell research. These treatments are tailored to the individual needs of patients, considering their unique genetic makeup, lifestyle, and specific health conditions. By leveraging the potential of stem cells, healthcare professionals can develop therapies that are not only more effective but also minimise adverse reactions typically associated with standardised treatments.

The integration of personalised medicine into stem cell therapies has opened new avenues for addressing degenerative diseases. Conditions such as Parkinson's and Alzheimer's, which have historically posed significant challenges to conventional treatment methods, can now be approached with innovative strategies involving patient-specific stem cells. This not only enhances the efficacy of the treatment but also aligns with the ethical considerations of utilising a patient's own cells, thereby reducing the risk of immune rejection.

Ethical considerations remain paramount in the field of stem cell research, especially as customised treatments gain prominence. Healthcare professionals must navigate the complex landscape of ethical guidelines while ensuring that patients are fully informed about the implications of their treatment options. This includes discussions surrounding consent, the use of embryonic stem cells, and the need for ongoing research to establish the safety and efficacy of these bespoke therapies.

Advancements in stem cell technology have significantly contributed to the feasibility of customised treatments. Innovations such as CRISPR gene editing and induced pluripotent stem cells (iPSCs) are at the forefront of this evolution, enabling scientists to create patient-specific stem cells that can be used in therapies. These advancements not only enhance the precision of treatments but also facilitate the exploration of new applications in regenerative medicine and genetic disorders.

As customised treatments continue to evolve, the public's perception and understanding of stem cell research play a crucial role in its acceptance and integration into mainstream medicine. Education is key to dispelling misconceptions and fostering trust between healthcare professionals and patients. By addressing concerns and highlighting the successes of stem cell therapies, the medical community can pave the way for broader adoption of these innovative treatments, ultimately transforming the landscape of personalised medicine.

Pharmacogenomics

Pharmacogenomics is a pivotal field that explores the interplay between genetics and drug response, particularly in the context of stem cell therapies. It focuses on how genetic variations among individuals can influence their reactions to medications, including those derived from or involving stem cells. With the advent of personalised medicine, pharmacogenomics aims to tailor treatments based on an individual's genetic makeup, thereby maximising efficacy and minimising adverse effects. This approach is particularly relevant in the treatment of degenerative diseases, where stem cells can play a transformative role in patient outcomes.

In the realm of stem cell research, ethical considerations are paramount, especially when it comes to pharmacogenomics. The manipulation of genetic information raises significant moral questions about consent, privacy, and the potential for discrimination based on genetic profiles. Health care professionals must navigate these ethical waters carefully, ensuring that patients are fully informed and treated with the utmost respect. This ethical framework is essential not only for advancing research but also for maintaining public trust in stem cell therapies.

As advances in technology continue to enhance our understanding of the genome, the role of pharmacogenomics in regenerative medicine becomes increasingly vital. By integrating genetic testing into the clinical setting, healthcare providers can identify which patients are most likely to benefit from specific stem cell treatments. This not only optimises therapeutic strategies but also reduces the risk of ineffective treatments, paving the way for more successful outcomes in regenerative medicine.

Moreover, the implications of pharmacogenomics extend beyond individual patients to broader public health considerations. Effective stem cell therapies can significantly alleviate the burden of genetic disorders, offering new hope to patients and their families. As research progresses, pharmacogenomics can facilitate the development of targeted therapies that address the root causes of these conditions, transforming the landscape of treatment and care.

Lastly, the public perception of pharmacogenomics and stem cell research is crucial for its acceptance and implementation. Education and outreach are necessary to dispel misconceptions and inform the public about the benefits and risks associated with these advancements. By fostering a well-informed dialogue, healthcare professionals can contribute to a more nuanced understanding of how pharmacogenomics intersects with stem cell therapies, ultimately enhancing patient care and advancing medical science.

Patient-Derived Stem Cells

Patient-derived stem cells represent a pivotal advancement in the field of regenerative medicine, as they provide a unique opportunity to understand and treat various degenerative diseases. These cells are harvested from patients, allowing for the creation of personalised therapies that are tailored to individual genetic profiles. This approach not only enhances the efficacy of treatments but also minimises the risk of immune rejection, a common challenge in traditional stem cell therapies. By utilising a patient's own tissues, the potential for adverse reactions is significantly reduced, paving the way for safer and more effective medical interventions.

The ethical considerations surrounding patient-derived stem cells are substantial and multifaceted. As these cells are obtained directly from individuals, it is crucial to ensure that informed consent is obtained, and that patients are fully aware of the implications of their contribution. Furthermore, the discussion extends to the moral responsibilities of researchers in handling these cells, particularly in terms of privacy and the potential for exploitation. Addressing these ethical concerns is vital for maintaining public trust and advancing stem cell research in a responsible manner.

In the realm of personalised medicine, patient-derived stem cells hold immense potential for treating genetic disorders. By studying these cells, researchers can gain insights into the underlying mechanisms of various diseases, leading to the development of targeted therapies. This strategy not only enhances our understanding of disease pathology but also facilitates the creation of bespoke treatments that are more effective for individual patients. As a result, the potential for breakthroughs in the management of genetic disorders is significant, offering hope for many affected individuals.

Moreover, patient-derived stem cells are increasingly being integrated into clinical practices, with ongoing studies exploring their applications in veterinary medicine as well. The use of these cells in animals has the potential to revolutionise treatment protocols, providing new avenues for addressing chronic conditions and injuries in pets and other animals. This cross-disciplinary approach not only enhances veterinary care but also contributes valuable insights that can inform human medicine, creating a symbiotic relationship between the two fields.

Lastly, public perception and misconceptions surrounding stem cell research play a critical role in its advancement. Education and transparency are essential in dispelling myths and fostering a more informed dialogue about the potential benefits and risks associated with patient-derived stem cells. By engaging with the public and addressing concerns, healthcare professionals and researchers can build greater acceptance and support for stem cell research, ultimately leading to improved patient outcomes and advancements in medical science.

The Impact of Stem Cells on Genetic Disorders

Understanding Genetic Disorders

Genetic disorders represent a significant area of concern within the field of medicine, affecting millions of individuals worldwide. They arise from alterations in the DNA sequence, which can occur due to hereditary factors or environmental influences. Understanding the genetic basis of these disorders is crucial for healthcare professionals and biomedical scientists, as it lays the groundwork for potential interventions, including stem cell therapies. The intricate relationship between genetics and stem cells opens new avenues for research and treatment, offering hope for those affected by these conditions.

Stem cells have the unique ability to differentiate into various cell types, making them a valuable resource in the treatment of genetic disorders. By harnessing their regenerative properties, researchers are exploring innovative methods to correct genetic defects at the cellular level. This approach not only aims to alleviate symptoms but also targets the root cause of the disorder. The potential for personalised medicine, where treatments are tailored to the individual's genetic makeup, is particularly promising in this context, enhancing the efficacy of stem cell therapies.

Ethical considerations play a pivotal role in the discourse surrounding stem cell research, particularly when it comes to genetic disorders. The use of embryonic stem cells raises significant moral questions, while advancements in induced pluripotent stem cells (iPSCs) offer an alternative that sidesteps some of these ethical dilemmas. Healthcare professionals must navigate these complexities, balancing the need for scientific advancement with ethical responsibility. A clear understanding of the ethical landscape is essential for fostering public trust and supporting continued research in this vital area.

Advancements in stem cell technology have accelerated the pace of research and development in addressing genetic disorders. Techniques such as genome editing, particularly CRISPR-Cas9, have revolutionised the ability to modify genes with precision. This has significant implications for stem cell therapies, as researchers can now potentially correct genetic mutations in stem cells before reintroducing them into the patient. The integration of these technologies into clinical practice holds great promise for treating previously intractable genetic conditions, although careful consideration of long-term effects and safety remains paramount.

The impact of stem cells on genetic disorders is multifaceted, encompassing not only therapeutic applications but also potential avenues for prevention and diagnosis. Stem cell banking is emerging as a key component in this field, providing a resource for future therapies and research. As our understanding of genetics and stem cell biology deepens, the prospects for improving outcomes for individuals with genetic disorders become increasingly viable. Engaging with the scientific community and the public is essential to demystifying stem cell research and highlighting its potential benefits, ultimately paving the way for innovative treatments that could transform the lives of those affected.

Gene Therapy and Stem Cells

Gene therapy represents a revolutionary approach in medicine, aiming to treat or prevent diseases by directly modifying the genetic material within an individual's cells. This innovative technique often intersects with stem cell research, as stem cells possess unique properties that make them ideal candidates for gene therapy applications. By integrating therapeutic genes into stem cells, it is possible to create a source of cells that can continuously produce the desired proteins or factors needed to combat genetic disorders, thereby offering a potential cure rather than merely alleviating symptoms.

The ethical considerations surrounding gene therapy and stem cell research are significant and multifaceted. Healthcare professionals and researchers must navigate the complexities of informed consent, potential long-term effects, and the implications of altering human genetics. Additionally, the use of embryonic stem cells in gene therapy raises further ethical dilemmas regarding the moral status of embryos and the extent to which they should be utilised in research and treatment. Addressing these concerns is crucial for fostering public trust and ensuring the responsible advancement of these technologies.

Stem cell therapies have shown promise in treating degenerative diseases, such as Parkinson's disease, spinal cord injuries, and certain types of cancer. By employing gene therapy in conjunction with stem cell treatments, researchers can enhance the efficacy of these therapies. For instance, genetically modified stem cells can be directed to repair damaged tissues or produce neuroprotective factors that may halt or reverse the progression of neurodegenerative conditions. This synergistic approach holds the potential to transform the landscape of regenerative medicine, offering hope to patients with previously untreatable ailments.

Advancements in stem cell technology have opened new avenues for personalised medicine, as treatments can be tailored to an individual's genetic makeup. By combining patient-specific stem cells with gene therapy techniques, healthcare providers can develop bespoke treatments that are more effective and have fewer side effects. This personalised approach not only improves clinical outcomes but also enhances patient engagement and satisfaction, as individuals are more likely to respond positively to therapies designed specifically for their unique genetic profiles.

In summary, the intersection of gene therapy and stem cells represents a frontier of medical innovation with vast potential. As research continues to evolve, it will be essential for healthcare professionals to stay informed about the latest advancements and ethical considerations. The future of medicine may very well hinge on the ability to harness these powerful technologies, ultimately leading to transformative treatments for genetic disorders and degenerative diseases alike.

Case Studies: Cystic Fibrosis

Cystic fibrosis (CF) is a genetic disorder that primarily affects the lungs and digestive system, leading to significant morbidity and mortality. Advances in our understanding of the underlying genetic mechanisms have paved the way for novel therapeutic approaches, particularly those involving stem cell technology.

By examining case studies, we can begin to uncover the potential of stem cells in treating this debilitating condition, offering hope to patients and their families.

One notable case study involves the use of induced pluripotent stem cells (iPSCs) derived from patients with cystic fibrosis. Researchers have successfully created organoids that mimic the intestinal epithelium, allowing for in-depth studies of CF pathology. These organoids not only provide insights into disease mechanisms but also serve as a platform for drug testing, enabling the identification of therapies that could ameliorate symptoms or potentially correct the underlying genetic defect.

Another compelling example is the exploration of gene editing technologies, such as CRISPR/Cas9, in conjunction with stem cell therapy. A case study involving the application of these techniques to patient-derived stem cells demonstrates the feasibility of correcting mutations associated with cystic fibrosis. This innovative approach could lead to personalised medicine strategies, where treatments are tailored to the specific genetic profiles of individual patients, representing a significant advancement in the management of CF.

Moreover, the ethical considerations surrounding stem cell research are highlighted in the context of cystic fibrosis. As healthcare professionals and researchers navigate the complexities of stem cell applications, it is crucial to strike a balance between scientific advancement and ethical responsibility. Case studies provide valuable insights into how ethical frameworks can guide research practices while ensuring that patient welfare remains a priority.

Finally, the impact of stem cell banking on cystic fibrosis research cannot be overstated. With an increasing number of biobanks focusing on CF, researchers have access to a wealth of genetic material that can facilitate ongoing studies. This accessibility not only accelerates research efforts but also enhances collaboration across institutions, ultimately driving forward the development of effective stem cell therapies for cystic fibrosis and similar genetic disorders.

Stem Cell Banking and Its Implications

Types of Stem Cell Banking

Stem cell banking has emerged as a vital component in the field of regenerative medicine, offering various types of banking options that cater to different needs and preferences. The most known form is umbilical cord blood banking, which involves collecting and storing the blood from the umbilical cord after childbirth. This type of banking is particularly valuable due to the rich source of haematopoietic stem cells it provides, which can be used in treatments for various blood disorders and certain cancers.

Another significant type is adult stem cell banking, which typically involves the collection of stem cells from sources such as bone marrow or peripheral blood. These cells are often used in therapies for degenerative diseases and injuries, making their availability crucial for patients requiring immediate treatment. Adult stem cell banking, however, presents challenges related to the extraction process and the limited quantity of stem cells that can be harvested, which can impact their therapeutic potential.

Induced pluripotent stem cell (iPSC) banking is another innovative approach that has gained popularity in recent years. iPSCs are generated by reprogramming somatic cells, allowing for an unlimited source of stem cells that can be tailored to match the genetic profile of the patient. This type of banking holds immense promise for personalised medicine, as it allows for the development of patient-specific therapies while circumventing some ethical concerns associated with embryonic stem cell research.

Moreover, there is a growing interest in veterinary stem cell banking, which provides similar benefits for animals. This type of banking allows for the storage of stem cells derived from pets, enabling the treatment of various conditions such as osteoarthritis and other degenerative diseases. The expansion of stem cell banking into veterinary medicine highlights the versatility and potential of stem cell therapies across species, fostering advancements in animal health care.

In summary, the various types of stem cell banking not only reflect the diversity in sources and applications but also underscore the ethical considerations and technological advancements in the field. As stem cell research continues to evolve, the implications of these banking methods will play a crucial role in the future of regenerative medicine and personalised therapies. Understanding these types can empower healthcare professionals and researchers to make informed decisions in their practice, ensuring better outcomes for patients and advancing the field.

Ethical and Legal Considerations

The ethical and legal considerations surrounding stem cell research are paramount in guiding the direction of scientific inquiry and clinical application. As stem cells hold immense potential for treating degenerative diseases and contributing to regenerative medicine, the implications of their use raise profound moral questions. Health care professionals and biomedical scientists must navigate the complex landscape of ethical dilemmas, including the source of stem cells, informed consent, and the potential for exploitation of vulnerable populations. The principles of beneficence and non-maleficence must be at the forefront of discussions regarding the appropriate use of stem cell therapies.

Legislation varies significantly across countries, influencing the progress and acceptance of stem cell research. In some regions, strict regulations limit the types of stem cells that can be used, while others adopt a more permissive approach. This disparity creates challenges for researchers aiming to collaborate internationally, as differing legal frameworks can hinder the sharing of knowledge and resources. It is crucial for health care professionals and those in training to understand the legal context within which they operate, ensuring compliance with local laws and ethical guidelines to foster responsible research and application.

Public perception plays a critical role in shaping the landscape of stem cell research. Misconceptions regarding the nature and potential of stem cells can lead to fear and resistance from the community. Educational initiatives that inform the public about the scientific basis and potential benefits of stem cell therapies are vital in addressing these concerns. Health care professionals must be equipped to engage in conversations with patients and the public, dispelling myths and fostering a more informed understanding of stem cell applications in personalised medicine and treatment of genetic disorders.

Furthermore, the issue of stem cell banking introduces additional ethical and legal dimensions. The storage and use of stem cells for future therapies raise questions about ownership, consent, and the rights of donors. It is essential for health care professionals to advocate for transparent policies that protect individuals' rights while maximising the potential benefits of stem cell research. Ethical frameworks should be established to guide practices in stem cell banking, ensuring that the focus remains on patient welfare and scientific integrity.

In conclusion, the intersection of ethics and law in stem cell research demands ongoing dialogue among health care professionals, scientists, and policymakers. As advancements in stem cell technology continue to unfold, it is imperative that ethical considerations remain central to the discourse. By fostering a culture of ethical awareness and legal compliance, the medical community can fully realise the promise of stem cells while maintaining public trust and safeguarding human dignity in the pursuit of scientific progress.

Future of Stem Cell Banking

The future of stem cell banking holds significant promise for both regenerative medicine and personalised healthcare. As our understanding of stem cells continues to evolve, the banking of these cells for future use is becoming an increasingly viable option for patients with degenerative diseases. The ability to store stem cells from various sources, including umbilical cord blood and adult tissues, allows for a personalised approach to treatment. This proactive measure not only safeguards the potential for future therapies but also opens avenues for innovative research into the applications of stem cells.

Ethical considerations remain at the forefront of discussions surrounding stem cell banking. As healthcare professionals, it is crucial to navigate the ethical landscape carefully, ensuring that practices comply with regulations and respect the rights of donors. The debate surrounding the use of embryonic stem cells versus adult stem cells exemplifies the complexities involved. Ensuring informed consent and maintaining transparency in the banking process will be vital to fostering public trust and acceptance of stem cell therapies.

Advancements in stem cell technology and techniques are rapidly transforming the field, enhancing the efficiency and efficacy of stem cell therapies. With innovations such as induced pluripotent stem cells (iPSCs), researchers are now able to generate patient-specific stem cells that can be used for personalised treatments. This advancement not only minimises the risk of rejection but also allows for tailored therapies that address the unique genetic makeup of individuals, thus revolutionising the approach to regenerative medicine.

Public perception and misconceptions surrounding stem cell research pose challenges to the field's advancement. As health care professionals, it is essential to engage in effective communication, educating the public about the potential benefits and limitations of stem cell banking. By addressing misconceptions and providing accurate information, professionals can help cultivate a more informed discourse, ultimately leading to greater acceptance of stem cell therapies in mainstream medicine.

In conclusion, the future of stem cell banking is intertwined with the advancements in stem cell research and technology. As we continue to explore the therapeutic potential of stem cells, it is imperative to consider ethical practices, public perception, and the personalised nature of emerging treatments. The potential impact on genetic disorders and regenerative medicine is profound, making stem cell banking not just a preservation method, but a critical component of future healthcare strategies.

Stem Cell Applications in Veterinary Medicine

Veterinary Uses of Stem Cells

The application of stem cells in veterinary medicine has emerged as a transformative approach to treating various health conditions in animals. These cells, with their unique ability to differentiate into different cell types, offer promising solutions for regenerative therapies. This potential is particularly valuable in treating degenerative diseases that are common in companion animals, such as osteoarthritis and certain types of heart disease. By harnessing the power of stem cells, veterinarians are beginning to provide more effective treatments that enhance the quality of life for their patients.

One notable use of stem cells in veterinary practice is in the treatment of joint injuries and diseases. Stem cell therapies have been shown to promote healing and regeneration of damaged cartilage, significantly alleviating pain and improving mobility in affected animals. This is especially pertinent for older pets who suffer from chronic conditions, as they can benefit immensely from these advanced therapeutic options. Additionally, the minimally invasive nature of stem cell injections makes them an attractive alternative to traditional surgical interventions.

Furthermore, stem cells are being explored for their potential in treating a range of other conditions, including neurological disorders and skin ailments. For instance, conditions such as spinal cord injuries and certain autoimmune diseases are being targeted with stem cell therapies that aim to repair or regenerate affected tissues. The versatility of stem cells continues to open new avenues for research and treatment, fostering hope for conditions that were once considered untreatable in veterinary medicine.

However, the use of stem cells in animals is not without its ethical considerations. As with human applications, there are ongoing discussions regarding the sourcing of stem cells and the implications of their use. Ensuring that the methods employed are ethical and transparent is crucial for maintaining public trust and advancing the field responsibly. As veterinary professionals advocate for the responsible use of stem cells, it is essential to balance scientific progress with ethical accountability.

In conclusion, the veterinary uses of stem cells represent a significant advancement in medical treatment for animals. As research progresses, the potential for stem cells to revolutionise veterinary medicine continues to grow. With increasing acceptance and understanding of these therapies, the future holds great promise for the enhancement of animal health and welfare, paving the way for innovative treatment options that can lead to longer and healthier lives for our beloved pets.

Success Stories in Animal Treatment

The integration of stem cell technology into veterinary medicine has yielded remarkable success stories that highlight the potential of this innovative approach. One notable case involved the treatment of a racehorse suffering from severe tendon injuries. Traditional therapies had failed to provide relief, but the application of stem cell therapy facilitated an unprecedented recovery, allowing the horse to return to competitive racing. This success not only underscores the efficacy of stem cells in healing but also illuminates their role in enhancing the quality of life for animals.

In the realm of companion animals, stem cell therapies have shown promising results in treating osteoarthritis in dogs. A clinical study demonstrated that administering stem cells derived from the dog's own fat tissue resulted in significant improvements in mobility and reduction of pain. Pet owners reported a marked enhancement in their dogs' overall happiness and activity levels, showcasing the emotional and physical benefits of such treatments. This case exemplifies how stem cell therapies can provide a new lease of life to beloved pets, reinforcing the importance of continued research in this field.

Another remarkable success story involves the use of stem cells in treating feline chronic gingivostomatitis, a painful inflammatory condition affecting cats. Conventional treatments often proved ineffective; however, veterinarians successfully implemented stem cell injections to regenerate damaged tissues in the affected areas. The outcomes were astounding, with many cats experiencing complete resolution of symptoms and a return to normalcy. This case highlights the versatility of stem cell applications and their potential to transform veterinary medicine by addressing conditions that have long posed challenges.

Moreover, advancements in stem cell banking have opened new avenues for veterinary medicine. By preserving stem cells from healthy animals, veterinarians can create a reservoir of regenerative therapies ready for use in future treatments. This proactive approach not only enhances the treatment options available but also fosters a deeper understanding of genetic disorders in various species. The implications for animal health are profound, suggesting a future where personalised medicine becomes the norm in veterinary practices.

As these success stories accumulate, public perception of stem cell research in veterinary medicine is evolving. Once shrouded in scepticism, awareness of the tangible benefits of stem cell therapies is fostering greater acceptance among pet owners and the broader community. Continued education and transparency regarding ethical considerations and scientific advancements are essential in sustaining this momentum. As we witness the unfolding narrative of stem cells in animal treatment, it becomes clear that the potential for innovation and healing is vast and exciting for both animal and human health.

Regulatory Considerations

Regulatory considerations play a crucial role in the field of stem cell research and therapy. As the understanding of stem cells evolves, so too does the need for comprehensive regulations that ensure both the ethical application and the safety of stem cell therapies. Governments and regulatory bodies worldwide are tasked with creating frameworks that balance innovation with public safety, which is particularly important given the rapid advancements in stem cell technology.

One of the primary concerns in stem cell research is the ethical implications associated with the sourcing of stem cells. Regulations often focus on the sources of these cells, particularly embryonic stem cells, which raise moral and ethical questions. Health care professionals and biomedical scientists must navigate these complex issues, ensuring that their work complies with local laws and ethical standards while also considering the potential benefits for patients suffering from degenerative diseases.

Clinical applications of stem cell therapies present additional regulatory challenges. The approval process for new treatments can be lengthy and complex, requiring extensive preclinical and clinical data to demonstrate safety and efficacy. This process is vital for ensuring that stem cell therapies are not only effective but also do not pose undue risks to patients. As such, ongoing collaboration between researchers, regulatory agencies, and medical personnel is essential to facilitate the translation of stem cell research into clinical practice.

Furthermore, public perception plays a significant role in shaping regulatory policies. Misconceptions about stem cell research can lead to public resistance or support for certain types of therapies. Regulatory bodies must engage with the public to educate and inform about the benefits and risks associated with stem cell applications. This is particularly important in the context of personalised medicine, where the potential for tailored therapies could greatly enhance treatment outcomes for individuals with genetic disorders.

Finally, the implications of stem cell banking also warrant careful regulatory oversight. As more individuals consider stem cell banking for future medical needs, regulations must address the ethical, legal, and practical aspects of this practice. Ensuring that stem cell banking operates within a framework that protects patient rights while promoting scientific advancement is critical for the future of regenerative medicine. Health care professionals and researchers alike must remain informed about these evolving regulations to effectively contribute to the field and advocate for their patients.

Public Perception and Misconceptions of Stem Cell Research

Media Influence on Public Opinion

The media plays a crucial role in shaping public opinion, particularly in sensitive fields such as stem cell research. Health care professionals and biomedical scientists must understand that the portrayal of stem cells in news outlets, documentaries, and social media can influence perceptions among the general public. This influence can either foster support for innovative therapies or generate fear and misconceptions, which are often rooted in ethical debates surrounding the origins and applications of stem cells.

One significant aspect of media influence is the framing of stem cell research in terms of potential benefits versus ethical dilemmas. Reports that highlight the success stories of stem cell therapies for degenerative diseases can inspire hope and optimism. Conversely, negative framing, such as focusing on ethical controversies or highlighting the risks involved, can lead to public scepticism. It is essential for health care professionals to engage with the media proactively to ensure accurate representation of the scientific realities of stem cells.

Public perception is also heavily influenced by the accessibility of information. In the digital age, the rapid dissemination of information through social media platforms can result in widespread misconceptions about stem cell applications. Misleading narratives can lead to a lack of understanding regarding the potential of stem cells in personalised medicine or their role in treating genetic disorders. Health professionals must advocate for clear communication and education to counteract misinformation.

Furthermore, the implications of stem cell banking and its benefits are often misunderstood. The media can either perpetuate myths about the ineffectiveness of stored stem cells or provide a balanced view that highlights their potential in future therapies. By collaborating with journalists and engaging in public discussions, biomedical scientists can help demystify stem cell banking and clarify its significance in regenerative medicine.

In conclusion, the media's influence on public opinion regarding stem cell research is profound and multifaceted. Health care professionals and medical personnel in training must be equipped to navigate this landscape effectively. By fostering informed discussions and engaging with the media, they can help shape a more accurate public understanding of stem cells, their origins, and their potential applications in various fields, including veterinary medicine.

Addressing Common Misconceptions

Stem cell research is often surrounded by several misconceptions that can hinder public understanding and acceptance. One prevalent myth is that all stem cells come from embryos, which leads to confusion regarding the ethical implications of this research. In reality, stem cells can be derived from various sources, including adult tissues and umbilical cord blood, allowing for significant advancements without the ethical dilemmas often associated with embryonic stem cell use. This understanding is crucial for healthcare professionals and biomedical scientists as they navigate discussions about stem cell therapies and their applications.

Another common misconception is that stem cell therapies are a panacea for all diseases, leading to unrealistic expectations among patients and the general public. While stem cells hold immense potential for regenerating damaged tissues and treating degenerative diseases, they are not a cure-all solution. Each therapy must be tailored to the individual patient, and the effectiveness can vary widely depending on the condition being treated and the patient's overall health. It is essential for medical personnel in training to communicate these nuances effectively to manage patient expectations and foster informed decision-making.

Furthermore, many people believe that stem cell research is largely unregulated and lacks scientific validity. This notion undermines the rigorous protocols and ethical guidelines that govern stem cell research and clinical applications. In fact, extensive research and clinical trials are required to ensure the safety and efficacy of stem cell therapies before they can be widely adopted. Healthcare professionals should be well-versed in these regulations to educate patients and the public accurately and help dispel any fears surrounding the legitimacy of stem cell treatments.

Public perception of stem cell research is also clouded by sensationalised media reports, which can exaggerate the potential benefits while downplaying the risks. This can lead to a misinformed public that may be wary of legitimate advancements in regenerative medicine. It is crucial for healthcare professionals to engage with the public through transparent communication, providing clear and factual information about the current state of stem cell research and its implications for personalised medicine.

Lastly, misconceptions about stem cell banking often arise, particularly regarding its necessity and efficacy. Many assume that banking stem cells is a guaranteed insurance policy against future health problems. However, the reality is that while stem cell banking can offer options for certain conditions, it does not guarantee treatment for all genetic disorders or diseases. Professionals in the biomedical field must strive to clarify these points to ensure that families make informed decisions regarding stem cell banking and its potential implications for their health.

Strategies for Public Engagement

Engaging the public in the discourse surrounding stem cells is crucial for fostering understanding and dispelling misconceptions. Health care professionals and biomedical scientists have a unique role in this landscape, as their expertise can guide informed discussions about the potential of stem cells and their applications. By actively participating in community outreach initiatives, workshops, and seminars, these professionals can bridge the gap between scientific advancements and public perception, ensuring accurate information is disseminated to a wider audience.

Utilising social media platforms effectively is another strategy for public engagement. These platforms allow for the rapid sharing of information and can be tailored to address specific concerns or questions raised by the public. Health care professionals can leverage social media to highlight breakthroughs in stem cell research, share success stories of stem cell therapies, and clarify ethical considerations, thereby creating a more informed public. Engaging with followers through Q&A sessions can also demystify complex topics and encourage dialogue.

Educational partnerships with schools and universities can further enhance public understanding of stem cell research. By collaborating on curriculum development or offering guest lectures, health care professionals can introduce students to the foundational concepts of stem cells early on. This proactive approach not only cultivates interest in the field but also empowers future generations to engage thoughtfully with emerging biotechnologies and their implications for society.

Public forums and discussion panels provide platforms for open dialogue about stem cell research and its ethical considerations. These events can be designed to include a diverse range of voices, including scientists, ethicists, patients, and advocates. By facilitating these conversations, health care professionals can ensure that multiple perspectives are considered, fostering a more comprehensive understanding of the implications of stem cell therapies and research.

Finally, transparency in research and clinical practices is essential for building trust within the community. By openly sharing research findings, funding sources, and the processes behind stem cell therapies, health care professionals can help demystify the field. This transparency not only addresses public concerns but also enhances the credibility of the scientific community, encouraging a more supportive environment for stem cell research and its potential benefits for regenerative medicine and personalised healthcare.

Pause For Thought

- Life ends when degeneration exceeds regeneration thus the role of embryonic stem cells in regenerative medicine is welcomed as they can lead to breakthroughs in tissue engineering and organ replacement. This possibility has led to the investigation of ways to harness the regenerative capabilities of embryonic stem cells to repair damaged tissues and to develop therapies that can restore function in degenerative diseases.

- Advances in stem cell technology have moved the field of medicine forward. Techniques such as CRISPR gene editing and advanced cell culture methods have enabled researchers to manipulate embryonic stem cells thus facilitating the study of genetic disorders and the development of personalised medicine

- Despite the progress made in this field public perception can place a damper to the speed of progress. Misinformation can hinder funding and support for research initiatives making it crucial for health care professionals to communicate the relevant information clearly.

- Adult stem cells, also known as somatic stem cells, are undifferentiated cells found throughout the body. These cells play a crucial role in tissue haemostasis and repair, providing a reservoir of cells that can replenish damaged or lost tissues. Adult stem cells are limited in the ability to differentiate into various cell types. This intrinsic limitation highlights their role in maintaining the functionality of adult organs, thus giving insight into the potential role of stem cells in regenerative medicine.

- The potential of adult stem cells in regenerative medicine is extensive, specifically in treating degenerative diseases as Parkinson's, diabetes and various forms of arthritis. The use of those cells to replace damaged cells in affected tissues can potentially restore function and improve patient outcomes.

- The capability of adult stem cells is further advanced through the development of induced pluripotent stem cells, which essentially reprograms adult stem cells allowing them to regain pluripotency making them particularly appealing to personalised medicine.

- Stem cells because of their unique properties of self-renewal and the ability to differentiate into various cell types have characteristics that enable them to play crucial roles in tissue repair and regeneration. Stem cells secrete a range of bioactive factors. These factors can modulate immune response, promote cell survival, and stimulate the repair of damaged tissues – a feature which is essential in regenerative medicine, as stem cells are able to influence their microenvironment and facilitate healing.

- When exposed to specific stimuli, stem cells can differentiate into specialised cells, such as neurons, cardiomyocytes or insulin producing cells. This differentiation is influenced by intrinsic factors, such as genetic programming and extrinsic factors such as growth factors and extracellular matrix components.

- Tissue engineering represents a pioneering frontier in the realm of regenerative medicine. Here principles of biology and engineering are intertwined to create functional tissues that can restore or replace damaged biological structures. The harnessing of unique properties of stem cells, tissues can be fabricated to mimic the natural architecture of human organs which can integrate seamlessly with the host biological systems. This offers hope in the treatment of degenerative diseases where traditional therapies fall short.

- Advancement in stem cell technology and techniques have led to significant progress in tissue engineering. Techniques such as 3Dbioprinting and scaffolding technologies are paving the way for the creation of complex tissue structures that can be used in both research and clinical applications. These innovations not only enhance the functional capabilities of engineered tissues but also improves their visibility and integration within the host organism, thus offering new hope for patients with conditions that currently lack effective treatment options.

Take Home Nuggets

- Stem cell transplantation is a significant advancement in modern medicine offering hope for patients with various degenerative diseases. This involves the transfer of stem cells into a patient's body to replace damaged or diseased cells.

- Stem cells play a major role in repairing and regenerating damaged tissues. The advent of stem cell banking has been significant, allowing for the preservation of stem cells for future use. Public perception and misconception surrounding stem cell research can greatly influence funding and support for on going studies. Community engagement and dissemination of accurate information is essential about benefits and limitations of stem cell transplantation

- Stem cell therapy has also found some utility in veterinary medicine. Here they are used to treat a variety of conditions such as osteoarthritis and tendon injuries.

- CRISPR has virtually revolutionised the field of gene editing, with precision and efficiency in modifying genetic material. This allows for the targeting of specific DNA sequences which allows for effective manipulation of genes associated with various diseases.

- The emergence of 3D cell cultures has led to significant advancement in biomedical research. 3D cultures provide a more physiologically relevant environment than the traditional 2D cultures, thus allowing for better mimicry of in vivo conditions, allowing for observation within a more natural context.

- The use of 3Dcultures allow for the creation of organoids that closely resemble real organs, thus offering a unique platform for investigating various degenerative diseases allowing for insights into disease mechanisms and potential therapeutic targets.

- With bioprinting of tissues comes the potential to create functional living tissues that can be used for transplantation and drug testing. This technique utilises bioinks which have the capacity to support cell growth and mimic, natural extracellular matrix. With the precise deposition of these bioinks layer by layer, tissues can be engineered which closely resemble their natural counterparts and thus enhance the availability of tissue spare parts.

- Bioprinting allows for the customisation of tissue for individual patients an asset in the treatment of degenerative diseases, since such tailored solutions can enhance treatment efficiency. Innovations of 3D printing combined with stem cell technology allows for the creation of more sophisticated tissue structures which can better mimic the physiological properties of human tissues. These advancements have the potential to revolutionise regenerative as well as pharmacological testing thus allowing more accurate assessments of drug efficiency and safety.

- Pharmacogenomics, an evolving field that explores the interplay between genetics and drug response in the context of stem cell therapies. It focuses on how genetic variations among individuals can influence their reactions to medications, including those derived from or involving stem cells.

- Gene therapy is a revolutionary approach in medicine which aims to treat or prevent diseases by directly modifying the genetic material within an individual cell. By integrating therapeutic genes into stem cells, it is possible to create a source of cells that can continuously produce a desired protein or factors needed to combat genetic disorders and thereby offer a potential cure, not merely alleviation of symptoms.rd

Chapter 3
Significance of Stem Cell Research

Historical Context

The historical context of stem cell research provides a foundational understanding of its significance in the field of tissue engineering. The journey began in the late 20th century when scientists first isolated stem cells, leading to breakthroughs in our understanding of cellular differentiation and regeneration. This era marked a pivotal shift in biomedical research, as the potential for stem cells to repair or replace damaged tissues became evident, igniting interest among healthcare professionals and biomedical scientists alike.

In the early 2000s, advancements in stem cell technology further propelled the field forward. The discovery of induced pluripotent stem cells (iPSCs) revolutionised the landscape, allowing researchers to reprogram adult cells into a pluripotent state. This breakthrough not only offered a new source of stem cells for research and therapy but also raised ethical questions surrounding the use of embryonic stem cells, prompting a re-evaluation of research practices and policies governing stem cell use in various countries.

The role of stem cells in tissue engineering emerged as a central theme in the dialogue surrounding regenerative medicine. By harnessing the unique properties of stem cells, researchers began to develop innovative approaches to create functional tissues and organs. This integration of stem cells into tissue engineering highlighted the interdisciplinary nature of the field, drawing expertise from biology, engineering, and medicine to address complex health challenges.

Funding and policy issues have played a critical role in shaping the trajectory of stem cell research. In many regions, government regulations and financial support have fluctuated, impacting the pace of discovery and application. The interplay between scientific innovation and policy frameworks continues to influence the availability of resources for stem cell research, thus affecting the progress of tissue engineering initiatives.

Finally, a comparative analysis of stem cell types, particularly embryonic and adult stem cells, reveals significant differences in their applications and ethical considerations. While embryonic stem cells offer greater pluripotency, adult stem cells present a more ethically acceptable alternative, albeit with limitations in differentiation potential. This ongoing debate underscores the need for continued research and dialogue within the scientific community to explore the full potential of stem cells in advancing tissue engineering and regenerative therapies.

Ethical Considerations

Ethical considerations in stem cell research are paramount, particularly as advancements in technology enable more complex manipulations of stem cells. Health care professionals and biomedical scientists must navigate these ethical waters carefully, balancing the potential benefits of stem cell therapies against the moral implications of their sources. The use of embryonic stem cells, for instance, raises significant ethical questions regarding the status of the embryo and the rights of potential life. Such dilemmas necessitate a robust ethical framework that can guide research and clinical applications in a responsible manner.

The role of ethics in tissue engineering extends beyond the choice of stem cell sources to include issues surrounding consent, particularly in the case of obtaining samples from donors. It is crucial that health care professionals ensure that all research adheres to strict ethical guidelines, including obtaining informed consent from donors. This practice not only protects the rights of individuals but also fosters public trust in the scientific community, which is essential for the ongoing support of stem cell research initiatives.

Funding for stem cell research is significantly influenced by ethical considerations, as public and private funding bodies often have strict policies that reflect societal values. Health care professionals must advocate for funding that supports ethically sound research while also addressing the pressing health needs that stem cell therapies can fulfil. Engaging with policymakers to create supportive frameworks can help secure necessary resources while maintaining ethical integrity in research practices.

Comparative analysis of embryonic and adult stem cells also involves ethical scrutiny, as each type presents different ethical challenges and advantages. Embryonic stem cells offer greater pluripotency, which can lead to breakthroughs in treatment, but their use remains controversial. Alternatively, adult stem cells, while less versatile, present fewer ethical dilemmas and have gained acceptance in clinical therapies, making them a focal point for ethically conscious researchers.

Ultimately, the ethical landscape surrounding stem cell research and tissue engineering is complex and constantly evolving. Health care professionals and biomedical scientists must remain engaged in ongoing discussions about these ethical implications, ensuring that their work not only advances scientific knowledge but also upholds the highest ethical standards. This commitment to ethics will be essential in determining the future trajectory of stem cell research and its applications in health care.

Impact on Regenerative Medicine

The field of regenerative medicine has witnessed transformative changes in recent years, largely driven by advancements in stem cell research. Stem cells possess unique properties that enable them to differentiate into various cell types, making them invaluable for repairing damaged tissues and organs. This versatility not only enhances our understanding of developmental biology but also opens new avenues for treating previously incurable diseases. As healthcare professionals and biomedical scientists delve deeper into stem cell applications, the potential for regenerating human tissues becomes increasingly tangible, providing hope for patients with chronic conditions.

Recent advances in stem cell technology have significantly improved the efficacy of regenerative therapies. Innovations such as induced pluripotent stem cells (iPSCs) and the refinement of mesenchymal stem cell (MSC) isolation techniques have expanded the toolkit available for researchers. These developments enable the creation of patient-specific stem cells, thus minimising the risk of immune rejection during transplantation. Moreover, the ability to manipulate stem cells genetically enhances their therapeutic potential, allowing for targeted treatments that are tailored to individual patient needs.

The role of stem cells in tissue engineering is pivotal, as they serve as the foundational elements for constructing functional tissues. Through the combination of stem cells with biomaterials, researchers are developing scaffolds that mimic the natural extracellular matrix, promoting cell growth and tissue regeneration. This synergy between stem cells and engineering principles catalyses the creation of complex tissues that can be used for transplantation or as models for drug testing. Consequently, regenerative medicine stands at the forefront of personalised medicine, aligning treatment strategies more closely with the biological needs of patients.

Funding and policy for stem cell research play a crucial role in the advancement of regenerative medicine. As this field continues to evolve, securing adequate funding remains a challenge, particularly in the face of ethical concerns surrounding embryonic stem cell research. Policymakers must navigate these complexities to establish supportive frameworks that foster innovation while addressing public apprehensions. Increased investment in stem cell research not only accelerates scientific discoveries but also catalyses collaborations between academia, industry, and healthcare providers, thereby enhancing the translation of research findings into clinical applications.

Finally, the comparative analysis of stem cell types, including embryonic and adult stem cells, reveals significant implications for regenerative medicine. While embryonic stem cells offer pluripotency, adult stem cells provide a more ethically acceptable alternative with proven capabilities in tissue repair. Understanding the strengths and limitations of each stem cell type is essential for optimising therapeutic strategies. As researchers continue to explore these differences, the integration of various stem cell types may yield synergistic effects, further advancing the field of regenerative medicine and improving patient outcomes.

Potential for Disease Treatment

The potential for disease treatment through tissue engineering and stem cell technology is profoundly significant in the medical field. With the ability to regenerate damaged tissues and organs, stem cells provide a revolutionary approach to curing diseases that were once deemed incurable. Research has shown that stem cells can differentiate into various cell types, making them invaluable in treating conditions such as diabetes, neurodegenerative diseases, and heart diseases. This capacity to regenerate tissues opens new avenues for therapies that can restore function and improve the quality of life for patients.

Advances in stem cell technology have led to the development of innovative techniques such as induced pluripotent stem cells (iPSCs), which are derived from adult cells and possess the ability to develop into any cell type. This advancement not only circumvents ethical concerns associated with embryonic stem cells but also enhances the feasibility of personalised medicine. By using a patient's own cells, the risk of immune rejection is significantly reduced, allowing for tailored treatment strategies that are both effective and safe. This technological progress is paving the way for new clinical applications in disease management.

The role of stem cells in tissue engineering extends beyond mere regeneration; it also includes the potential for creating complex tissue structures that can mimic natural organs. This capability is crucial for developing functional replacements for tissues damaged by injury or disease. For instance, researchers are exploring the use of stem cells to engineer heart tissues that can be used in transplant procedures or to repair damaged myocardial tissue. Such advancements could drastically alter the landscape of organ transplantation, reducing the dependency on donor organs and waiting lists.

Funding and policy for stem cell research play a pivotal role in realising the potential of these therapies. Increased investment in stem cell research is essential for driving innovation and ensuring that breakthroughs can transition from the laboratory to clinical applications. Policymakers must navigate the ethical considerations surrounding stem cell use while promoting an environment conducive to research and development. Adequate funding not only supports scientific discovery but also fosters collaboration between academic institutions, private sector companies, and government agencies.

Finally, a comparative analysis of stem cell types, particularly embryonic versus adult stem cells, highlights the unique advantages and limitations of each. While embryonic stem cells hold immense potential due to their pluripotency, adult stem cells are more readily available and pose fewer ethical dilemmas. Understanding the strengths and weaknesses of these cell types is crucial for developing effective treatments. As research progresses, the integration of both stem cell types may provide comprehensive solutions for a range of diseases, ultimately enhancing therapeutic outcomes for patients.

Advances in Stem Cell Technology

Induced Pluripotent Stem Cells (iPSCs)

Induced pluripotent stem cells (iPSCs) represent a remarkable advancement in the field of regenerative medicine and tissue engineering. These cells, which can be generated from adult somatic cells, exhibit properties akin to embryonic stem cells, including the ability to differentiate into any cell type. The significance of iPSCs lies in their potential to provide a limitless source of cells for therapeutic applications, circumventing the ethical issues associated with embryonic stem cell research. This breakthrough not only enhances our understanding of developmental biology but also opens new avenues for personalised medicine.

The process of generating iPSCs involves reprogramming somatic cells through the introduction of specific transcription factors. This technology has evolved significantly, with advances such as improved reprogramming techniques and the development of non-integrative methods that enhance safety profiles. As a result, iPSCs can be derived from a variety of tissues, making them a versatile tool in biomedical research. The ability to create patient-specific iPSCs facilitates the study of diseases at a cellular level, allowing for tailored therapeutic strategies based on individual genetic backgrounds.

In the context of tissue engineering, iPSCs are invaluable for constructing complex tissues and organs. Their pluripotent nature provides the flexibility needed to generate diverse cell types required for functional tissue replacement. Furthermore, iPSCs can be used to create disease models, offering insights into the pathophysiology of various conditions. This capability is particularly crucial for conditions that currently lack effective treatments, as it allows researchers to test new drugs and therapies in a human cell context.

Funding and policy frameworks surrounding stem cell research, particularly iPSCs, are crucial for advancing this innovative field. As the potential applications of iPSCs expand, it is essential for governments and institutions to support research initiatives that explore their capabilities. Ethical considerations continue to play a significant role in shaping policy, emphasising the need for balanced regulations that promote scientific progress while safeguarding moral standards.

A comprehensive comparative analysis of stem cell types highlights the unique advantages of iPSCs over traditional embryonic and adult stem cells. While embryonic stem cells possess inherent pluripotency, the ability to generate iPSCs from adult cells presents a less controversial and more ethically acceptable alternative. This comparative perspective not only underscores the significance of iPSCs in contemporary biomedical research but also reinforces their potential to revolutionise therapeutic strategies in tissue engineering and regenerative medicine.

Gene Editing Techniques

Gene editing techniques have revolutionised the field of biomedical science, particularly in the realm of stem cell research. Techniques such as CRISPR-Cas9 enable precise modifications to the genetic material of stem cells, allowing for tailored therapies to combat various diseases. This capability is significant as it paves the way for advancements in tissue engineering, where the creation of functional tissues can be achieved through genetically modified stem cells that have enhanced regenerative properties.

The application of gene editing in stem cell technology not only improves the efficacy of treatments but also minimises the risk of immune rejection. By editing the genes of stem cells to make them more compatible with the recipient's immune system, healthcare professionals can enhance patient outcomes significantly. Furthermore, this technology allows for the correction of genetic defects at the source, offering a potential cure rather than merely treating symptoms.

In the context of tissue engineering, gene editing techniques facilitate the generation of specific cell types that are essential for constructing complex tissues. For instance, researchers can engineer stem cells to differentiate into cardiomyocytes for heart tissue or neurons for nerve regeneration. This specificity is crucial in developing personalised medicine approaches, where therapies can be tailored to the individual's genetic makeup, thereby improving the effectiveness of interventions.

Funding and policy considerations play a vital role in the advancement of gene editing and stem cell research. As breakthroughs emerge, it is essential for policymakers to ensure that ethical guidelines keep pace with scientific progress. This includes addressing concerns surrounding the implications of modifying human germline cells and ensuring that research is conducted responsibly while fostering innovation in therapeutic applications.

A comparative analysis of stem cell types—embryonic versus adult—reveals the advantages of utilising gene editing in both categories. Embryonic stem cells offer pluripotency, allowing for a broader range of applications, while adult stem cells present ethical advantages. Gene editing techniques can enhance the capabilities of both types, making them more versatile for use in regenerative medicine and tissue engineering, ultimately leading to more effective treatments for patients with various conditions.

Bioprinting and 3D Tissue Models

Bioprinting is revolutionising the field of tissue engineering by offering innovative methods to create three-dimensional tissue models that closely mimic human biology. This technology utilises a combination of living cells and bio-inks to fabricate complex structures layer by layer. By precisely controlling the placement of cells, researchers can replicate the architecture of native tissues, paving the way for improved drug testing and disease modelling. As such, bioprinting represents a significant advancement in stem cell technology, enabling the development of personalised medicine approaches that cater to individual patient needs.

The integration of stem cells in bioprinting facilitates the generation of functional tissues that can be used for regenerative medicine. Stem cells possess the unique ability to differentiate into various cell types, making them ideal candidates for creating tissue models that can mimic the function of specific organs or systems. For instance, researchers are exploring the potential of printing cardiac tissue models to study heart diseases and evaluate treatment strategies. This application showcases the vital role of stem cells in enhancing the efficacy of bioprinting techniques.

Moreover, the advancements in bioprinting technology have led to significant improvements in the scalability and efficiency of tissue production. This is particularly important for healthcare professionals and biomedical scientists who require reliable and reproducible tissue models for research and clinical applications. With the ongoing development of bioprinting platforms, there is a growing potential for creating off-the-shelf tissue products that can be used in therapeutic settings, thereby addressing the current limitations in organ transplantation and donor availability.

Funding and policy support play a crucial role in advancing bioprinting research. As the technology continues to evolve, securing investment for both basic and applied research is essential to foster innovation in this field. Policymakers must also navigate the ethical considerations surrounding the use of stem cells, ensuring that research is conducted responsibly while promoting the translation of bioprinted tissues into clinical practice. This balance between innovation and regulation is vital for the future of regenerative medicine.

In conclusion, bioprinting and 3D tissue models represent a promising frontier in tissue engineering, driven by the significant advancements in stem cell technology. As healthcare professionals and biomedical scientists embrace these innovative approaches, the potential to create functional tissues for therapeutic interventions becomes increasingly tangible. The synergy between bioprinting and stem cell research not only enhances our understanding of human biology but also opens new avenues for personalised medicine, ultimately improving patient outcomes in the future.

Cell Reprogramming Innovations

Cell reprogramming innovations have emerged as a groundbreaking frontier in stem cell research, significantly influencing the landscape of tissue engineering. These advancements allow for the conversion of somatic cells into induced pluripotent stem cells (iPSCs), offering immense potential for regenerative medicine. This technology not only facilitates the creation of patient-specific cell types but also enhances our understanding of cellular differentiation and disease modelling, thereby providing new avenues for therapeutic interventions.

Recent studies have demonstrated the efficacy of novel reprogramming techniques that utilise small molecules and non-viral methods. These innovations reduce the risks associated with traditional viral reprogramming approaches, such as insertional mutagenesis. Furthermore, advancements in gene editing technologies, like CRISPR-Cas9, have enabled researchers to fine-tune the reprogramming process, ensuring higher efficiency and safety in generating iPSCs suitable for clinical applications.

The role of cell reprogramming in tissue engineering cannot be overstated. By harnessing the pluripotent nature of iPSCs, researchers can develop complex tissue structures that can mimic the functionality of native tissues. This capability is crucial for addressing tissue deficiencies caused by injury or disease, leading to improved outcomes in regenerative therapies. Additionally, reprogrammed cells can be utilised in drug screening and toxicity testing, offering a more relevant model compared to traditional methods.

Funding and policy frameworks play a critical role in advancing cell reprogramming innovations. As the field continues to evolve, it is essential for health care professionals and biomedical scientists to advocate for increased investment in stem cell research. Supportive policies can foster collaborations between academic institutions and industry partners, ultimately accelerating the translation of laboratory discoveries into clinical practice, thereby enhancing patient care.

In conclusion, the continual evolution of cell reprogramming technologies holds immense promise for the future of tissue engineering. By bridging the gap between basic research and clinical application, these innovations are poised to revolutionise the treatment of various diseases and injuries. As we further explore the potential of stem cells, it is imperative to remain informed of ongoing advancements to fully leverage their capabilities in regenerative medicine.

The Role of Stem Cells in Tissue Engineering

Mechanisms of Tissue Regeneration

Tissue regeneration is a complex biological process that involves the restoration of tissue architecture and function following injury or disease. Central to this process are stem cells, which possess the unique ability to differentiate into various cell types and self-renew. Understanding the mechanisms of tissue regeneration is crucial for developing effective therapeutic strategies in the realm of tissue engineering. Recent advances in stem cell technology have shed light on how these cells can be harnessed to facilitate regeneration in damaged tissues.

One key mechanism of tissue regeneration is the role of stem cells in mediating inflammatory responses. Upon injury, stem cells can migrate to the site of damage, where they secrete various cytokines and growth factors that modulate the inflammatory response. This action not only helps to clear debris and pathogens but also sets the stage for tissue repair. Furthermore, the interaction between stem cells and the local tissue environment, or niche, is vital in determining the fate of stem cells and their ability to contribute to regeneration.

Another significant aspect of tissue regeneration involves the extracellular matrix (ECM). The ECM provides structural and biochemical support to surrounding cells, playing a crucial role in cell attachment, migration, and differentiation. Stem cells can interact with the ECM to receive signals that guide their regenerative capabilities. Advances in biomaterials have allowed researchers to create scaffolds that mimic the ECM, enabling more effective stem cell-based therapies by providing the necessary microenvironment for cell survival and function.

In addition to cellular mechanisms, the understanding of genetic and epigenetic factors influencing stem cell behaviour has advanced significantly. Research indicates that specific genes and their expression levels can dictate how stem cells respond to injury and the extent of tissue regeneration. Moreover, epigenetic modifications can influence stem cell pluripotency and lineage commitment, highlighting the importance of these factors in the development of targeted therapies for regenerative medicine.

Finally, ongoing research into the comparative analysis of stem cell types—such as embryonic versus adult stem cells—continues to reveal insights into their specific roles in tissue regeneration. Each stem cell type has distinct advantages and limitations, influencing their application in clinical settings. Understanding these differences is essential for optimising strategies in tissue engineering and ensuring that funding and policy frameworks support the advancement of this vital field.

Applications in Organ Replacement

The field of organ replacement has witnessed remarkable advancements through the application of stem cell technology, which holds the potential to revolutionise the way we approach transplantation medicine. Stem cells possess the unique ability to differentiate into various cell types, making them ideal candidates for regenerating damaged or diseased organs. With ongoing research focused on harnessing these cells, we are inching closer to creating functional organs in vitro that can be used in clinical settings, significantly reducing the reliance on donor organs' .

One of the most significant breakthroughs in this arena is the development of bioengineered tissues derived from stem cells. These engineered constructs can mimic the mechanical and biological properties of native tissues, thus providing a viable option for organ replacement. For instance, cardiac patches created from induced pluripotent stem cells have shown promise in restoring heart function in preclinical models, highlighting the potential for stem cell-derived constructs to address critical organ failures.

Furthermore, the integration of advanced technologies, such as 3D bioprinting, has catalysed the creation of complex organ structures. By layering stem cells in a controlled manner, researchers can fabricate tissues that not only replicate the architecture of natural organs but also maintain functionality. This innovative approach has opened new avenues for personalised medicine, wherein patient-specific tissues can be engineered, minimising the risk of rejection and the need for immunosuppressive therapies.

Despite the promising prospects, the journey towards widespread clinical application of stem cell-derived organs is fraught with challenges. Ethical considerations surrounding stem cell sourcing, particularly concerning embryonic stem cells, continue to spark debate among policymakers and the public. Moreover, securing adequate funding for research and development remains critical to advancing these technologies and ensuring they translate from the laboratory to the clinic.

In conclusion, the applications of stem cell technology in organ replacement present a groundbreaking shift in medical practice, offering hope for patients with end-stage organ failure. As researchers continue to navigate the complexities of stem cell biology and tissue engineering, the vision of lab-grown organs becoming a reality is no longer a distant dream but an achievable goal. Ongoing collaboration among healthcare professionals, scientists, and policymakers will be essential to foster an environment conducive to innovation and ethical research in this vital field.

Integration with Biomaterials

The integration of biomaterials in tissue engineering represents a pivotal advancement in the field, particularly when combined with the unique properties of stem cells. Biomaterials serve as scaffolds that provide structural support, facilitating the growth and differentiation of stem cells into specialised tissues. This synergy not only enhances the mechanical stability of engineered tissues but also influences cellular behaviour, promoting the regeneration of damaged or diseased tissues in a clinically relevant manner.

One of the primary functions of biomaterials in tissue engineering is to mimic the natural extracellular matrix (ECM), which is crucial for stem cell attachment and proliferation. The composition, architecture, and surface properties of these materials can be engineered to create optimal conditions that favour stem cell differentiation. Recent advances in biomaterial science have led to the development of innovative materials that can respond to biological signals, further enhancing their compatibility with stem cells and improving the overall efficacy of tissue engineering applications.

Additionally, the integration of biomaterials with stem cells has opened new avenues for the treatment of various conditions, including degenerative diseases and injuries. For instance, hydrogels and nanofibrous scaffolds have been employed to deliver stem cells directly to the site of injury, where they can exert their regenerative potential. This targeted approach not only increases the likelihood of successful integration but also minimises the risks associated with more invasive surgical procedures.

Funding and policy support have also evolved to accommodate the burgeoning field of biomaterials and stem cell integration. As researchers demonstrate the efficacy of these technologies in preclinical and clinical settings, there is a growing recognition of the need for increased investment in this area. Policymakers are beginning to understand the potential of these advancements to address significant healthcare challenges, thereby driving increased funding opportunities and fostering collaboration between academia and industry.

In conclusion, the integration of biomaterials with stem cells is at the forefront of tissue engineering breakthroughs. This collaboration enhances the potential for successful tissue regeneration, providing hope for patients with previously untreatable conditions. As research continues to unfold, the need for interdisciplinary approaches combining biomaterials, stem cell technology, and clinical applications will only become more critical, ensuring that the next generation of therapies is both effective and accessible to those in need.

Case Studies of Successful Tissue Engineering

Tissue engineering has witnessed remarkable progress, with various case studies illustrating the successful application of stem cells to overcome significant medical challenges. One notable example is the development of bioengineered skin for patients suffering from severe burns. Researchers utilised a combination of stem cells and biomaterials to create a living skin substitute, enabling faster healing and improved outcomes for patients. This case study exemplifies how integrating stem cell technology with tissue engineering can lead to innovative solutions in regenerative medicine.

Another successful application of tissue engineering involves the regeneration of cartilage using stem cells. In one groundbreaking study, scientists harvested mesenchymal stem cells from patients' bone marrow and cultured them to form cartilage-like tissues. These engineered tissues were then implanted into patients suffering from osteoarthritis, resulting in reduced pain and improved joint function. This case study underscores the significance of stem cell research in addressing degenerative conditions and enhancing patients' quality of life.

Furthermore, the field of dental tissue engineering has also benefitted from advances in stem cell technology. Researchers have successfully utilised stem cells from dental pulp to regenerate dentin and pulp tissues. In clinical trials, these engineered tissues have shown promising results in restoring tooth vitality and function. This case study highlights the potential for stem cell applications in dental medicine, providing new avenues for treating dental injuries and diseases.

In addition to these specific applications, funding and policy support play a crucial role in advancing tissue engineering research. For instance, significant government and private investments have facilitated the exploration of various stem cell types, including embryonic and adult stem cells. The comparative analysis of these stem cell sources has led to important discoveries, guiding researchers in selecting the most suitable cells for specific tissue engineering projects. This case study illustrates how financial backing and supportive policies can drive innovation in the field.

Lastly, the integration of stem cells in developing organoids has emerged as a revolutionary approach in tissue engineering. Researchers have created miniaturised organ models that mimic the structure and function of human organs using pluripotent stem cells. These organoids serve as valuable tools for drug testing and disease modelling, significantly advancing personalised medicine. This case study demonstrates the transformative impact of stem cell technology on the future of healthcare, paving the way for tailored therapies and improved patient outcomes.

Funding and Policy for Stem Cell Research

Overview of Funding Sources

The landscape of funding sources for stem cell research is diverse and multifaceted, reflecting the critical importance of this field in advancing medical science. Government grants have historically been a significant source of funding, particularly in the United States, where initiatives like the National Institutes of Health (NIH) have allocated substantial resources to support innovative research projects. These funding bodies often prioritise studies that promise to translate into clinical applications, thereby driving the advancement of stem cell technologies.

In addition to government funding, private sector investment plays a crucial role in the financial ecosystem of stem cell research. Pharmaceutical companies and biotechnology firms recognise the potential of stem cells in developing new therapies and are increasingly contributing to research funding. This investment not only accelerates the development of products but also fosters collaborations between academia and industry, which can lead to groundbreaking discoveries in tissue engineering.

Non-profit organisations and philanthropic foundations also significantly impact the funding landscape. These entities often focus on specific diseases or conditions that could benefit from stem cell therapies, providing targeted support for research initiatives. Their contributions are vital, as they can fund high-risk, high-reward projects that might not secure traditional grants due to perceived uncertainties in outcomes.

Furthermore, international collaborations and funding sources have become increasingly prominent, particularly as the field of stem cell research transcends national borders. Collaborative efforts can lead to shared resources and knowledge, enhancing the quality and reach of research. This global perspective allows researchers to access a wider array of funding opportunities, thereby broadening the scope and impact of their work in tissue engineering.

Finally, the role of public policy cannot be overlooked in shaping the funding landscape for stem cell research. Legislative decisions can either facilitate or hinder funding opportunities, influencing the direction and pace of research. Advocacy for supportive policies is essential to ensure that funding continues to flow into this vital area of medical science, enabling ongoing advancements in the application of stem cells in tissue engineering and beyond.

Governmental and Non-Governmental Support

Governmental and non-governmental support play a crucial role in advancing the field of stem cell research and tissue engineering. In many countries, government funding is essential for enabling researchers to explore innovative therapies and technologies that utilise stem cells. Grants from national health institutes and research councils provide the financial backing necessary for scientific studies, clinical trials, and the establishment of research facilities focused on stem cell applications. This financial support allows biomedical scientists to push the boundaries of knowledge and develop new treatments that can significantly impact patient care.

Non-governmental organisations (NGOs) and private foundations also play a pivotal role in the landscape of stem cell research. These entities often focus on specific diseases or conditions, funding targeted research that aligns with their mission. By providing grants and resources, they not only supplement governmental funding but also foster collaboration among researchers, clinicians, and industry partners. This synergy can accelerate the pace of discovery and lead to breakthroughs that might otherwise be delayed due to financial constraints.

Moreover, advocacy groups contribute to the visibility and importance of stem cell research in the public domain. They raise awareness about the potential benefits of stem cell therapies and the need for continued investment in this area. By mobilising public support and lobbying for favourable policies, these organisations can influence government funding decisions and help create a more supportive environment for researchers. Public engagement is crucial, as it helps to demystify stem cell research and emphasise its significance in advancing medical science.

Funding policies and regulatory frameworks established by governments significantly impact the direction of stem cell research. Clear and supportive policies can facilitate innovation, while restrictive regulations may hinder progress. It is essential for health care professionals and biomedical scientists to stay informed about these policies and actively participate in discussions about them. By advocating for balanced regulations that promote research while ensuring ethical standards, they can help shape a future where stem cell technologies can be fully realised in clinical settings.

In conclusion, the interplay between governmental and non-governmental support is vital for the success of stem cell research and its applications in tissue engineering. As researchers navigate the complexities of funding and policy, the collective efforts of various stakeholders—ranging from government bodies to private organisations—will determine the trajectory of this promising field. By fostering an environment of collaboration and support, we can unlock the full potential of stem cells to revolutionise healthcare and improve patient outcomes.

Policy Frameworks and Regulations

The policy frameworks and regulations governing stem cell research are pivotal in shaping the future of tissue engineering. These regulations ensure that research is conducted ethically and that the potential benefits of stem cell therapies are realised while minimising risks to patients. In recent years, various countries have developed their own legislative approaches, reflecting their unique social and ethical values regarding stem cell use. This divergence highlights the importance of international collaboration to harmonise standards, which can facilitate advancements in the field while maintaining public trust.

Significant advancements in stem cell technology have emerged as a response to evolving policy frameworks. Governments and funding bodies are increasingly recognising the therapeutic potential of stem cells, leading to increased investment and support for research initiatives. This funding is crucial for driving innovation, particularly in areas such as regenerative medicine and tissue engineering, where the application of stem cells can lead to groundbreaking treatments for previously incurable conditions. As a result, researchers are often required to navigate complex regulations to secure the necessary funding and approval for their projects.

The role of stem cells in tissue engineering is underscored by the regulatory landscape that governs their application. Policies aimed at safeguarding ethical practices often dictate the types of stem cells that can be used, influencing the direction of research. For instance, while embryonic stem cells offer extensive potential due to their pluripotency, their use is heavily regulated in many countries. In contrast, adult stem cells, which pose fewer ethical concerns, are gaining popularity and support within regulatory frameworks, leading to a shift in focus among researchers and investors alike.

Comparative analysis of stem cell types reveals differing regulatory challenges that affect research outcomes. Embryonic stem cells are often subject to stringent regulations, which can impede scientific progress and limit the scope of research.

Conversely, adult stem cells, despite their limitations in versatility, are more readily accessible under current policies, allowing for a broader range of applications in clinical settings. Understanding these distinctions is vital for healthcare professionals and biomedical scientists as they navigate the landscape of tissue engineering and its associated regulations.

As the field of stem cell research continues to evolve, so too must the policy frameworks that govern it. Ongoing dialogue between scientists, policymakers, and the public is essential to ensure that regulations remain relevant and conducive to innovation. By fostering a collaborative environment, stakeholders can work together to establish guidelines that not only protect ethical standards but also encourage the advancement of stem cell technologies that hold the promise of transforming healthcare for future generations.

International Collaboration in Research

International collaboration in research has become increasingly vital in the field of tissue engineering, particularly in the realm of stem cell research. The complexity of biological systems and the multifaceted challenges of diseases require a diverse array of expertise and resources. By pooling knowledge and facilities from across the globe, researchers can accelerate advancements, share innovative methodologies, and enhance the quality of scientific inquiry. This cooperative approach not only fosters a richer understanding of stem cell biology but also promotes the development of novel therapies that can be translated into clinical practice.

One significant advantage of international collaboration is the ability to access a wider range of funding opportunities. Various global initiatives and governmental bodies provide grants and support for collaborative projects aimed at advancing stem cell technology. Such funding is crucial for high-impact research that might be too ambitious or expensive for individual institutions to undertake alone. Moreover, collaborative networks can attract significant investments from private sectors eager to capitalise on cutting-edge research, thus benefiting all parties involved.

In addition to financial support, collaboration facilitates the sharing of diverse scientific perspectives and expertise. Researchers from different countries bring unique insights that can lead to innovative approaches in tissue engineering. For instance, while some regions may excel in the development of advanced biomaterials, others may be pioneers in stem cell differentiation techniques. This exchange of knowledge not only enriches the research environment but also cultivates a culture of innovation that is essential for breakthroughs in stem cell applications.

Furthermore, international partnerships can expedite the translation of research findings into clinical applications. By uniting scientists, healthcare professionals, and regulatory bodies, collaborative efforts can streamline the pathways to clinical trials and approval processes. This is particularly important in stem cell research, where regulatory frameworks can vary significantly across borders. A unified approach can help harmonise standards, ensuring that promising therapies can be developed and made available to patients more swiftly and efficiently.

Finally, the ethical considerations surrounding stem cell research can benefit from international collaboration. Different countries have varying regulations and ethical guidelines governing stem cell use, particularly regarding embryonic stem cells. By engaging in dialogue and sharing best practices, researchers can develop a more comprehensive understanding of these issues. This collective effort can lead to the establishment of globally accepted ethical standards that respect diverse cultural perspectives while advancing scientific knowledge and patient care.

Comparative Analysis of Stem Cell Types: Embryonic vs. Adult

Definitions and Characteristics

In the realm of tissue engineering, the definitions and characteristics of stem cells are pivotal to understanding their potential applications. Stem cells are unique in that they possess the ability to differentiate into various cell types and have the capacity for self-renewal. This intrinsic property distinguishes them from other cell types and underpins their significance in regenerative medicine and tissue engineering. As health care professionals and biomedical scientists explore these characteristics, they unveil the myriad possibilities for treating complex diseases and injuries.

Embryonic stem cells (ESCs) and adult stem cells (ASCs) represent the two primary categories of stem cells, each with distinct characteristics. ESCs, derived from the early embryo, are pluripotent and can give rise to any cell type in the body. In contrast, ASCs are multipotent, typically restricted to differentiating into cell types of their tissue of origin. This fundamental difference in potency influences their applications in tissue engineering, where the choice of stem cell type can dictate the success of the engineered tissues.

The advances in stem cell technology have accelerated the field of tissue engineering, with researchers developing innovative methods for stem cell isolation, culture, and differentiation. Techniques such as induced pluripotent stem cells (iPSCs) have revolutionised the landscape by allowing adult cells to be reprogrammed back into a pluripotent state. These advances not only enhance the versatility of stem cells but also mitigate ethical concerns associated with using embryonic sources, thereby broadening the scope of research and clinical applications.

Funding and policy frameworks play a crucial role in shaping the trajectory of stem cell research. Government and private sector investments are essential for supporting innovative research initiatives and overcoming regulatory hurdles. As health care professionals and scientists advocate for robust funding mechanisms, they must also navigate the complex landscape of ethical considerations surrounding stem cell research, ensuring that scientific progress aligns with societal values and expectations.

Lastly, a comparative analysis of embryonic and adult stem cells reveals important insights into their respective advantages and limitations. While ESCs offer unparalleled versatility, ethical concerns regarding their use persist. On the other hand, ASCs, although limited in their differentiation potential, provide a more ethically acceptable option for many researchers. Understanding these characteristics is vital for health care professionals and biomedical scientists as they strive to harness the power of stem cells for revolutionary advancements in tissue engineering and regenerative medicine.

Advantages and Disadvantages

The advantages of stem cell research in tissue engineering are manifold, particularly in the ability to regenerate damaged tissues and organs. Stem cells possess the unique ability to differentiate into various cell types, making them invaluable in creating functional tissue constructs. This potential allows for targeted therapies that can address specific ailments, leading to improved patient outcomes. Furthermore, the use of stem cells in regenerative medicine could significantly reduce the burden of organ shortages, offering hope to patients awaiting transplants.

On the other hand, there are notable disadvantages and ethical considerations surrounding stem cell research. The use of embryonic stem cells, in particular, raises moral dilemmas that can hinder funding and public support. Additionally, the process of isolating and culturing stem cells can be complex and costly, presenting financial barriers for many research institutions. These challenges may slow the pace of advancements in stem cell technology and its application in clinical settings.

Another advantage of stem cell technology is the potential for personalised medicine. By harvesting a patient's own stem cells, clinicians can create tailored treatments that minimise the risk of rejection and adverse reactions. This personalised approach not only enhances the effectiveness of therapies but also fosters a deeper understanding of individual health conditions. As research progresses, it is likely that more customised solutions will emerge, paving the way for breakthroughs in chronic disease management.

However, the comparative analysis of different stem cell types, such as embryonic versus adult stem cells, presents its own set of challenges. While embryonic stem cells have greater plasticity, adult stem cells are often more ethically acceptable and easier to obtain. This dichotomy can complicate the decision-making process for researchers and policymakers alike, as they weigh the benefits of scientific advancement against ethical responsibilities. The ongoing debate underscores the necessity for clear regulatory frameworks that can support research while addressing ethical concerns.

In conclusion, while the advantages of stem cell research in tissue engineering are promising, they are counterbalanced by significant disadvantages that require careful consideration. The field is at a critical juncture where advancements in technology must be matched with ethical and funding policies that support sustainable research. As healthcare professionals and biomedical scientists navigate these complexities, a balanced approach is essential for harnessing the full potential of stem cells in improving healthcare outcomes.

Current Research Trends

Current research trends in the field of stem cell technology are shaping the future of tissue engineering. Health care professionals and biomedical scientists are increasingly recognising the significance of stem cell research as it holds the potential to revolutionise regenerative medicine. Recent advancements have led to the development of novel techniques for stem cell differentiation, enhancing our ability to generate specific cell types for therapeutic applications. These advancements not only improve our understanding of cellular mechanisms but also facilitate the creation of tailored treatments for various degenerative diseases.

The role of stem cells in tissue engineering cannot be overstated. With the capacity to self-renew and differentiate into multiple cell types, stem cells are integral to constructing functional tissues and organs. Researchers are exploring various sources of stem cells, including embryonic and adult stem cells, each offering unique advantages and challenges. The comparative analysis of these stem cell types is crucial, as it informs the selection of the most suitable cells for specific tissue engineering applications, ultimately impacting patient outcomes.

Funding and policy frameworks play a pivotal role in advancing stem cell research. As government and private institutions invest more resources into this field, the potential for breakthroughs increases significantly. Current trends indicate a growing acceptance of stem cell research within regulatory bodies, leading to more streamlined processes for clinical trials. This supportive environment encourages innovative research and allows scientists to explore the full potential of stem cells in treating a wide array of medical conditions.

Moreover, interdisciplinary collaborations are becoming increasingly common in stem cell research. By bringing together experts from diverse fields such as bioengineering, molecular biology, and clinical medicine, researchers are able to tackle complex challenges in tissue engineering. These collaborative efforts foster a more holistic understanding of stem cell biology and drive forward the development of effective therapies. Such synergies are essential for translating laboratory findings into clinical applications that can benefit patients.

In conclusion, current research trends in stem cell technology are advancing at a remarkable pace. The significance of stem cell research, coupled with technological innovations, is driving progress in tissue engineering. As funding increases and policy frameworks evolve, the future of regenerative medicine looks promising. Continuous comparative analyses of stem cell types will further enhance our understanding, paving the way for breakthrough therapies that could change lives. The collaborative spirit within the scientific community will undoubtedly accelerate these advancements, leading to a new era in healthcare.

Future Directions in Stem Cell Utilisation

As we look towards the future of stem cell utilisation, it is evident that the potential applications of this technology will expand significantly over the coming years. The significance of stem cell research has already transformed our understanding of regenerative medicine, and continued advancements in this field promise to unlock even greater therapeutic possibilities. Researchers are exploring innovative methods to harness the regenerative capabilities of stem cells, which could lead to breakthroughs in treating a range of conditions, from degenerative diseases to traumatic injuries.

Advances in stem cell technology are paving the way for more efficient and reliable applications. Techniques such as CRISPR gene editing and induced pluripotent stem cells (iPSCs) are revolutionising the landscape, allowing for customised therapies tailored to individual patient needs. These advancements not only enhance the efficacy of stem cell therapies but also minimise ethical concerns associated with embryonic stem cells, making them more accessible in clinical settings.

The role of stem cells in tissue engineering cannot be overstated, as they serve as the foundational building blocks for developing functional tissues and organs. Future research is likely to focus on creating bioengineered constructs that mimic natural tissue environments, utilising stem cells to promote integration and functionality. This will not only improve outcomes for patients undergoing transplantation but also reduce the reliance on donor organs, addressing a critical shortage in many healthcare systems.

Funding and policy for stem cell research will play a crucial role in shaping the future landscape of this field. As more governments and private organisations recognise the potential benefits of stem cell therapies, increased investment is expected. However, it is essential to establish ethical frameworks and regulatory guidelines to ensure that research is conducted responsibly and that the rights of patients are safeguarded. This will help maintain public trust and encourage further financial backing for innovative stem cell projects.

Lastly, a comparative analysis of stem cell types, specifically embryonic versus adult stem cells, will continue to be a focal point in future research. Each type presents unique advantages and limitations that must be understood to optimise their use in clinical applications. As stem cell science progresses, it is vital for healthcare professionals and biomedical scientists to stay informed about these differences to make informed decisions regarding patient care and treatment options.

Pause for Thought

- Stem cells were first isolated in the late 20th century and led to break throughs in our understanding of cellular differentiation and regeneration. This led to a pivotal shift in biomedical research as stem cells potential to repair or replace damaged tissues became increasingly evident.

- The ability to reprogram adult cells into a pluripotent state, revolutionised the research landscape in both tissue engineering and regenerative medicine. The involvement of stem cells into tissue engineering argued for a multi-disciplinary approach drawing on expertise from biology, engineering and medicine to address complex health challenges.

- Stem cells have a role in tissue engineering as they serve as the foundational elements for constructing functional tissues. The combination of stem cells with biomaterials, allows for the development of scaffolds that mimic the natural extracellular matrix promoting cell growth and tissue regeneration. This leads to the development of complex tissues that can be used for transplantation or as models for drug testing.

- Stem cells with their ability to regenerate damaged tissues and organs provide a revolutionary approach to curing diseases that were once considered incurable. As a result of their pluripotency, stem cells are invaluable in treating conditions such as diabetes, neurodegenerative diseases and heart diseases. This capacity to regenerate tissues opens new avenues for therapies that can restore function and improve the quality of life for patients.

- Induced pluripotent stem cells can develop into any cell type. Since these cells are derived from adult tissue, they can bypass much of the ethical concerns.

- An exciting role of stem cells is that through tissue engineering, there is the potential for creating complex tissue structures that can mimic natural organs. This provides the capability for developing functional replacements for tissue damaged by injury or disease; for instance, stem cells are now being engineered with the hope of producing heart tissues that can be used in transplant procedures or to repair damaged myocardial tissue.

- The process of generating induced pluripotent stem cells (iPSC) involves reprogramming somatic cells through the introduction of specific transcription factors. Ipsccan be derived from a variety of tissues, thus making them versatile tools in biomedical research.

- The iPSC can be used to generate disease models and thus offer insights into the pathophysiology of various conditions. This capacity allows researchers to explore therapy for conditions that currently lack effective treatment by allowing for the testing of new drugs and therapies in a human cell context.

- Gene editing techniques have revolutionised the field of biomedical science particularly as it relates to stem cell research. Techniques such as CRISPR-Cas 9 enable precise modifications to the genetic material of stem cells, allowing for tailored therapies to combat various diseases. The application of gene editing in stem cell therapy improves the efficacy of treatment and minimises the risk of immune rejection.

- Researchers can engineer stem cells to differentiate into cardiomyocytes for heart tissue or neurons for nerve regeneration. This is crucial in developing personalised medical approaches where therapies can be tailored to the individual genetic make-up, thus improving the effectiveness of interventions.

Take Home Nuggets

- Tissue regeneration is a complex biological process that involves the restoration of tissue architecture and function following injury as well as self-renewal or disease. Central to this process are stem cells because of their unique ability to differentiate into various cell types and self-renew.

- Stem cells play a role in mediating inflammatory responses. Upon injury stem cells can migrate to the site of the injury where they secrete various cytokines and growth factors that modulate the inflammatory response, this sets the stage for tissue repair.

- Specific genes and their expression levels can dictate how stem cells respond to injury and the extent of tissue regeneration. Epigenetic modifications can influence stem cells pluripotency and lineage commitment.

- Each stem cell type has distinct advantages and limitations, influencing their application in clinical settings

- The pluripotency of stem cells allows them the unique ability to differentiate into various cell types which makes them ideal candidates for regenerating damaged or diseased organs. By harnessing these cells, progress is made to the creation of functional organs in vitro that can be used in clinical settings and significantly reduces the reliance on donor organs and waiting lists.

- The application of gene editing in stem cell technology not only improves the efficacy of treatments but also minimises the risk of immune rejection. By editing the genes of stem cells, they can be made more compatible with the recipient's immune system. This technique also has the potential to correct genetic defects at the source, thus giving hope for a potential cure.

- Bioprinting is an advanced layer-by-layer additive manufacturing technique that uses bioinks- mixture of living cells, growth factors and biomaterials to create 3D, functional, tissue -like structures. It allows precise control over cell distribution and scaffolding architecture to build human tissue, cartilage, skin, and vascular structures for medical research and regenerative medicine.

- Bioprinting and 3D tissue models have offered innovative methods to create 3-dimensional tissue models which closely mimic human biology. This technology utilized a combination living cells and bioinks to fabricate complex structures layer by layer. With bioprinting researchers can replicate the architecture of native tissues, paving the way for improved drug testing and disease modelling. Bioprinting thus represents a significant advancement in stem cell technology enabling the development of personalised medical approaches that cater to individual patient needs.

- Hydrogels and nanofibrous scaffolds have been employed to deliver stem cells directly to the site of injury, where they can exert their regenerative potential. The advantage of this targeted approach is that it increases the likelihood of successful integration and minimises the risk associated with more invasive procedures.

- Tissue engineering has made remarkable progress with various studies illustrating the successful application of stem cells to overcome significant medical challenges; for example, in skin, it has rejuvenated areas after severe burns which led to faster healing and improve outcomes for patients. This technology has led to the regeneration of cartilage-like tissue which when implanted in patients suffering from osteoarthritis resulted in reduced pain and improved joint function. This benefit has also been extended to dental tissue engineering in which stem cells from dental pulp has been used to regenerate dentin and pulp tissue.

Chapter 4
The Promise of Regeneration

Introduction to Stem Cell Therapy

Stem cell therapy represents a paradigm shift in the field of medicine, offering unprecedented opportunities for regeneration and repair of damaged tissues. This innovative approach leverages the unique properties of stem cells, which possess the ability to differentiate into various cell types and self-renew, making them invaluable in treating a range of health conditions. As health care professionals and biomedical scientists delve into this burgeoning field, understanding the fundamentals of stem cell therapy is essential for harnessing its full potential.

The dawn of promise in regenerative medicine is marked by significant advancements in stem cell research, particularly in the treatment of neurodegenerative diseases. Conditions such as Parkinson's disease and Alzheimer's are being explored for therapeutic interventions that utilise stem cells to restore lost functions and improve patient outcomes. By advancing our knowledge in this area, we empower ourselves to develop targeted therapies that could potentially alter the course of these debilitating diseases.

Ethical considerations in stem cell research play a crucial role in shaping the landscape of therapy applications. The debate surrounding the sourcing of stem cells, particularly embryonic stem cells, raises important questions about the moral implications of such research. Engaging in thoughtful dialogue and establishing ethical guidelines is paramount to ensuring that the advancements in stem cell therapy are conducted responsibly and with respect for human dignity.

In orthopaedic treatments, stem cells are increasingly being used to promote healing and regeneration of musculoskeletal tissues. From cartilage repair to bone regeneration, the application of stem cells offers promising outcomes that could enhance recovery times and improve the quality of life for patients suffering from injuries or degenerative conditions. As research continues to evolve, the integration of stem cell therapy in orthopaedics represents a significant milestone in enhancing patient care.

Finally, the role of stem cells in managing autoimmune diseases and their applications in paediatric medicine cannot be overlooked. Emerging studies indicate that stem cell therapy may offer new avenues for treating conditions such as lupus and rheumatoid arthritis, as well as providing potential treatments for childhood disorders. As we embrace these innovations, it is vital to consider public perception and acceptance of stem cell therapies, which will ultimately influence the trajectory of research and clinical application in this exciting field.

Historical Context and Advances

The landscape of medicine has been profoundly transformed by the advances in stem cell therapy, which have roots tracing back to early discoveries in the field of cellular biology. The 20th century heralded significant milestones, such as the identification of stem cells and their unique properties, paving the way for innovative treatments. As researchers began to comprehend the potential of these cells, the foundation was laid for what is now regarded as a revolutionary approach to regenerative medicine. This historical context is crucial for understanding the trajectory of stem cell therapies and their implications for various medical disciplines.

In the decades that followed, breakthroughs in biotechnology and genetic engineering catalysed the development of stem cell applications. The advent of techniques such as induced pluripotent stem cells (iPSCs) in the early 2000s marked a significant turning point, allowing for the reprogramming of somatic cells into a pluripotent state. This innovation not only expanded the potential sources of stem cells but also raised ethical considerations that prompted ongoing debates within the scientific community and the public sphere. Such advances have made it possible to explore therapies for conditions once deemed untreatable, including neurodegenerative diseases and certain types of cancer.

As the field matured, regulatory frameworks began to evolve, ensuring that stem cell research and therapies adhered to ethical standards while promoting innovation. In many countries, guidelines were established to oversee clinical trials involving stem cells, balancing the need for scientific progress with the imperative of patient safety. This regulatory landscape is essential for fostering trust among healthcare professionals and the public, as it provides a framework for evaluating the efficacy and safety of emerging treatments. The dynamic interplay between innovation and regulation continues to shape the future of stem cell therapy.

The application of stem cell therapy has shown promise across a myriad of medical specialties, from orthopaedics to cardiovascular disorders. In orthopaedic treatments, for instance, stem cells have been utilised to regenerate cartilage and repair joint injuries, demonstrating significant clinical outcomes. Similarly, advancements in cellular therapies for cardiovascular disorders have opened new avenues for addressing heart diseases, which remain a leading cause of mortality worldwide. As research progresses, the potential for stem cells to revolutionise treatment paradigms continues to expand, offering hope to patients and practitioners alike.

As we look to the future, the integration of stem cell therapies into mainstream medicine will require a commitment to ongoing research, ethical considerations, and public education. The promise of regeneration through stem cells is immense, yet it is accompanied by the responsibility to ensure that such therapies are accessible, safe, and effective. Engaging with the public to enhance understanding and acceptance of these therapies will be crucial, as it fosters a supportive environment for continued innovation in regenerative medicine.

Current Landscape of Regenerative Medicine

The current landscape of regenerative medicine is marked by rapid advancements and a growing body of research that highlights the potential of stem cell therapies. As healthcare professionals and biomedical scientists continue to explore the capabilities of stem cells, innovative treatments are emerging for various conditions, including neurodegenerative diseases, cardiovascular disorders, and autoimmune diseases. These breakthroughs promise not only to enhance patient care but also to shift the paradigm of traditional medical approaches, fostering hope for many patients who previously faced limited options.

In the realm of neurodegenerative diseases, stem cell therapy is demonstrating transformative potential. Research has begun to unveil how stem cells can be utilised to repair damaged neural tissue and restore function in conditions such as Parkinson's and Alzheimer's diseases. The integration of stem cells into treatment regimens could lead to significant improvements in the quality of life for patients, thereby marking a pivotal moment in the field of neurobiology and regenerative medicine.

Moreover, the application of stem cell therapy in orthopaedic treatments is gaining traction. Techniques such as using mesenchymal stem cells to heal bone and cartilage injuries showcase the versatility of stem cells in addressing musculoskeletal disorders. These advancements not only enhance recovery times but also promote the long-term health of patients, making stem cell therapy an attractive option within orthopaedics.

Ethical considerations remain a crucial aspect of stem cell research, especially considering the complex nature of sourcing stem cells. As public perception evolves, ongoing dialogue surrounding the ethical implications of stem cell use is essential to ensure responsible research practices. Engaging with the community and educating stakeholders about the benefits and risks associated with regenerative medicine will be vital in garnering support for future innovations.

Finally, the promise of stem cell therapies extends to paediatric applications, cancer treatment, and diabetes management. As research progresses, there is a burgeoning interest in how these therapies can be tailored to meet the unique needs of children and individuals battling chronic diseases. The landscape of regenerative medicine is undoubtedly dynamic, offering a glimpse into a future where stem cell therapies could revolutionise treatment paradigms across various medical fields.

Regenerative Medicine Innovations

Breakthrough Technologies in Stem Cell Research

Breakthrough technologies in stem cell research are reshaping the landscape of regenerative medicine and offering new hope for patients suffering from a variety of ailments. Recent advancements in gene editing techniques, such as CRISPR-Cas9, allow scientists to precisely modify the genetic makeup of stem cells. This capability not only enhances the potential for developing personalised therapies but also addresses ethical concerns by reducing the dependency on embryonic stem cells. As research progresses, these technologies promise to unlock new pathways for treating conditions like neurodegenerative diseases and cardiovascular disorders.

Another significant development is the use of induced pluripotent stem cells (iPSCs), which are derived from adult cells and can differentiate into any cell type. iPSCs have revolutionised the field by providing a more ethical alternative to traditional stem cells. They offer immense potential for patient-specific therapies, particularly in the treatment of autoimmune diseases and cancer. The ability to generate iPSCs from a patient's own cells minimises the risk of rejection and enhances treatment efficacy, marking a pivotal shift in how stem cell therapies are approached.

In the realm of orthopaedic treatments, advancements in 3D bioprinting technology are enabling the creation of complex tissue structures that can be used for regenerative purposes. This innovative approach allows for the fabrication of customised scaffolds that can support stem cell growth and facilitate tissue regeneration. As a result, patients with severe injuries or degenerative conditions may experience improved recovery times and outcomes. The integration of bioprinting with stem cell therapy is paving the way for groundbreaking solutions in orthopaedics.

Furthermore, researchers are exploring the application of stem cells in paediatric medicine, particularly for congenital disorders and genetic conditions. The ability to harness the regenerative properties of stem cells in children opens new avenues for early intervention and treatment strategies. This emerging focus on paediatric applications underscores the importance of tailoring therapies to the unique needs of younger patients, ensuring that they receive the most effective care possible.

Finally, public perception and acceptance of stem cell therapies remain crucial for the future of this field. As breakthrough technologies continue to evolve, it is essential for healthcare professionals and scientists to engage with the community and address concerns around ethical implications and treatment efficacy. Transparency and education will play vital roles in fostering trust and understanding, ultimately enabling more widespread adoption of these promising therapies in clinical practice.

The Role of Bioprinting in Regeneration

Bioprinting has emerged as a revolutionary technology in regenerative medicine, offering innovative solutions for tissue engineering and organ regeneration. At its core, bioprinting involves the layer-by-layer deposition of bioinks, which are composed of living cells and biomaterials, to create complex three-dimensional structures that mimic the natural architecture of tissues. This capability enables researchers and clinicians to fabricate tissues that can potentially replace damaged or diseased organs, and thus address the critical shortage of organ donors and improving patient outcomes in various medical fields.

The application of bioprinting in stem cell therapy is particularly promising. By integrating stem cells within bioprinted constructs, scientists can harness the regenerative properties of these cells to enhance tissue repair and regeneration. For instance, bioprinted scaffolds embedded with stem cells can promote the growth of new cartilage in orthopaedic treatments, offering hope to patients suffering from degenerative joint diseases. This synergy between bioprinting technology and stem cell biology not only optimises the therapeutic potential of stem cells but also paves the way for personalised medicine approaches in regenerative therapies.

Moreover, bioprinting can address the ethical concerns associated with stem cell research. The ability to create tissues from induced pluripotent stem cells (iPSCs) allows for the development of patient-specific models without the ethical dilemmas that accompany the use of embryonic stem cells. This advancement is crucial for advancing research in areas such as neurodegenerative diseases and cancer treatment, where patient-derived models can provide insights into disease mechanisms and facilitate the development of targeted therapies. By circumventing ethical issues, bioprinting strengthens the legitimacy and acceptance of stem cell therapies in the public eye.

In addition to its ethical advantages, bioprinting holds significant potential for treating autoimmune diseases. By producing tissues that can modulate the immune response, researchers can explore new therapeutic avenues for conditions like rheumatoid arthritis and lupus. Bioprinted constructs can be designed to release immuno-regulatory factors that promote tolerance and reduce inflammation, thereby providing a novel strategy for managing autoimmune disorders. This innovative approach exemplifies how bioprinting can transform the landscape of regenerative medicine, offering hope for conditions previously deemed difficult to treat.

Ultimately, the role of bioprinting in regeneration underscores a paradigm shift in how medical professionals approach tissue repair and organ replacement. As this technology continues to evolve, it will undoubtedly enhance the field of stem cell therapy and regenerative medicine, bringing us closer to the realisation of fully functional engineered tissues. By embracing the potential of bioprinting, health care professionals and biomedical scientists can together forge a new frontier in patient care, ensuring that the promise of regeneration is not just a dream but a tangible reality.

Gene Editing and Stem Cells

Gene editing, particularly through techniques like CRISPR-Cas9, has revolutionised the landscape of stem cell research and therapy. This powerful tool allows for precise modifications to the genome, enabling scientists to correct genetic defects and enhance the therapeutic potential of stem cells. By integrating gene editing with stem cell technology, researchers are exploring innovative treatments for a range of conditions, from genetic disorders to degenerative diseases, thereby paving the way for regenerative medicine innovations that promise to transform patient outcomes.

Stem Cell Therapy for Neurodegenerative Diseases

Mechanisms of Neurodegeneration

Neurodegeneration encompasses a range of disorders characterised by the progressive degeneration of the structure and function of the nervous system. This process is often initiated by a variety of factors, including genetic mutations, environmental toxins, and inflammation. These triggers can lead to cellular stress, resulting in the death of neurons and their supporting cells. Understanding the mechanisms behind neurodegeneration is crucial for developing effective stem cell therapies that can mitigate or reverse the damage done to neural tissues.

One key mechanism of neurodegeneration is the accumulation of misfolded proteins within neuronal cells. Proteins such as amyloid-beta and tau in Alzheimer's disease, for instance, can form toxic aggregates that disrupt cellular function. This accumulation not only leads to neuronal cell death but also triggers inflammatory responses that exacerbate the condition. Targeting these misfolded proteins through innovative stem cell strategies may pave the way for potential therapeutic interventions.

Another significant aspect is the role of oxidative stress in neurodegeneration. Reactive oxygen species (ROS) can cause cellular damage and impair mitochondrial function, which is vital for energy production in neurons. As oxidative stress increases, it can lead to a cascade of events that culminate in neuronal death. Stem cell therapies that enhance antioxidant defence mechanisms or replace damaged neurons with healthy stem cell-derived cells could offer promising avenues for treatment.

Furthermore, neuroinflammation plays a critical role in the progression of neurodegenerative diseases. Activated microglia and astrocytes release pro-inflammatory cytokines that can further damage neurons and disrupt the blood-brain barrier. By harnessing the potential of stem cells to modulate inflammatory responses, researchers aim to create therapies that not only replace lost neurons but also restore a healthy neuroinflammatory environment.

Lastly, the interplay between genetic and epigenetic factors cannot be overlooked in the context of neurodegeneration. Genetic predispositions, combined with environmental influences, can lead to changes in gene expression that promote disease. Stem cell research is exploring ways to correct these epigenetic changes, offering hope for targeted therapies that could potentially alter the course of neurodegenerative diseases. As advancements continue, a comprehensive understanding of these mechanisms will be essential for the successful application of stem cell therapies in treating neurodegenerative conditions.

Current Applications and Research

The field of stem cell therapy has witnessed remarkable advancements, leading to various current applications that showcase its potential in regenerative medicine. Healthcare professionals and biomedical scientists are increasingly exploring the therapeutic possibilities stem cells offer in treating a range of conditions, including neurodegenerative diseases, cardiovascular disorders, and autoimmune diseases. These applications not only highlight the versatility of stem cells but also their promise in revolutionising treatment methodologies across different medical disciplines.

Research into stem cell therapy for neurodegenerative diseases, such as Parkinson's and Alzheimer's, is a focal point of current studies. Scientists are investigating how stem cells can repair damaged neural tissues and restore function, providing hope for patients suffering from these debilitating conditions. Clinical trials are underway to evaluate the efficacy and safety of these therapies, with preliminary results indicating positive outcomes in some cases, thus paving the way for future innovations in this area.

Moreover, the application of stem cells in orthopaedic treatments has shown significant progress. Regenerative techniques involving stem cells are being employed to heal cartilage injuries and degenerative joint diseases. By harnessing the body's natural repair mechanisms, these therapies aim to reduce pain and improve mobility, offering an alternative to traditional surgical interventions. This approach not only enhances patient recovery but also has the potential to transform the management of musculoskeletal disorders.

In the realm of cancer treatment, stem cell therapy is emerging as a vital component in combating various malignancies. Researchers are exploring the use of stem cells for targeted delivery of therapies and for regenerating healthy tissues post-chemotherapy. The integration of stem cell technology into oncology is opening new avenues for personalised medicine, allowing for tailored treatments that align with the unique genetic profiles of patients, thereby improving therapeutic outcomes and minimising side effects.

While the promise of stem cell therapy is vast, ethical considerations remain pivotal in guiding research and clinical applications. The dialogue surrounding stem cell research is crucial, particularly regarding the sourcing of stem cells and the implications for patients and society. As public perception evolves, it is essential for healthcare professionals to engage in transparent discussions about the benefits and risks associated with stem cell therapies, ensuring informed decision-making and fostering trust within the community.

Future Directions in Treatment

As we look to the future of stem cell therapy, several exciting directions are emerging that promise to revolutionise the treatment landscape. Advances in regenerative medicine innovations are paving the way for more effective therapies targeting neurodegenerative diseases such as Alzheimer's and Parkinson's. Enhanced understanding of stem cell biology is leading to the development of tailored treatments that hold the potential to significantly improve patient outcomes and quality of life. This evolution is not just limited to the central nervous system but extends into various fields, including orthopaedics and cardiovascular disorders, where regenerative strategies are showing remarkable promise.

The application of stem cells in orthopaedic treatments is particularly noteworthy, as researchers are exploring ways to utilise mesenchymal stem cells to repair cartilage and bone injuries. Techniques such as tissue engineering and the use of biomaterials are being combined with stem cell therapies to create functional tissues that can restore mobility and alleviate pain in patients suffering from degenerative joint diseases. These advancements not only enhance the efficacy of treatments but also have the potential to reduce the need for invasive surgical procedures, thereby improving patient recovery times and overall satisfaction.

In the realm of cardiovascular disorders, stem cell therapy is emerging as a transformative approach to regenerate damaged heart tissue following events such as myocardial infarction. Ongoing clinical trials are investigating the efficacy of various stem cell types, including induced pluripotent stem cells (iPSCs) and cardiac progenitor cells, in promoting cardiac repair and improving heart function. As these therapies advance through clinical stages, there is a growing optimism about their potential to significantly reduce the burden of heart disease, which remains a leading cause of mortality worldwide.

However, as the field progresses, ethical considerations in stem cell research must remain at the forefront of our discussions. The necessity for robust ethical frameworks to guide researchers and clinicians cannot be overstated. Public perception and acceptance of stem cell therapies play a crucial role in their adoption, and ongoing dialogue about the ethical implications of stem cell use is essential to foster trust and understanding within the community. Engaging stakeholders, including patients and advocacy groups, is vital in shaping a responsible path forward that respects both scientific advancement and ethical standards.

Finally, the future of stem cell therapy also holds significant promise for paediatric applications, particularly in the treatment of genetic disorders and autoimmune diseases. The ability to harness the regenerative capabilities of stem cells in younger populations offers hope for early intervention and improved long-term outcomes. As research in this area continues to expand, the integration of stem cell therapies into standard care protocols may soon become commonplace, heralding a new era in paediatric medicine that prioritises regeneration and healing over traditional, more invasive treatments.

Ethical Considerations in Stem Cell Research

Ethical Frameworks and Guidelines

The landscape of stem cell therapy is rapidly evolving, promising revolutionary advancements in regenerative medicine. However, as these innovations unfold, they bring forth a myriad of ethical considerations that must be addressed by health care professionals and biomedical scientists alike. The ethical frameworks guiding stem cell research are essential for ensuring that scientific progress does not come at the expense of moral integrity. This subchapter explores these frameworks, emphasising the importance of ethical guidelines in fostering responsible research and application of stem cell therapies across various medical fields.

At the core of ethical frameworks in stem cell research is the principle of respect for persons, which acknowledges the rights and dignity of all individuals involved in research processes. This principle extends to the informed consent of donors, who must be fully aware of the implications and potential risks associated with stem cell donation. Furthermore, the principle of beneficence requires that researchers and clinicians strive to maximise benefits while minimising harm. These ethical considerations are particularly pertinent in areas such as paediatric applications of stem cell therapy, where vulnerable populations are involved.

Another key component of ethical frameworks is justice, which addresses the fair distribution of the benefits and burdens of research. In the context of stem cell therapy, this means ensuring equitable access to treatments, particularly for underserved populations. The promise of regeneration through stem cell therapy should not be limited to those who can afford it; rather, ethical guidelines must advocate for inclusivity in research designs and clinical applications. This commitment to justice is critical as the public perception and acceptance of stem cell therapies hinge on the belief that these advancements are accessible to all.

Moreover, ethical frameworks in stem cell therapy also encompass considerations regarding the use of embryonic stem cells and the moral status of embryos. Ongoing debates surrounding these issues necessitate a nuanced understanding of cultural, religious, and personal beliefs. Health care professionals must navigate these complexities delicately, balancing scientific inquiry with respect for diverse perspectives. This dialogue is crucial for advancing regenerative medicine innovations while fostering public trust and support.

In conclusion, ethical frameworks and guidelines are indispensable in the realm of stem cell therapy. They ensure that research is conducted responsibly and that the potential benefits of regenerative medicine are realised in a manner consistent with moral values. As health care professionals and biomedical scientists continue to explore the possibilities offered by stem cells in treating various conditions, adherence to these ethical principles will be vital in shaping a future where stem cell therapies are both innovative and ethically sound.

Controversies Surrounding Stem Cell Sources

The debate surrounding stem cell sources is a complex and multifaceted issue that has garnered significant attention within the medical and scientific communities. Central to this discussion is the distinction between embryonic stem cells and adult stem cells, each offering unique advantages and ethical dilemmas. Embryonic stem cells, derived from early-stage embryos, have the potential to differentiate into any cell type, making them invaluable for research and therapeutic applications. However, the use of these cells raises profound ethical questions about the status of the embryo and the moral implications of its destruction.

On the other hand, adult stem cells, which can be sourced from tissues such as bone marrow or adipose tissue, present a less controversial alternative. These cells have demonstrated considerable promise in treating a variety of conditions, including cardiovascular disorders and orthopaedic injuries. The relative ease of obtaining adult stem cells contributes to their appeal, yet their limited ability to differentiate compared to embryonic stem cells poses challenges in their application for regenerative medicine.

Induced pluripotent stem cells (iPSCs) have emerged as a revolutionary solution that bridges the gap between embryonic and adult stem cells. These cells are reprogrammed from somatic cells and possess pluripotency, allowing them to develop into various cell types. The ethical implications are significantly reduced since iPSCs do not involve the destruction of embryos. However, concerns regarding the potential for genetic mutations and long-term effects remain a critical area of research that must be addressed before iPSCs can be widely adopted in clinical settings.

Public perception plays a crucial role in the ongoing discourse about stem cell sources. Misinformation and sensationalism often cloud understanding, leading to hesitancy in embracing stem cell therapies. Education is paramount in dispelling myths and providing clear information regarding the benefits and risks associated with different stem cell sources. Health care professionals and biomedical scientists must advocate for informed discussions to foster acceptance and support for stem cell research and its applications.

In conclusion, the controversies surrounding stem cell sources are emblematic of the broader ethical and scientific dilemmas faced in regenerative medicine. As research progresses, it is imperative to continue exploring innovative solutions like iPSCs while ensuring ethical standards are upheld. Balancing the potential benefits of stem cell therapies with ethical considerations will be vital in advancing this promising field, ultimately leading to improved treatment options for patients suffering from various diseases.

Informed Consent and Patient Autonomy

Informed consent is a foundational principle in the practice of medicine, particularly in the realm of stem cell therapy. It ensures that patients are fully aware of the procedures, potential risks, and benefits involved in their treatment. This principle underlines the importance of transparency between healthcare providers and patients, fostering a relationship built on trust. As stem cell therapies evolve, the complexity of procedures necessitates even greater emphasis on informed consent, especially given the innovative nature of these treatments for conditions that were previously deemed untreatable.

Patient autonomy is closely linked to informed consent, as it empowers individuals to make decisions regarding their healthcare. In the context of stem cell therapy, this autonomy becomes increasingly critical, as patients may face various treatment options with differing implications. Healthcare professionals must guide patients through the intricacies of their choices, ensuring they understand the ethical considerations and scientific realities behind stem cell treatments. This support helps patients to feel more confident in their decisions, aligning their treatment plans with personal values and preferences.

The ethical considerations surrounding stem cell research and therapy also play a significant role in informed consent. Healthcare providers must navigate a landscape where scientific advancements often outpace regulatory frameworks. This can lead to uncertainty regarding the ethical implications of certain stem cell procedures. It is essential for professionals to stay informed about regulations and ethical guidelines, ensuring they communicate these factors effectively to patients. By doing so, they uphold the integrity of the informed consent process and respect patient autonomy.

Furthermore, the public perception of stem cell therapies can influence patients' willingness to engage in informed consent discussions. As healthcare professionals, it is crucial to address misconceptions and educate patients about the realities of stem cell therapy. Engaging in open conversations helps demystify the subject and encourages patients to ask questions, thereby enhancing their understanding and involvement in the treatment process. This proactive approach not only supports informed consent but also promotes a more informed patient population.

In conclusion, informed consent and patient autonomy are vital components in the evolving field of stem cell therapy. As healthcare professionals, it is our responsibility to ensure that patients are not only informed but also empowered to make decisions that reflect their individual needs and values. By fostering an environment of trust, transparency, and education, we can navigate the complexities of stem cell therapy and uphold the ethical standards that govern our practice. This commitment ultimately enhances patient care and promotes a more ethical approach to regenerative medicine.

Stem Cells in Orthopaedic Treatments

Stem Cell Applications in Bone Healing

Stem cell therapy has emerged as a revolutionary approach in the field of regenerative medicine, particularly in the context of bone healing. The unique properties of stem cells, including their ability to differentiate into various cell types and their potential to modulate immune responses, make them ideal candidates for enhancing bone repair processes. In recent years, significant advancements have been made in understanding the mechanisms through which stem cells contribute to fracture healing, offering new avenues for clinical application in orthopaedic treatments.

One of the primary applications of stem cells in bone healing is their use in treating non-union fractures, which are a significant challenge in orthopaedic surgery. By isolating stem cells from sources such as bone marrow or adipose tissue, clinicians can create a cellular environment conducive to bone regeneration. These stem cells can differentiate into osteoblasts, the cells responsible for new bone formation, thus accelerating the healing process and improving outcomes for patients.

Moreover, stem cell therapy also holds promise for enhancing the efficacy of existing surgical techniques, such as bone grafting. The integration of stem cells into grafts can improve the biological activity of the graft material, leading to better incorporation and healing at the site of injury. This synergy not only reduces recovery times but also decreases the likelihood of complications associated with traditional grafting procedures.

Clinical trials are currently underway to evaluate the safety and effectiveness of various stem cell therapies for bone healing. Initial results have been promising, indicating that patients receiving stem cell treatments often experience quicker healing times and improved functional outcomes compared to those receiving standard care. These findings underscore the potential of stem cell applications to transform the landscape of orthopaedic medicine and provide new hope for patients suffering from complex bone injuries.

Despite the exciting prospects of stem cell therapy in bone healing, ethical considerations remain paramount. It is crucial for healthcare professionals and researchers to navigate the complexities of stem cell research responsibly, ensuring that advancements are made with due consideration for ethical standards and patient safety. As the field of regenerative medicine continues to evolve, the commitment to ethical practices will be essential in maintaining public trust and acceptance of stem cell therapies.

Cartilage Regeneration and Repair

Cartilage plays a crucial role in joint health, acting as a cushion between bones and facilitating smooth movement. However, its limited regenerative capacity poses significant challenges in treating cartilage injuries and degenerative diseases. Recent advancements in stem cell therapy present promising avenues for enhancing cartilage repair and regeneration. By harnessing the potential of stem cells, researchers are exploring innovative approaches to restore cartilage function and alleviate pain in patients suffering from osteoarthritis and other joint disorders.

One of the most exciting developments in this field involves the use of mesenchymal stem cells (MSCs), which can differentiate into chondrocytes, the cells responsible for cartilage formation. Studies have shown that MSCs can be isolated from various sources, including bone marrow, adipose tissue, and even umbilical cord blood. These cells can be expanded in vitro and subsequently delivered to the damaged cartilage site, where they may promote healing by regenerating the cartilage matrix and reducing inflammation.

Additionally, tissue engineering techniques are being employed to create scaffolds that support the growth and integration of stem cells into the existing cartilage. These biomaterials can provide a conducive environment for cell proliferation and differentiation, mimicking the natural extracellular matrix. Combined with stem cell therapy, these scaffolds hold the potential to enhance the overall efficacy of cartilage regeneration strategies, offering hope for patients with severe cartilage damage.

Ethical considerations remain paramount in the discussion of stem cell therapies. The source of stem cells, particularly embryonic stem cells, has raised significant ethical debates within the medical community. However, the use of adult stem cells and induced pluripotent stem cells (iPSCs) has alleviated some concerns, allowing researchers to focus on the therapeutic potential without compromising ethical standards. Ongoing public education and transparency in research practices will be essential to gain wider acceptance of these innovative treatments.

As we continue to uncover the mechanisms behind cartilage regeneration, it is crucial for healthcare professionals and researchers to collaborate and share knowledge. By integrating advancements in stem cell therapy with clinical practices, we can pave the way for novel treatments that not only repair damaged cartilage but also improve the quality of life for patients suffering from musculoskeletal disorders. The promise of regeneration through stem cells is not merely a theoretical concept; it is rapidly becoming a tangible reality in modern medicine.

Clinical Outcomes and Case Studies

Clinical outcomes in stem cell therapy have evolved significantly, showcasing remarkable advancements in regenerative medicine. Numerous case studies highlight the potential benefits of stem cell applications across various medical fields, including orthopaedics, cardiovascular disorders, and neurodegenerative diseases. For health care professionals and biomedical scientists, these outcomes provide a compelling narrative about the transformative potential of stem cells in clinical practice.

One noteworthy case study involved the use of mesenchymal stem cells (MSCs) in patients with osteoarthritis. The results demonstrated significant improvements in joint function and pain reduction, illustrating the effectiveness of stem cell therapy in orthopaedic treatments. Such findings encourage further exploration into the mechanisms by which stem cells may regenerate damaged tissues and improve quality of life for patients suffering from chronic conditions.

In the realm of cardiovascular disorders, stem cell therapy has shown promise in repairing myocardial damage following heart attacks. Several clinical trials have reported enhanced cardiac function and reduced scar tissue formation after stem cell injections. These advancements highlight the potential of regenerative medicine to address some of the most pressing health concerns, offering hope for patients who previously faced limited treatment options.

Neurodegenerative diseases, such as Parkinson's and Alzheimer's, present unique challenges for treatment. Case studies involving stem cell therapy in these areas have revealed encouraging results, with patients experiencing improved cognitive function and motor skills. These outcomes underscore the necessity for continued research into the ethical considerations surrounding stem cell research, as well as the importance of public perception and acceptance of these innovative therapies.

Overall, the clinical outcomes and case studies surrounding stem cell therapy illustrate a promising frontier in medicine. For stem cell enthusiasts and professionals alike, the potential to harness the power of stem cells for regenerative medicine is an exciting prospect, paving the way for future innovations and improved patient care across a variety of medical conditions.

Advances in Stem Cell Therapy for Cardiovascular Disorders

Mechanisms of Cardiac Stem Cell Function

Cardiac stem cells (CSCs) play a pivotal role in the homeostasis and repair of the heart. These cells are unique in their ability to regenerate cardiac tissue following injury, such as myocardial infarction. Research has shown that CSCs can differentiate into various cardiac cell types, including cardiomyocytes, endothelial cells, and smooth muscle cells, thus contributing to cardiac tissue regeneration. Understanding the mechanisms underlying CSC function is crucial for harnessing their potential in regenerative medicine, particularly in the treatment of cardiovascular disorders.

The functional capacity of cardiac stem cells is modulated by various intrinsic and extrinsic factors. Intrinsically, CSCs possess unique molecular markers and signalling pathways that govern their proliferation and differentiation. Extrinsically, the cardiac microenvironment, including cytokines and extracellular matrix components, significantly influences CSC behaviour. For instance, growth factors such as fibroblast growth factor (FGF) and vascular endothelial growth factor (VEGF) have been implicated in promoting CSC survival and enhancing their regenerative capabilities, highlighting the importance of the niche in stem cell biology.

Recent advances in regenerative medicine have focused on optimising the use of CSCs for therapeutic applications. Techniques such as cardiac tissue engineering and the application of biomaterials aim to create supportive environments that enhance CSC function. Furthermore, the integration of CSCs with gene therapy approaches has shown promise in augmenting their regenerative potential. By manipulating specific signalling pathways, researchers aim to improve the survival and functionality of CSCs in vivo, thereby enhancing tissue repair and regeneration after cardiac injury.

Ethical considerations surrounding cardiac stem cell research continue to be a topic of significant debate. While the promise of regenerative therapies is immense, concerns related to the source of stem cells, potential for tumour formation, and long-term effects of therapy must be addressed. Ensuring that research adheres to ethical standards is crucial for gaining public trust and acceptance of stem cell therapies. This includes transparent communication about the risks and benefits associated with CSC-based treatments and the importance of informed consent in clinical applications.

In conclusion, the mechanisms of cardiac stem cell function are complex and multifaceted, encompassing a range of biological processes that contribute to heart repair and regeneration. As research continues to unfold, it holds the potential to revolutionise the management of cardiovascular diseases through innovative therapies. By deepening our understanding of CSC biology, we can unlock new avenues for treatment that not only improve patient outcomes but also advance the field of regenerative medicine.

Clinical Trials and Efficacy

Clinical trials are the cornerstone of validating the efficacy of stem cell therapies, serving as the bridge between laboratory research and clinical application. They provide systematic evaluation of the safety and effectiveness of new treatments in diverse patient populations. Health care professionals must understand the rigorous methodologies employed in these trials, as they assess not only the therapeutic benefits, but also potential risks associated with stem cell interventions. As the field of regenerative medicine advances, the results of these trials are critical in shaping clinical guidelines and treatment protocols.

The landscape of clinical trials in stem cell therapy is marked by innovations tailored to specific conditions, including neurodegenerative diseases, cardiovascular disorders, and autoimmune diseases. Each trial is designed with unique endpoints, focusing on functional improvements and quality of life enhancements for patients. For instance, trials targeting neurodegenerative diseases like Alzheimer's often measure cognitive function and daily living activities as primary outcomes. This tailored approach ensures that the therapies developed are not only effective but also relevant to patient needs.

Moreover, ethical considerations play a pivotal role in the design and conduct of clinical trials involving stem cells. The use of human subjects necessitates stringent ethical oversight to ensure informed consent and the minimisation of risks. Health care professionals are encouraged to engage with the ethical dimensions of stem cell research, as public perception can significantly influence the acceptance and funding of clinical trials. Transparency in trial outcomes and ethical compliance builds trust among stakeholders and the broader community.

The results of these clinical trials are paramount in establishing the therapeutic potential of stem cell applications in various fields, including orthopaedics and cancer treatment. Positive outcomes not only bolster confidence in stem cell therapies but also pave the way for regulatory approvals. As these therapies transition from experimental to standard practice, it is essential for biomedical scientists and health care professionals to remain updated on the latest findings and advancements in the field, ensuring that they provide the best possible care to their patients.

In conclusion, clinical trials serve as a vital component in the journey of stem cell therapies from bench to bedside. They embody the promise of regeneration and the potential to transform treatment paradigms across numerous medical disciplines. As the evidence base grows, it is crucial for health care professionals to advocate for ongoing research and to participate in shaping the future of regenerative medicine, ultimately enhancing patient outcomes and quality of life.

Prospects for Cardiovascular Health

The prospects for cardiovascular health through stem cell therapy are both promising and complex. With the increasing prevalence of cardiovascular diseases worldwide, innovative treatment approaches are paramount. Stem cell therapy presents a revolutionary avenue, aiming to repair damaged heart tissue and improve overall cardiac function. Recent advancements in regenerative medicine indicate that harnessing the power of stem cells could transform the landscape of cardiovascular treatment options, offering hope to millions affected by these conditions.

Ongoing research is revealing the potential of various stem cell types, including embryonic stem cells, induced pluripotent stem cells, and mesenchymal stem cells, in treating cardiovascular disorders. These cells can differentiate into cardiac cell types, promoting regeneration of damaged myocardium and improving heart function. Additionally, novel techniques such as 3D bioprinting and gene editing are being explored to enhance the efficacy of stem cell therapies, paving the way for personalised medicine approaches in cardiovascular health.

However, along with the promise of these therapies comes a host of ethical considerations that must be addressed. The utilisation of embryonic stem cells, for instance, raises significant moral questions that need careful deliberation. Ensuring that research and clinical applications are conducted ethically is vital for maintaining public trust and acceptance. As healthcare professionals and researchers, it is our responsibility to navigate these ethical landscapes while pursuing advancements that could save lives.

Public perception and acceptance of stem cell therapies will play a crucial role in their future implementation in cardiovascular health. Engaging with communities to educate them about the science behind stem cells and their potential benefits can help alleviate fears and misconceptions. Transparent communication regarding the research process, potential risks, and expected outcomes will contribute to a more informed public, ultimately fostering a supportive environment for these innovative therapies.

In conclusion, as we look ahead, the integration of stem cell therapy into cardiovascular health management appears to be a beacon of hope. The convergence of scientific innovation, ethical practice, and public engagement will determine the extent to which these therapies can be successfully adopted. With continued research and collaboration among healthcare professionals, biomedical scientists, and policymakers, the future of cardiovascular health may indeed be revitalised through the promise of regeneration.

Stem Cells and Autoimmune Disease Management

Understanding Autoimmune Disorders

Autoimmune disorders represent a complex group of conditions where the body's immune system mistakenly attacks its own tissues. These disorders can affect various systems within the body, leading to a wide range of symptoms and complications. Understanding the underlying mechanisms of these diseases is crucial for healthcare professionals and biomedical scientists, as it informs both diagnosis and treatment strategies. The role of stem cells in managing autoimmune diseases has emerged as a promising area of research, indicating potential pathways for regeneration and healing.

Research into autoimmune disorders has illuminated the intricate interplay between genetic predisposition and environmental factors. This understanding is vital not only for developing targeted therapies but also for creating preventative strategies. The promise of stem cell therapy lies in its ability to modulate immune responses and repair damaged tissues. By harnessing the regenerative potential of stem cells, researchers are exploring innovative treatments that could significantly improve the quality of life for patients suffering from these debilitating conditions.

Particularly in cases of severe autoimmune diseases, such as systemic lupus erythematosus or multiple sclerosis, traditional therapies may fall short. Stem cell therapy offers a novel approach by aiming to reset the immune system and promote tissue regeneration. Clinical trials are currently underway, testing various stem cell types and their efficacy in treating these disorders. Such advancements highlight the importance of interdisciplinary collaboration among health care professionals, researchers, and ethicists to ensure the responsible development of these therapies.

Ethical considerations also play a critical role in the advancement of stem cell therapies for autoimmune diseases. The source of stem cells, whether derived from embryos or adult tissues, raises important questions about consent, moral implications, and public acceptance. Addressing these concerns is essential to foster trust and transparency within the medical community and among patients. As researchers continue to explore the frontiers of regenerative medicine, ethical frameworks must evolve alongside scientific progress to guide responsible practices.

In summary, understanding autoimmune disorders and the potential of stem cell therapy in their management represents a frontier of regenerative medicine. As healthcare professionals and biomedical scientists delve deeper into this field, the hope is to not only alleviate symptoms but to achieve lasting remission and recovery for patients. Continued research and ethical discourse will be paramount in unlocking the full promise of stem cells in treating autoimmune conditions and enhancing patient outcomes.

Role of Stem Cells in Modulating Immune Response

Stem cells possess unique properties that allow them to modulate the immune response, making them a focal point in regenerative medicine. These cells can differentiate into various types of tissues and modulate the immune environment by secreting various cytokines and growth factors. By doing so, they can promote tissue repair and reduce inflammation, offering a promising avenue for treating autoimmune diseases and other conditions associated with dysfunctional immune responses.

The interaction between stem cells and the immune system is complex and multi-faceted. Stem cells can exert immunosuppressive effects, which can be beneficial in preventing tissue rejection during transplantation or in managing autoimmune disorders. This immunomodulation occurs through various mechanisms, including the alteration of dendritic cell maturation and the induction of regulatory T cells, which play a crucial role in maintaining immune tolerance.

In the context of neurodegenerative diseases, stem cell therapy has shown potential in not only replacing damaged neurons but also in modulating the immune response to reduce neuroinflammation. Studies indicate that stem cells can influence the activity of microglia, the resident immune cells of the central nervous system, thereby creating a more favourable environment for neuronal survival and regeneration. This dual role highlights the therapeutic promise of stem cells in conditions such as multiple sclerosis and Alzheimer's disease.

Moreover, stem cells are being explored for their applications in cardiovascular disorders, where they can help in repairing damaged heart tissue and modulating the inflammatory response following myocardial infarction. This regenerative capability, coupled with their ability to modulate immune response, positions stem cells as a vital component in the future treatment of heart diseases, offering hope for enhanced recovery and improved patient outcomes.

As research progresses, ethical considerations surrounding stem cell therapy continue to evolve. The manipulation of immune responses raises important questions regarding safety, efficacy, and the potential for unintended consequences. Therefore, it is crucial for healthcare professionals and biomedical scientists to navigate these ethical landscapes carefully while exploring the vast potential of stem cells in medical therapies, ensuring that advancements are both scientifically grounded and ethically sound.

Case Studies and Clinical Applications

The exploration of stem cell therapy has led to remarkable advancements, particularly evident in various case studies that highlight its clinical applications. One notable example is the use of stem cells in treating neurodegenerative diseases such as Parkinson's and Alzheimer's. Clinical trials have demonstrated the potential to restore lost function and improve quality of life for patients suffering from these debilitating conditions. These cases not only showcase the promise of regeneration but also the necessity for ongoing research and refinement of methodologies to optimise outcomes.

In the realm of orthopaedic treatments, stem cell therapy has shown significant promise in the management of joint disorders and injuries. Case studies involving patients with osteoarthritis have revealed that stem cell injections can reduce pain and enhance mobility, offering an innovative alternative to traditional surgical interventions. This approach highlights the role of regenerative medicine in not just alleviating symptoms but also addressing the underlying causes of musculoskeletal diseases, thereby changing the landscape of orthopaedic care.

Cardiovascular disorders represent another critical area where stem cell therapy has made strides. Clinical applications have included the use of stem cells to repair damaged heart tissue post-myocardial infarction. Case studies indicate that patients receiving stem cell transplants often exhibit improved cardiac function and reduced incidence of heart failure. These findings underscore the potential for stem cell therapy to transform cardiovascular treatment paradigms, providing hope for patients with previously limited options.

Moreover, the ethical considerations surrounding stem cell research and therapy cannot be overlooked. Case studies often serve as a foundation for discussions about the moral implications of using embryonic versus adult stem cells. By examining historical and contemporary cases, healthcare professionals can navigate the complexities of patient consent, sourcing of stem cells, and the impact of public perception on research funding and policymaking.

Lastly, paediatric applications of stem cell therapy are witnessing encouraging results, particularly in conditions such as juvenile diabetes and certain cancers. The outcomes reported in case studies suggest that early intervention using stem cell therapy can lead to significant improvements in long-term health and disease management. This emerging field exemplifies the potential of regenerative medicine to not only heal but also enhance the lives of younger patients, ensuring a brighter future for those affected by chronic illnesses.

Paediatric Applications of Stem Cell Therapy

Unique Considerations in Paediatric Patients

In the realm of paediatric patients, the application of stem cell therapy presents a unique set of considerations that differ significantly from those encountered in adults. The developmental stage of children means that their physiological responses to treatment can vary widely. This variability necessitates careful consideration of dosage, delivery methods, and the timing of interventions to ensure optimal outcomes. Furthermore, the potential for growth and development during treatment introduces complexities that require ongoing monitoring and adjustments to therapy as the child matures.

Ethical considerations play a pivotal role in the implementation of stem cell therapies in paediatric populations. Informed consent processes must be adapted to accommodate the understanding of both the child and their guardians. It is crucial to engage families in discussions about the benefits, risks, and uncertainties associated with stem cell treatments, particularly as many therapies are still experimental. The decision-making process must balance the potential for significant health benefits against the ethical implications of intervening in a developing child's biology.

Moreover, the long-term implications of stem cell therapy in children remain largely unexplored. Given that children are still undergoing development, there is a pressing need for research into the long-term effects of stem cell interventions on growth, cognitive development, and overall health. This lack of data creates a challenge for healthcare professionals in making evidence-based recommendations and raises questions about the sustainability of positive outcomes achieved through such therapies.

Additionally, the psychological and emotional aspects of receiving stem cell therapy should not be overlooked. Paediatric patients may experience anxiety or fear related to their condition and the treatments they undergo. Support systems involving family, peers, and healthcare providers are essential in addressing these emotional needs. Providing a comprehensive care approach that includes psychological support can enhance the overall experience and improve adherence to treatment protocols.

Finally, the integration of stem cell therapy into existing paediatric practices necessitates collaboration among various healthcare professionals. Paediatricians, haematologists, and other specialists need to work together to develop protocols that are tailored to the unique needs of children. This interdisciplinary approach not only fosters innovation in treatment strategies but also ensures a holistic focus on the child's health, encompassing both physical and emotional wellbeing as they navigate their treatment journey.

Stem Cell Therapy for Genetic Disorders

Stem cell therapy represents a groundbreaking approach in the treatment of genetic disorders, harnessing the potential of stem cells to repair or replace damaged tissues and cells. These therapies are particularly promising for conditions that have long been deemed incurable, offering hope to patients with genetic anomalies. The underlying mechanism involves utilising the unique properties of stem cells, which can differentiate into various cell types and contribute to tissue regeneration. Her we will explore the latest advancements in stem cell therapy specifically targeting genetic disorders, highlighting the techniques employed and the outcomes observed in clinical settings.

One of the most significant applications of stem cell therapy for genetic disorders is in the treatment of inherited metabolic diseases. Conditions such as cystic fibrosis and phenylketonuria are characterised by specific genetic mutations that hinder normal cellular function. By employing gene editing techniques alongside stem cell therapy, researchers have been able to correct these mutations at the cellular level. This innovative approach not only addresses the symptoms of the disorders but also targets the root cause, leading to more sustainable outcomes for patients.

Moreover, the field of regenerative medicine has seen substantial progress in utilising induced pluripotent stem cells (iPSCs) for genetic therapy. iPSCs, derived from adult cells, can be reprogrammed to acquire the properties of embryonic stem cells, allowing for the development of patient-specific therapies. This personalised medicine approach has opened new avenues for treating genetic disorders, as it minimises the risk of immune rejection and enhances the compatibility of the therapy with the patient's biological makeup. Recent studies have demonstrated successful applications of iPSCs in modelling genetic diseases, paving the way for tailored treatment strategies.

Ethical considerations remain a crucial aspect of stem cell research, especially concerning genetic manipulation. The prospect of modifying human genetics raises profound ethical questions about the implications of such interventions. Healthcare professionals and researchers must navigate these complexities, ensuring that advancements in stem cell therapy align with ethical standards and societal values. Engaging in public discourse and fostering transparency in research processes will be vital in shaping the future of genetic therapies and maintaining public trust.

In conclusion, stem cell therapy holds immense promise for addressing genetic disorders, with ongoing research revealing new possibilities for treatment. As advancements continue to unfold, collaboration among healthcare professionals, scientists, and ethicists will be essential in overcoming challenges and realising the full potential of this innovative field. The journey towards effective and ethical stem cell therapies for genetic disorders is a testament to human ingenuity and the relentless pursuit of medical excellence.

Success Stories and Challenges

Stem cell therapy has made significant strides in recent years, with numerous success stories emerging from various fields of medicine. One notable case involves the use of stem cells in treating neurodegenerative diseases such as Parkinson's and Alzheimer's. In clinical trials, patients have shown remarkable improvements in their motor function and cognitive abilities, providing hope to countless individuals and their families. These successes underscore the potential of regenerative medicine to transform the treatment landscape for conditions once deemed untreatable.

However, the journey towards widespread acceptance and application of stem cell therapies is fraught with challenges. Ethical concerns surrounding the use of embryonic stem cells continue to spark debates in the medical community and among the public. Issues related to consent, the source of stem cells, and potential exploitation of vulnerable populations must be navigated carefully to ensure that advancements in this field are both scientifically sound and ethically responsible.

In orthopaedics, the application of stem cells for regenerative treatments has shown considerable promise, particularly in the repair of cartilage and bone injuries. Success stories of athletes returning to their sport after receiving stem cell injections highlight the potential of this innovative approach. Despite these positive outcomes, challenges such as standardising protocols and ensuring consistent results across diverse patient populations remain a significant hurdle in advancing these therapies.

The landscape of stem cell therapy is also evolving rapidly in the realm of cardiovascular disorders. Clinical trials have demonstrated that stem cells can aid in repairing damaged heart tissue and improving overall cardiac function. Nevertheless, researchers face obstacles including the need for long-term studies to gauge the efficacy and safety of these treatments, as well as addressing patient variability in response to stem cell interventions.

Finally, public perception plays a crucial role in the future of stem cell therapies. While many individuals express enthusiasm about the potential benefits, misinformation and fear can hinder acceptance. It is vital for health care professionals and advocates to engage with the public, providing clear information and addressing concerns to foster a more informed dialogue about the promise and challenges of stem cell research and its applications in modern medicine.

Stem Cell Therapy in Cancer Treatment

Mechanisms of Action Against Cancer

The mechanisms of action by which stem cells combat cancer are multifaceted and complex, reflecting the intricate biology of both stem cells and tumours. Stem cells can differentiate into various cell types, providing a versatile approach to replace damaged tissues and potentially eliminate cancerous cells. This differentiation capacity allows for targeted therapy, where stem cells can be engineered to deliver cytotoxic agents directly to tumours, minimising damage to surrounding healthy tissues. Furthermore, the immunomodulatory properties of stem cells can enhance the body's natural response to cancer, promoting an environment that is less conducive to tumour growth.

One significant mechanism involves the secretion of bioactive molecules by stem cells. These molecules can induce apoptosis in cancer cells, inhibit tumour growth, and modulate the immune response. For instance, mesenchymal stem cells (MSCs) can release cytokines and growth factors that encourage the recruitment of immune cells to the tumour site. This not only helps in targeting cancer cells more effectively but also fosters a systemic immune response against the malignancy. The potential to harness these natural processes offers exciting avenues for innovative cancer therapies.

Moreover, stem cells possess the ability to migrate towards tumour sites, which can be exploited for targeted delivery of therapeutic agents. This homing ability is particularly advantageous in treating metastatic cancers, where the spread of cancer cells poses significant treatment challenges. By directing stem cells to the site of the tumour, clinicians can enhance the efficacy of localised treatments, ensuring that therapeutic agents are concentrated where they are needed most.

The role of stem cells in creating a supportive tumour microenvironment is also critical. Research indicates that stem cells can modify the extracellular matrix (ECM), influencing tumour behaviour and progression. By altering the ECM, stem cells can disrupt the pathways that cancer cells rely on for survival and growth. This interaction highlights the importance of understanding the stem cell-tumour dynamics, as it can lead to the development of novel therapeutic strategies that inhibit cancer progression while leveraging the regenerative capabilities of stem cells.

Finally, ethical considerations surrounding stem cell research must also be addressed in the context of cancer treatment. While the potential benefits are significant, the manipulation of stem cells for therapeutic use raises questions regarding safety, efficacy, and moral implications. It is essential for healthcare professionals and researchers to engage in ongoing discussions about these concerns, ensuring that advancements in stem cell therapy are pursued responsibly, with the well-being of patients and the integrity of scientific research at the forefront.

Current Therapeutic Strategies

In recent years, therapeutic strategies involving stem cell therapy have evolved significantly, positioning themselves at the forefront of regenerative medicine. These strategies encompass a wide variety of applications, including the treatment of neurodegenerative diseases, wherein stem cells are employed to replace damaged neurons and restore functionality. The promise of regeneration is not merely theoretical; clinical trials are yielding promising results, showcasing the potential of stem cells to transform the treatment landscape for conditions such as Alzheimer's and Parkinson's disease.

In the realm of orthopaedics, stem cell therapy has emerged as a revolutionary approach for managing musculoskeletal disorders. Techniques such as the injection of mesenchymal stem cells into damaged joints are being used to promote healing and regeneration of cartilage. This innovative strategy is being explored for its efficacy in osteoarthritis and other degenerative joint diseases, offering patients a less invasive alternative to traditional surgical interventions.

Cardiovascular disorders represent another critical area where stem cell therapy is making strides. The application of stem cells in repairing myocardial damage post-myocardial infarction is a focal point of current research. Studies indicate that stem cell-derived cardiomyocytes could facilitate heart tissue regeneration, potentially reducing the burden of heart disease and improving patients' quality of life.

Ethical considerations remain a central theme in the discourse surrounding stem cell research and its applications. While advancements are promising, the use of embryonic stem cells often raises moral questions. Ensuring that research adheres to ethical guidelines is paramount, as public perception can significantly influence funding and support for stem cell therapies. Engaging with the community to foster understanding and acceptance is vital for the advancement of these innovative treatments.

Finally, the paediatric applications of stem cell therapy are garnering attention, particularly in the treatment of congenital disorders and cancers. The potential for stem cells to correct genetic anomalies before they manifest into more severe health issues is a promising frontier. Continued research and clinical trials are essential to fully realise the benefits of these therapies in children, ensuring that the next generation can benefit from the advancements in regenerative medicine.

Future Directions in Oncology

The future of oncology is increasingly intertwined with advancements in stem cell therapy, signifying a transformative era in cancer treatment. As we explore the potential of regenerative medicine, it becomes evident that stem cells hold the key to novel therapeutic approaches. Innovations in this field are not only expected to enhance survival rates but also to improve the quality of life for patients undergoing cancer treatment. The integration of stem cell therapy into oncology promises to revolutionise the way we approach cancer, offering hope where traditional methods may have faltered.

One significant area of focus is the application of stem cells in treating neurodegenerative diseases that often co-occur with cancer. Research indicates that certain stem cell types can repair damaged neural tissues, offering profound implications for patients facing both cancer and neurological disorders. This intersection of oncology and regenerative medicine is paving the way for comprehensive treatment strategies that address multiple facets of patients' health, enhancing overall outcomes and minimising side effects associated with conventional therapies.

Ethical considerations surrounding stem cell research remain pivotal as we advance in this domain. Healthcare professionals and biomedical scientists must navigate the complex moral landscape that accompanies stem cell use, particularly regarding embryonic stem cells. Ongoing dialogue and transparent policies are essential to ensure that research progresses ethically and responsibly, fostering public trust and acceptance of these innovative therapies. The future of oncology will depend on our ability to address these ethical dilemmas while harnessing the potential of stem cells.

As we look towards the future, the potential applications of stem cell therapy in paediatric oncology warrant particular attention. Children diagnosed with cancer often have unique treatment needs, and advances in regenerative medicine can provide tailored solutions that minimise long-term side effects. By focusing on the specific characteristics of paediatric cancers, researchers aim to develop stem cell-based treatments that are not only effective but also safe for young patients, thereby laying the groundwork for a healthier generation.

In conclusion, the future directions in oncology are marked by the promise of stem cell therapy, with its potential to change the landscape of cancer treatment. By embracing innovations in regenerative medicine and addressing ethical considerations, we can move closer to realising the full benefits of these therapies. The collaboration between healthcare professionals, biomedical scientists, and stem cell enthusiasts is crucial for unlocking the transformative power of stem cells in oncology, ultimately leading to improved patient outcomes and a brighter future for cancer care.

The Role of Stem Cells in Diabetes Management

Pathophysiology of Diabetes

Diabetes mellitus is a complex metabolic disorder characterised by chronic hyperglycaemia resulting from defects in insulin secretion, insulin action, or both. The pathophysiology of diabetes is multifaceted, involving intricate interactions between genetic, environmental, and immunological factors. In type 1 diabetes, autoimmune destruction of pancreatic beta cells leads to an absolute deficiency of insulin, while type 2 diabetes is primarily linked to insulin resistance and relative insulin deficiency. Understanding these mechanisms is crucial for developing effective regenerative therapies aimed at restoring normal glucose homeostasis.

The role of the pancreatic islets in diabetes is central to its pathophysiology. In healthy individuals, beta cells within the islets of Langerhans secrete insulin in response to elevated blood glucose levels. However, in diabetes, particularly type 2, these beta cells undergo functional decline and apoptosis, leading to inadequate insulin production. This deficiency, compounded by the liver's unregulated glucose output and peripheral insulin resistance, creates a vicious cycle of hyperglycaemia that can result in severe complications. Stem cell therapy aims to regenerate or replace these dysfunctional beta cells, potentially restoring insulin production.

Moreover, inflammation plays a significant role in the pathophysiology of both types of diabetes. Chronic low-grade inflammation is prevalent in obese individuals, contributing to insulin resistance and beta-cell dysfunction. Pro-inflammatory cytokines can impair insulin signalling pathways, exacerbating the metabolic disturbances seen in diabetes. Investigating how stem cells can modulate the inflammatory response and protect beta cells from immune-mediated destruction presents a promising avenue for therapeutic intervention.

Another critical aspect of diabetes pathophysiology is the impact of glucotoxicity and lipotoxicity on beta-cell health. Prolonged exposure to high glucose and fatty acid levels can lead to beta-cell dysfunction and death, further complicating the disease's management. Strategies that utilise stem cells may help counteract these toxic effects, either by enhancing beta-cell regeneration or by improving the overall metabolic environment. Advances in the understanding of cellular reprogramming and stem cell differentiation are paving the way for innovative treatments.

Finally, the exploration of stem cell therapy's role in diabetes management highlights the need for ethical considerations and public acceptance. As regenerative medicine continues to advance, it is essential for healthcare professionals and researchers to address the concerns surrounding stem cell use, ensuring that therapies are safe, effective, and widely accepted. The promise of stem cell therapy in diabetes management not only holds potential for improving patient outcomes but also enhances our understanding of the underlying pathophysiological mechanisms that govern this challenging disease.

Stem Cell Approaches to Insulin Production

The advent of stem cell technology has opened new avenues in the quest for effective insulin production, particularly for individuals suffering from diabetes. Stem cells, with their unique ability to differentiate into various cell types, hold the potential to generate insulin-producing beta cells. This is particularly significant given the global rise in diabetes prevalence, which has necessitated innovative approaches to manage the condition more effectively and sustainably.

Recent advancements in regenerative medicine have demonstrated that pluripotent stem cells can be coaxed into becoming functional pancreatic beta cells. By understanding the precise cellular cues and environmental factors that govern this differentiation process, researchers are making strides toward developing a reliable source of insulin-producing cells. This breakthrough not only promises to alleviate the reliance on external insulin therapy but also aims to restore normal glucose homeostasis in patients.

Ethical considerations surrounding stem cell research remain a pertinent topic, particularly in the context of sourcing embryonic stem cells. However, the emergence of induced pluripotent stem cells (iPSCs) has provided an ethical alternative. iPSCs are derived from adult somatic cells, thus circumventing many ethical issues while still offering the flexibility of pluripotency. This shift in focus towards iPSCs has significant implications for the future of diabetes management, as it aligns with the growing demand for ethically responsible research.

Moreover, the application of stem cell therapy extends beyond mere insulin production. Researchers are exploring the potential of stem cells to modulate the immune response in autoimmune forms of diabetes, such as Type 1 diabetes. By harnessing the regenerative capabilities of stem cells, it may be possible not only to replace lost beta cells but also to promote an environment that prevents further autoimmune destruction, thereby offering a dual approach to treatment.

As these advancements progress, there is a growing need for increased public awareness and acceptance of stem cell therapies. Education and transparency regarding the potential benefits and ethical considerations of stem cell research are crucial in fostering trust within the community. As healthcare professionals, it is imperative to advocate for informed discussions surrounding the promise of stem cell approaches in insulin production, paving the way for transformative treatments in diabetes management.

Clinical Trials and Outcomes

Clinical trials represent a pivotal phase in the advancement of stem cell therapy, serving as the bridge between laboratory research and clinical application. These trials are meticulously designed to evaluate the safety and efficacy of stem cell interventions across various medical conditions. For healthcare professionals and biomedical scientists, understanding the nuances of clinical trials is essential for translating scientific innovations into therapeutic realities. The outcomes of these trials not only inform clinical practices but also shape the future landscape of regenerative medicine.

The promise of stem cell therapy is being actively explored in numerous clinical trials targeting neurodegenerative diseases. Conditions such as Parkinson's disease and amyotrophic lateral sclerosis (ALS) are at the forefront of this research. Outcomes from these trials are closely monitored to assess improvements in patient mobility, cognitive function, and overall quality of life. Each success or setback provides invaluable data that influences future studies and therapeutic strategies, highlighting the dynamic nature of clinical research in this field.

Ethical considerations play a critical role in the design and execution of clinical trials involving stem cells. Healthcare professionals must navigate complex ethical landscapes, ensuring that patient rights are upheld while advancing scientific knowledge. Informed consent, the use of embryonic versus adult stem cells, and the potential for exploitation are just a few of the ethical dilemmas faced. The integrity of clinical trials depends on transparent practices that respect both the scientific community and the patients involved.

Recent advancements in stem cell therapy are also being trialled for cardiovascular disorders. Research indicates that stem cells may facilitate the regeneration of damaged heart tissue, offering new hope for patients suffering from heart attacks or heart failure. Clinical outcomes from these trials are critical in establishing protocols for safe application in clinical settings. As results emerge, they pave the way for broader acceptance and integration of stem cell therapies into standard treatment regimens for cardiovascular health.

The public perception and acceptance of stem cell therapies are significantly influenced by the outcomes of clinical trials. Positive results can lead to increased funding and support for research, while negative outcomes may stifle progress. It is imperative for healthcare professionals to communicate these findings effectively to the public, fostering a well-informed dialogue about the potential and limitations of stem cell therapies. The future of regenerative medicine hinges not only on scientific breakthroughs but also on the collaborative engagement of the community in understanding and embracing these innovations.

Public Perception and Acceptance of Stem Cell Therapies

Influences on Public Attitudes

Public attitudes towards stem cell therapy are significantly influenced by various factors, including cultural beliefs, media representation, and personal experiences. Healthcare professionals and biomedical scientists play a crucial role in shaping these attitudes through their interactions with patients and the broader community. Education about the potential benefits and risks associated with stem cell treatments can help mitigate misconceptions and foster a more informed public perspective.

Media portrayals of stem cell research can either enhance or hinder public acceptance. Positive coverage highlighting successful treatments and breakthroughs can generate enthusiasm and support, while sensationalised reports focusing on ethical dilemmas or failures may provoke fear and scepticism. It is essential for health professionals to engage with the media constructively, providing accurate information and countering misinformation that can skew public perception.

Cultural and religious beliefs also shape how different communities view stem cell therapy. In some cultures, the idea of manipulating human cells can be seen as controversial, leading to resistance against therapies that rely on embryonic stem cells. Understanding these cultural sensitivities is vital for healthcare providers to approach discussions about stem cell therapies with respect and empathy, ensuring that they address concerns while promoting the potential benefits of regenerative medicine.

Personal experiences with illness and treatment can greatly influence individual attitudes towards stem cell therapies. Patients who have witnessed the positive impacts of such treatments on themselves or loved ones are often more open to exploring these options. Conversely, those who have faced negative outcomes may remain sceptical. Healthcare professionals must be aware of these narratives and incorporate them into their discussions, highlighting evidence-based successes while acknowledging the risks involved.

Finally, ethical considerations remain at the forefront of public discussions about stem cell research. Concerns regarding consent, the sourcing of stem cells, and potential exploitation must be addressed transparently to build trust within the community. Engaging stakeholders in ethical discourse can lead to a more nuanced understanding of the implications of stem cell therapies, ultimately fostering a more supportive environment for innovation in regenerative medicine.

Media Representation and Misinformation

Media representation plays a crucial role in shaping public understanding and perception of stem cell therapy. As advancements in regenerative medicine continue to emerge, the narratives presented by the media can either foster enthusiasm or instil fear among the general public and healthcare professionals alike. It is essential to critically analyse how these representations influence the acceptance and implementation of stem cell therapies in various medical fields, including neurodegenerative diseases, orthopaedics, and oncology.

Misinformation is rampant in discussions surrounding stem cell therapies, often exacerbated by sensationalist headlines and oversimplified explanations. The complexities of stem cell research and its ethical considerations are frequently overlooked, leading to misconceptions that hinder informed decision-making. Health care professionals must navigate this landscape carefully, ensuring that they communicate evidence-based information to patients and the public, thereby countering the pervasive myths associated with stem cell treatments.

Moreover, public perception is significantly impacted by the portrayal of stem cell therapies in popular media. While some coverage highlights the transformative potential of regenerative medicine, others focus on unverified claims and anecdotal successes that can mislead audiences. It is vital for biomedical scientists and health care practitioners to engage with media outlets, providing accurate insights that can help demystify the science behind stem cells and convey the true promise of these therapies.

The implications of misinformation extend beyond public understanding; they can also affect funding and research priorities within the biomedical community. As health care professionals advocate for stem cell research, they must confront the challenge of ensuring that the discourse surrounding these therapies is rooted in scientific credibility. This involves collaboration with journalists and policymakers to promote a balanced representation of stem cell advancements and their potential applications in treating various conditions, including autoimmune diseases and diabetes.

In conclusion, addressing media representation and misinformation is a critical component of the ongoing dialogue about stem cell therapy. By fostering a more accurate portrayal of regenerative medicine, health care professionals can help cultivate a more informed public and encourage ethical research practices. This, in turn, may facilitate greater acceptance and integration of stem cell therapies into mainstream medical practice, ultimately enhancing patient outcomes across diverse medical disciplines.

Strategies for Enhancing Public Understanding

Enhancing public understanding of stem cell therapy is crucial for its acceptance and successful implementation in clinical practice. Health care professionals and biomedical scientists must take the lead in demystifying the complex science behind stem cells, ensuring that accurate and accessible information is available to the public. This involves engaging with community outreach initiatives, where experts can explain the potential benefits and limitations of stem cell therapies in layman's terms, fostering a more informed discussion around regenerative medicine innovations.

Educational programmes targeting both the general public and specific interest groups, such as patients with neurodegenerative diseases or autoimmune disorders, can be instrumental in building understanding. These programmes should focus on the latest advancements in stem cell therapy and their applicability, such as treating conditions like diabetes or certain cancers. By tailoring information to the audience's needs, health care professionals can help dispel myths and clarify the ethical considerations involved in stem cell research, thereby enhancing trust and acceptance of these treatments.

Utilising digital platforms is another effective strategy for enhancing public understanding. Webinars, online courses, and social media campaigns can reach a wider audience, providing interactive and engaging content about the role of stem cells in various medical fields. These platforms can also facilitate discussions between experts and enthusiasts, creating a community of informed individuals who are passionate about regenerative medicine. The use of visual aids, such as infographics and videos, can further simplify complex concepts, making the information more digestible for the public.

Collaboration with patient advocacy groups is essential in tailoring communication strategies to address specific concerns and questions from the public. These groups can serve as a bridge between the scientific community and patients, ensuring that the information disseminated resonates with their experiences and needs. By actively involving patients in discussions about stem cell therapies, health care professionals can enhance transparency and build a supportive environment where patients feel empowered to make informed decisions regarding their treatment options.

Finally, continuous feedback from the community should be encouraged to refine strategies and improve understanding over time. Surveys, focus groups, and public forums can provide valuable insights into the public's perceptions and misconceptions about stem cell therapy. This iterative process not only helps in improving educational efforts but also fosters a sense of collaboration between scientists and the community, promoting a shared vision of advancing regenerative medicine for the benefit of society.

Pause for Thought

- Stem cells represent a paradigm shift in the field of medicine which offers a tremendous opportunity in the fields of tissue regeneration and repair of damaged tissues.

- The promise in regenerative medicine is marked by significant advancement in stem cell research, particularly in the treatment of neurodegenerative diseases. Conditions such as Alzheimer's and Parkinson's disease are explored for therapeutic that utilize stem cells to restore lost functions and improve patient outcomes. Knowledge in this area can help to develop targeted therapies that could potentially alter the course of these debilitating diseases.

- In orthopaedic treatments, stem cells are increasingly being used to promote healing and regeneration of musculoskeletal tissues. From cartilage repair to bone regeneration the application of stem cells offers promising outcomes that could enhance recovery times and improve the quality of life for patients suffering from injuries or degenerative conditions.

- Emerging research indicate that stem cell therapy may offer new avenues for treating autoimmune diseases such as lupus and rheumatoid arthritis as well as providing potential treatments for childhood disorders.

- The promise of regeneration through stem cells is immense, yet it is accompanied by the responsibility to ensure that such therapies are accessible, safe and effective.

- Bioprinting has emerged as a revolutionary tool in regenerative medicine by offering innovative solutions for tissue engineering and organ regeneration. It involves the layer-by-layer deposition of bioinks which are composed of living cells and biomaterials to create complex three-dimensional structures that mimic the natural architecture of tissues. This allows for the fabrication of tissues which can potentially replace damaged or diseased organs.

- Bioprinting can address ethical concerns associated with stem cell research. The ability to create tissues from induced pluripotential stem cells allows for the development of patient -specific models without the ethical dilemmas that are associated with the use of embryonic stem cells, whilst simultaneously paving the way for personalised medicine approaches in regenerative therapies.

- Cardiac stem cells play a pivotal role in the homeostasis and repair of the heart. These cells are unique in their ability to regenerate cardiac tissue following injury such as a myocardial infarction.

- Ethical considerations surrounding cardiac stem cell research continue to generate much debate. While the promise of regenerative therapies is immense, concerns related to the source of stem cells, potential for tumour formation and long-term effects of therapy must be addressed.

- The underlying mechanism for autoimmune is crucial for health care professionals and biomedical scientist as it informs both diagnosis and treatment strategies. The role of stem cells here has emerged as a promising area of research and indicates potential treatments for regeneration and healing.

Take Home Nuggets

- Stem cell therapy may find a useful home in the management of autoimmune disease because of its ability to modulate immune response and repair damaged tissues. By harnessing the regenerative potential of stem cells, researchers can explore innovative treatments that could significantly improve the quality of life for patients suffering from autoimmune disease.

- Ethical considerations play a critical role in the advancement of stem cell therapies for autoimmune disease. The source of stem cells, whether derived from embryos or adult tissue, raises important questions about consent, moral implications and public acceptance. It is essential that these concerns are addressed to foster trust and transparency within the medical community and among patients. Ethical frameworks must evolve alongside scientific progress to guide responsible practices.

- Stem cells can modulate immune response thus making them a focal point in regenerative medicine. These cells can differentiate into various tissue types and modulate the immune environment by secreting various cytokines and growth factors. By doing so, they can promote tissue repair and reduce inflammation offering a promising avenue for treating autoimmune disease and other dysfunctional immune responses.

- The interaction between stem cells and the immune system is complex and multifaceted. Stem cells can exert immunosuppressive effects which can be beneficial in preventing tissue rejection during transplantation or in managing autoimmune disease. Several mechanisms may be involved among which are alteration of dendritic cell maturation and the introduction of regulatory T-cells which are involved in maintaining immune tolerance.

- Studies indicate that stem cells can influence the activity of microglia, the resident immune cells of the CNS, thereby creating a more favourable environment for neuronal survival and regeneration. This dual role gives therapeutic promise for stem cell use in conditions such as multiple sclerosis and Alzheimer's

- With paediatric patients, the application of stem cell therapy presents a unique set of considerations that differ significantly from those encountered in adults. The developmental stage of children means that their physiological responses to treatment can vary widely as the potential for growth and development during treatment introduces complexities that require ongoing monitoring and adjustment to therapy as the child matures.

- The long-term implications of stem therapy in remain largely unexplored. Given that children are still undergoing development, there is a need for research into the long-term effects of stem cell interventions on growth, cognitive development and health.

- A significant application of stem cell therapy for genetic disorders is in inherited disorders characterised by specific genetic mutations that hinder normal cellular function. It is possible to correct these mutations at a cellular level using gene editing techniques in combination with stem cell therapy.

- Stem cells are also able to combat cancer through a multifaceted and complex mechanism which reflects the intricate biology of both stem cells and tumours. Stem cell's ability to differentiate into various cell types provides a versatile approach to replace damaged tissues and potentially eliminate cancerous cells. The capacity allows for targeted therapy where stem cells can be engineered to deliver cytotoxic agents directly to tumours minimising damage to surrounding healthy tissue. Additionally, immunomodulatory properties of stem cells can enhance the body's natural response to cancer, promoting an environment that is less conducive to tumour growth.

- One significant mechanism involves the secretion of bioactive molecules by stem cells. These molecules can induce apoptosis in cancer cells, inhibit tumour growth and modulate the immune response. This helps in targeting cancer cells more effectively and fosters a systemic immune response against malignancy.

Chapter 5
Introduction to Stem Cell Research and Regulations

Overview of Stem Cell Research

Stem cell research has emerged as a pivotal area in modern biomedical science, offering promising avenues for regenerative medicine and therapeutic interventions. The potential of stem cells to differentiate into various cell types provides unprecedented opportunities for treating diseases such as Parkinson's, diabetes, and spinal cord injuries. However, this promise is accompanied by complex ethical considerations that necessitate careful regulation and oversight to ensure responsible research practices. As such, stem cell research stands at the intersection of scientific innovation and moral inquiry, demanding a nuanced understanding of both scientific potential and ethical implications.

Attempts at establishing stem cell research regulations have varied widely across different countries, reflecting diverse cultural, ethical, and political landscapes. In some regions, stringent regulations limit research to certain types of stem cells, while others adopt a more permissive approach, encouraging innovation and exploration. This comparative analysis highlights the significant influence of national values on the regulatory framework, which in turn affects the pace and direction of stem cell research. Understanding these variations is crucial for researchers and ethicists alike, as they navigate the global landscape of stem cell science.

Public opinion plays a critical role in shaping the policies surrounding stem cell research regulations. The discourse surrounding stem cell research often polarises communities, with public sentiments influencing regulatory decisions and funding allocations. Education and engagement with the public are essential in demystifying stem cell research and addressing ethical concerns. Consequently, the relationship between public opinion and regulatory frameworks can create a dynamic interplay that affects the advancement of stem cell technologies and their applications in healthcare.

Governmental bodies are instrumental in shaping the legislation governing stem cell research, ensuring that ethical standards are upheld while fostering innovation. Their role encompasses not only the creation of laws but also the establishment of funding mechanisms that support research initiatives. The intersection of government policy and scientific inquiry requires continuous dialogue between regulatory agencies and the scientific community to adapt to new discoveries and societal needs. This collaborative approach is vital for developing a regulatory environment that both supports research and protects patient rights.

Finally, the influence of pharmaceutical companies on stem cell research regulations cannot be overlooked. As key players in the biomedical field, these companies often advocate for policies that promote their interests while navigating complex ethical landscapes. Innovations in stem cell technology present regulatory challenges that must be addressed to ensure compliance and uphold patient safety. The historical evolution of stem cell research regulations provides insights into the ongoing challenges faced by researchers and regulators, highlighting the need for adaptive frameworks that can accommodate rapidly advancing scientific frontiers.

Importance of Ethical Regulations

Ethical regulations play a crucial role in the realm of stem cell research, serving as a framework that guides scientists and healthcare professionals in their work. These regulations are designed to protect human dignity, ensure safety, and foster public trust in scientific endeavours. Without such ethical oversight, the potential for exploitation of vulnerable populations and the misuse of research findings could increase significantly. The importance of ethical regulations is underscored by the complex moral questions that surround stem cell research, necessitating a careful balance between scientific advancement and ethical responsibility.

One of the primary functions of ethical regulations is to delineate the boundaries of acceptable research practices. By establishing clear guidelines, these regulations help to mitigate risks associated with stem cell research, such as the procurement of stem cells from questionable sources or the potential for commercial exploitation. Health care personnel and researchers are therefore provided with a structured environment within which they can innovate while remaining accountable for their actions. This accountability not only protects participants but also enhances the integrity of the scientific community.

Comparative analysis of international stem cell research laws reveals significant variations in ethical standards and regulatory frameworks across different countries. Some nations have adopted permissive approaches, while others maintain stringent restrictions. This disparity highlights the influence of cultural, political, and social factors on ethical regulations. Understanding these differences is vital for researchers operating in a global context, as compliance with local laws is essential for ethical research conduct and international collaboration.

Public opinion also plays a significant role in shaping stem cell research regulations. As societal values evolve, so too do the expectations surround scientific research. Engaging with the public and understanding their concerns can lead to more informed and robust regulatory policies. This dynamic relationship between public sentiment and ethical regulations is crucial for fostering an environment where innovation can thrive without compromising ethical standards.

Finally, the role of governmental bodies and pharmaceutical companies in the regulatory landscape cannot be overstated. These entities often drive the formulation of ethical regulations, influencing funding opportunities and research priorities. As such, it is essential for stakeholders in the stem cell research community to advocate for transparency and accountability in the regulatory process. Innovations in stem cell technology present new regulatory challenges that necessitate ongoing dialogue among ethicists, researchers, and policymakers to ensure that ethical considerations remain at the forefront of scientific progress.

Goals and Objectives

The primary goal of, "Ethics at the Crossroads: The Moral Landscape of Stem Cell Research Regulations," is to provide a comprehensive exploration of the ethical, legal, and social implications surrounding stem cell research. This exploration is particularly pertinent given the rapid advancements in stem cell technology and the accompanying complexities in regulatory frameworks. The book aims to equip health care personnel, ethicists, and biomedical researchers with a nuanced understanding of the existing regulations and the varied ethical considerations that inform them. By addressing these aspects, the book seeks to promote informed dialogue among stakeholders involved in stem cell research and its governance.

Additionally, we intend to present a comparative analysis of international stem cell research laws, highlighting the differences and similarities across various jurisdictions. Understanding these regulatory landscapes is crucial for researchers who operate in a global context, as they must navigate a patchwork of laws and ethical norms. This analysis not only aids in compliance but also fosters collaboration among international research communities. By elucidating these legal frameworks, the book aspires to encourage harmonisation of regulations that can facilitate responsible research while respecting diverse ethical perspectives.

Another significant objective is to examine the impact of public opinion on stem cell regulation policies. Public perception plays a vital role in shaping legislative actions and funding decisions related to stem cell research. By analysing how societal beliefs influence regulatory environments, we aim to inform stakeholders about the importance of engaging with the public and addressing their concerns.

This engagement is essential for developing policies that are not only scientifically sound but also ethically acceptable to society at large.

Moreover, we will explore the influence of pharmaceutical companies on stem cell research regulations. The intersection of commercial interests and ethical considerations raises critical questions about the integrity of research and the prioritisation of patient rights. By scrutinising the role of the pharmaceutical industry, we seek to highlight potential conflicts of interest and the necessity for robust oversight to ensure that ethical standards are upheld in stem cell research initiatives.

Lastly, we will delve into the historical evolution of stem cell research regulations, providing context for current practices and challenges. Understanding the historical backdrop allows stakeholders to appreciate the complexities that have shaped today's regulatory frameworks. By reflecting on past developments, we aim to inspire future innovations in stem cell technology while ensuring that ethical governance remains at the forefront of research agendas. This holistic approach will ultimately contribute to a more responsible and ethically sound landscape for stem cell research.

Attempts at Stem Cell Research Regulations

Historical Context of Regulation Efforts

The historical context of regulation efforts in stem cell research reveals a complex interplay between scientific innovation and ethical considerations. In the early stages, the potential of stem cells was recognised, sparking enthusiasm within the biomedical community. However, this excitement was tempered by ethical concerns surrounding the source of stem cells, particularly those derived from human embryos. The need for regulatory frameworks became apparent as researchers sought to navigate these moral dilemmas while pursuing scientific advancements.

As stem cell research progressed, various attempts were made to establish guidelines that would govern its practice. In many countries, these regulations emerged in response to public outcry and ethical debates, reflecting societal values and fears. For instance, the United States witnessed a divided landscape, where federal funding for embryonic stem cell research was heavily restricted, prompting states to create more permissive environments. This patchwork of regulations highlighted the necessity for coherent policies that could balance innovation with ethical accountability.

Comparative analysis of international stem cell research laws reveals significant disparities in regulatory approaches. Some nations, like the UK, have developed robust frameworks that facilitate research while imposing strict ethical standards, whereas others maintain more lenient regulations. This divergence often results from cultural attitudes towards science and ethics, with public opinion playing a critical role in shaping legislation. Understanding these differences is essential for researchers and policymakers alike, as it informs the global dialogue on stem cell research ethics and regulation.

The influence of public opinion on stem cell regulation policies cannot be overstated. Advocacy groups, patient organisations, and the media have all contributed to shaping perceptions about the benefits and risks associated with stem cell research. As a result, regulatory bodies are often compelled to consider public sentiments when drafting legislation. This dynamic underscore the importance of transparency and engagement in the regulatory process, ensuring that the voices of all stakeholders are heard and considered.

Lastly, the evolving landscape of stem cell technologies presents new regulatory challenges that must be addressed. Innovations in this field are outpacing existing regulatory frameworks, creating potential gaps in oversight. Governmental bodies, alongside pharmaceutical companies, play a crucial role in adapting to these changes by developing comprehensive regulatory strategies that protect patient rights while promoting scientific advancement. The historical evolution of these regulations underscores the need for ongoing dialogue and adaptation as the field of stem cell research continues to grow and evolve.

Key Legislation and Policy Milestones

The landscape of stem cell research has been profoundly shaped by key legislation and policy milestones that have emerged over the past few decades. These legislative efforts often reflect a balancing act between scientific innovation and ethical considerations. The passage of the National Institutes of Health (NIH) guidelines in the United States in 2000 marked a significant step towards formal regulation, establishing parameters for federal funding of embryonic stem cell research. This was a pivotal moment that prompted discussions surrounding the moral implications of using human embryos, ultimately influencing public discourse and legislative frameworks across the globe.

Internationally, the approaches to stem cell research legislation vary widely, illustrating differing ethical perspectives and cultural attitudes. For instance, countries like Sweden and the United Kingdom have adopted more permissive regulations, allowing for extensive research and clinical applications, while others, such as Germany, enforce strict limitations. This comparative analysis reveals how public opinion, influenced by cultural and religious factors, plays a crucial role in shaping national policies. The divergent paths taken by these nations highlight the importance of understanding local contexts when discussing global stem cell research legislation.

The influence of governmental bodies cannot be understated in the evolution of stem cell regulations. Agencies such as the Food and Drug Administration (FDA) in the United States and the European Medicines Agency (EMA) in Europe have established rigorous frameworks for clinical trials involving stem cells, ensuring patient safety and ethical compliance. These regulatory bodies frequently engage with stakeholders, including researchers and ethicists, to refine policies that govern clinical applications. Their role is essential in navigating the complexities of scientific advancement while maintaining public trust in medical research.

Pharmaceutical companies also wield significant influence over stem cell research regulations, often lobbying for favourable policies that can accelerate the development of new therapies. Their investment in stem cell technologies can drive innovation, but it also raises ethical concerns regarding profit motives versus patient welfare. As these companies navigate the regulatory landscape, the potential for conflicts of interest necessitates robust oversight to ensure that ethical standards are upheld in research and clinical applications.

As stem cell technologies continue to evolve, so too do the regulatory challenges associated with them. Innovations such as induced pluripotent stem cells (iPSCs) present unique ethical and compliance considerations that existing frameworks may not adequately address. The historical evolution of stem cell research regulations serves as a backdrop for understanding these challenges, as policymakers strive to keep pace with rapid advancements. Ongoing dialogue among healthcare personnel, ethicists, and regulatory bodies will be crucial in shaping a future where stem cell research can thrive ethically and responsibly.

Challenges in Implementing Regulations

The implementation of regulations surrounding stem cell research presents numerous challenges that can impede progress in this vital field. One of the primary obstacles lies in the complexity and variability of existing laws across different jurisdictions. This inconsistency creates confusion among researchers and healthcare personnel, who may struggle to navigate the regulatory landscape. As a result, the potential for innovative therapies can be stifled, as researchers may hesitate to pursue projects that could be deemed non-compliant with local regulations.

Ethical considerations also play a significant role in the challenges faced when implementing stem cell research regulations. The moral implications of using human embryonic stem cells, for instance, raise complex questions that are often subject to intense debate. This discourse can lead to polarised views within the scientific community and among the public, complicating efforts to establish universally accepted regulatory frameworks. As ethicists grapple with these dilemmas, the resulting guidelines may be slow to evolve, hindering timely advancements in research.

Public opinion is another critical factor influencing the regulatory landscape of stem cell research. As societal values shift, regulations must adapt to reflect these changes, which can be a daunting task for governmental bodies. The influence of advocacy groups and public sentiment can lead to increased pressure on policymakers to enact stricter regulations, often in response to moral concerns. This dynamic can create a delicate balancing act, as regulators must consider both ethical implications and the need to promote scientific advancement.

Moreover, the financial aspect of stem cell research cannot be overlooked when discussing regulatory challenges. Funding for research is frequently contingent upon compliance with specific regulations, which can vary significantly between countries. This situation can lead to disparities in research capabilities, where nations with more flexible regulatory environments may attract greater investment and talent. Consequently, researchers may find themselves at a disadvantage if they operate in a more restrictive regulatory landscape, ultimately affecting the overall progress of stem cell research.

Lastly, the role of pharmaceutical companies in shaping stem cell research regulations adds another layer of complexity. These companies often have substantial resources and lobbying power, which can influence the development of regulations in ways that may not always align with ethical considerations. As they seek to protect their interests, the potential for conflicts of interest arises, further complicating the regulatory environment. It is essential for oversight committees to remain vigilant and ensure that the primary focus of regulations is on patient rights and the advancement of ethical research practices.

Ethical Considerations in Stem Cell Research Regulations

Moral Status of Stem Cells

The moral status of stem cells is a pivotal topic in the realm of biomedical ethics, particularly in the context of stem cell research regulations. Central to this discourse is the question of when life begins and the ethical implications of manipulating cellular materials that have the potential to develop into human beings. Various ethical frameworks, including utilitarianism, deontology, and virtue ethics, provide different perspectives on the moral consideration owed to stem cells, complicating the regulatory landscape surrounding their use in research and therapy.

Different countries approach the moral status of stem cells in varied ways, influenced by cultural, religious, and philosophical beliefs. For instance, some jurisdictions allow the use of embryonic stem cells under stringent conditions, while others impose strict bans due to the belief that human life begins at conception. This comparative analysis highlights the necessity for harmonised international regulations that respect diverse moral viewpoints while promoting scientific advancement and public health.

Public opinion plays a significant role in shaping stem cell research regulations, often swaying governmental policies and funding decisions. Surveys indicate that public sentiment can be influenced by awareness and understanding of the potential benefits of stem cell therapies, as well as ethical concerns surrounding their derivation. Consequently, policymakers must navigate the delicate balance between promoting scientific innovation and addressing public apprehensions about the moral implications of stem cell research.

The involvement of governmental bodies is crucial in establishing clear regulatory frameworks for stem cell research. These bodies must consider not only the ethical dimensions but also the scientific validity and safety of stem cell applications. Regulatory compliance is essential for fostering a research environment where patient rights are protected and where innovations can be pursued responsibly, ensuring that advancements in stem cell technology do not outpace ethical considerations.

Lastly, pharmaceutical companies exert considerable influence on stem cell research regulations, often driven by the potential for profit from novel therapies. This relationship can lead to ethical dilemmas, particularly if profit motives overshadow patient welfare and ethical standards. It is essential for regulatory bodies to remain vigilant against such influences, ensuring that ethical governance prevails in the pursuit of scientific and medical breakthroughs in stem cell research.

Informed Consent and Autonomy

Informed consent is a fundamental ethical principle in healthcare and biomedical research, underscoring the importance of autonomy for patients and research participants. When it comes to stem cell research, the complexities surrounding informed consent become particularly pronounced due to the nature of stem cells and the potential implications for individuals and society. Researchers and healthcare professionals must ensure that participants are fully aware of the risks, benefits, and alternatives associated with stem cell procedures, thereby empowering them to make informed decisions about their involvement.

The ethical considerations of autonomy in stem cell research are amplified by the diverse cultural, legal, and social perspectives that exist globally. In some jurisdictions, the regulatory frameworks have been designed to prioritise patient autonomy, while in others, the approach may focus more on collective societal benefits. This comparative analysis highlights the necessity for researchers and ethics committees to navigate these varying standards, ensuring that consent processes are not only compliant with local laws but also respect the rights and values of individuals.

Public opinion plays a critical role in shaping stem cell research regulations, as it can influence policy decisions made by governmental bodies. When the public is informed and engaged in discussions about stem cell research, it can lead to more robust regulations that reflect societal values and ethical considerations. Consequently, researchers must be adept at communicating their work and the implications of stem cell research to the public, fostering an environment where informed consent is valued and upheld.

Additionally, the influence of pharmaceutical companies on stem cell research regulations cannot be overlooked. These entities often have significant resources that can impact the regulatory landscape, leading to potential conflicts of interest. It is essential for ethics committees and regulatory bodies to remain vigilant and ensure that patient rights are not compromised in the pursuit of innovation and profit, thereby maintaining the integrity of the informed consent process.

In conclusion, the historical evolution of stem cell research regulations reveals a continual balancing act between scientific advancement and ethical considerations surrounding informed consent and autonomy. As stem cell technologies continue to innovate, regulatory frameworks must adapt to address the challenges that arise while prioritising the rights and autonomy of individuals involved. By fostering a culture of informed consent, stakeholders can ensure that stem cell research progresses in a manner that is ethically sound and respects the dignity of all participants.

Equity and Access to Treatments

Equity in access to treatments derived from stem cell research is a pressing issue that demands thorough consideration within the framework of ethical regulations. As advancements in stem cell technology promise revolutionary therapies, disparities in access based on socioeconomic status, geographic location, and healthcare infrastructure become increasingly evident. It is essential for regulatory bodies to ensure that ethical principles guide the distribution of these treatments, promoting fairness and justice in healthcare access for all patients.

The regulatory landscape surrounding stem cell therapies varies significantly across countries, reflecting differences in public opinion, cultural attitudes, and governmental policies. In some regions, stringent regulations may limit access to potentially life-saving treatments, while in others, a more permissive approach may lead to exploitation and inequity. A comparative analysis of international laws reveals the need for harmonisation of regulations that prioritise both innovation and equitable access, ensuring that all patients benefit from scientific advances in stem cell research.

Public opinion plays a critical role in shaping stem cell research regulations. Societal attitudes towards stem cell treatments influence legislative decisions and funding allocations, impacting the availability of these therapies. Engaging with the public through education and dialogue is vital for fostering an informed consensus that balances ethical considerations with the demand for access to innovative treatments, ultimately guiding policymakers in their decisions.

The influence of pharmaceutical companies on stem cell research regulations cannot be underestimated. These entities often have significant power in shaping the regulatory environment through lobbying and funding strategies. While their involvement can drive innovation and expedite development, it also raises concerns about profit-driven motives overshadowing patient rights and equitable access. Regulatory frameworks must therefore be designed to mitigate undue influence and ensure that the focus remains on patient welfare and ethical governance.

As the field of stem cell research continues to evolve, the challenges surrounding equity and access to treatments will persist. Innovations in technology must be accompanied by robust regulatory frameworks that prioritise the rights of patients and the ethical distribution of therapies. By addressing these issues head-on, stakeholders, including healthcare personnel, ethicists, and researchers, can work together to ensure that the benefits of stem cell research are accessible to all, paving the way for a more equitable future in healthcare.

Comparative Analysis of International Stem Cell Research Laws

Overview of Global Regulatory Approaches

The landscape of stem cell research regulations varies significantly across the globe, with countries adopting diverse approaches influenced by cultural, ethical, and political factors. In the United States, for instance, the regulatory framework is largely shaped by the National Institutes of Health (NIH) and the Food and Drug Administration (FDA), which govern funding allocations and clinical trials respectively. This dual oversight creates a complex environment where ethical considerations must balance against scientific advancement and public opinion, often leading to contentious debates about the moral implications of stem cell research.

Conversely, European countries generally adopt a more precautionary stance toward stem cell research. The European Union has established rigorous guidelines that prioritise ethical considerations, often limiting the use of embryonic stem cells. Countries like Germany and Italy have particularly stringent regulations, reflecting historical sensitivities surrounding bioethics. This regulatory caution can impact the speed of innovation in these countries, as researchers navigate a landscape that is often more restrictive than in the US.

In Asia, the regulatory approaches to stem cell research are equally varied, with countries like Japan and South Korea showing a more permissive attitude. Japan, for instance, has made significant investments in stem cell technology, driven by a government that actively supports research while ensuring ethical oversight. South Korea has established a robust regulatory framework that encourages innovation, balancing the need for ethical governance with the desire to remain competitive in the global biomedical research arena.

Public opinion plays a crucial role in shaping the regulatory landscape of stem cell research. Societal attitudes towards stem cell research can influence legislative actions and funding decisions. In regions where public support is strong, regulations tend to be more favourable towards research initiatives. Conversely, in areas where ethical concerns dominate public discourse, regulations may become more restrictive. This dynamic interplay between public opinion and regulatory frameworks highlights the necessity for ongoing dialogue between scientists, ethicists, and the public.

Finally, the influence of pharmaceutical companies cannot be overlooked in the context of stem cell research regulations. These corporations often advocate for more flexible regulations that facilitate clinical trials and expedite the development of new therapies. However, this influence raises ethical concerns regarding the prioritisation of profit over patient rights and the potential for conflicts of interest. As innovations in stem cell technology continue to evolve, so too must the regulatory frameworks that govern them, ensuring that they remain responsive to both scientific advancements and ethical imperatives.

Case Studies: United States, United Kingdom, and Japan

In the United States, stem cell research regulations have evolved significantly over the past two decades. The landscape is shaped by a combination of federal and state laws, with a notable influence from public opinion and advocacy groups. The National Institutes of Health (NIH) plays a central role in overseeing funding and guidelines, yet the patchwork of state regulations can lead to inconsistencies in research practices across the nation. Ethical considerations, particularly regarding embryonic stem cells, remain contentious issues that frequently spark public debate and affect legislative outcomes.

In contrast, the United Kingdom has established a more cohesive regulatory framework for stem cell research. Governed by the Human Fertilisation and Embryology Authority (HFEA), the UK's approach prioritises ethical oversight while promoting scientific advancement. The regulatory body ensures that all research complies with strict ethical guidelines, reflecting the public's cautious support for stem cell research. This balance between innovation and ethical responsibility is evident in the UK's commitment to transparency and public engagement in the decision-making processes around stem cell research.

Japan presents a unique case, having historically maintained a more conservative stance on stem cell research. However, recent advancements and a growing recognition of the potential benefits have prompted a shift in regulatory attitudes. The Japanese government has introduced new policies aimed at fostering research while addressing ethical concerns. The regulatory framework is evolving, with an emphasis on patient rights and safety, while navigating the complexities of public opinion and cultural attitudes towards stem cell use.

Comparative analysis of these three countries reveals distinct approaches to stem cell research regulations, influenced by cultural, ethical, and political factors. The United States showcases a fragmented system where state-level variations can complicate uniformity, while the UK's structured oversight reflects a prioritisation of ethical considerations. Japan, on the other hand, illustrates a transitional phase where historical caution is giving way to a more proactive regulatory environment that encourages innovation while safeguarding ethical standards.

Ultimately, the interplay between governmental bodies, public opinion, and the influence of pharmaceutical companies shapes the regulatory landscape for stem cell research. Each country's case study highlights the importance of balancing ethical considerations with the need for scientific progress. As innovations in stem cell technology continue to emerge, the challenge remains to adapt regulatory frameworks that ensure patient safety and ethical integrity while fostering an environment conducive to research and development in this critical field.

Lessons Learned from International Practices

The landscape of stem cell research is profoundly influenced by international practices that highlight the complexities and ethical considerations inherent in this field. By examining various regulatory frameworks across countries, we can identify lessons that help shape more effective and ethically sound policies. Countries such as the United States, the United Kingdom, and Japan have implemented diverse approaches to stem cell regulations, providing a rich comparative analysis that can inform future developments. Each of these nations has faced unique challenges and public sentiments that have inevitably influenced their legislative processes.

One critical lesson learned from international practices is the importance of engaging with public opinion while formulating regulations. In many instances, public perception has either expedited or hindered the progress of stem cell research legislation. For instance, in the U.S., the polarized views on stem cell research have led to fluctuating funding and regulatory environments. In contrast, countries with more uniform public support have been able to establish clearer and more stable regulatory frameworks that foster innovation while ensuring ethical compliance.

Another key takeaway from global examples is the significant role of governmental bodies in shaping the regulatory landscape. In countries like Canada and Australia, governmental oversight committees have been instrumental in creating robust frameworks that prioritise patient rights and ethical considerations. These committees often provide crucial oversight on clinical trials, ensuring that stem cell research aligns with ethical standards and public expectations. This governance not only safeguards patient rights but also bolsters public trust in the scientific community.

The influence of pharmaceutical companies on stem cell research regulations is another crucial aspect that merits attention. Various nations have witnessed the impact of private sector interests on regulatory policies, which can both drive innovation and raise ethical concerns. Regulatory bodies must navigate these relationships carefully, ensuring that funding and support from private entities do not compromise the integrity of research or undermine patient welfare. Learning from international practices can provide insights into balancing commercial interests with ethical responsibilities.

Finally, the historical evolution of stem cell research regulations reveals a pattern of learning and adaptation. As innovations in stem cell technology emerge, regulatory frameworks must continuously evolve to address new challenges. By reflecting on the successes and failures of international practices, policymakers can develop a more nuanced understanding of how to regulate this rapidly advancing field. Ultimately, the lessons learned from international practices underscore the necessity for a collaborative approach that integrates ethical considerations, public engagement, and sound governance in stem cell research regulations.

Impact of Public Opinion on Stem Cell Regulation Policies

Public Perception and Understanding of Stem Cell Research

The public perception of stem cell research plays a crucial role in shaping the regulatory landscape surrounding this field. Many individuals hold strong opinions influenced by ethical, religious, and personal beliefs, which can significantly impact funding and legislative initiatives. Understanding these perceptions is essential for health care personnel, ethicists, and researchers, as they navigate the complexities of regulatory compliance and public sentiment. Public opinion often reflects broader societal values, making it imperative that stakeholders engage in meaningful dialogue with the community to address concerns and misconceptions about stem cell research.

Historically, various events and breakthroughs in stem cell science have shaped public understanding and acceptance. For instance, the discovery of induced pluripotent stem cells (iPSCs) has provided a new avenue for research that is perceived as more ethically acceptable by some segments of the public. However, misinformation and fear surrounding embryonic stem cells continue to persist, necessitating clear communication from scientists and policymakers. Public education initiatives can help demystify the science, thus fostering a more informed public discourse and potentially influencing regulatory frameworks in a positive direction.

The impact of public opinion on stem cell regulation policies cannot be overstated. Policymakers often respond to public sentiment through legislation that reflects the collective values and concerns of society. This responsiveness can lead to more stringent regulations or, conversely, to a more permissive environment for research, depending on the prevailing attitudes. Engaging with the public through surveys, forums, and educational programmes can provide valuable insights into their concerns, allowing for better alignment of research initiatives with societal expectations.

Moreover, the interplay between pharmaceutical companies and public perception of stem cell research is significant. These companies are often at the forefront of funding and innovation in this field; however, their influence can sometimes lead to scepticism among the public regarding the motivations behind stem cell research. Transparency in funding sources and research goals is crucial to building trust. Both the pharmaceutical industry and researchers must work collaboratively to ensure that the public understands the benefits and risks associated with stem cell therapies, fostering a climate of trust that can enhance regulatory support.

In conclusion, enhancing public understanding of stem cell research and addressing ethical considerations are vital for the advancement of this field. The role of governmental bodies in shaping regulations is heavily influenced by societal attitudes, which are often reflected in public opinion. By prioritising education and open dialogue, stakeholders can work towards a more informed public that supports innovative research while maintaining ethical standards. This collaborative approach will ultimately facilitate the development of effective and responsive regulatory frameworks that govern stem cell research.

The Role of Advocacy Groups

Advocacy groups play a pivotal role in shaping the landscape of stem cell research regulations. These organisations, often comprising patients, scientists, and concerned citizens, strive to ensure that ethical considerations are at the forefront of policy discussions. They work tirelessly to educate both the public and lawmakers about the potential benefits and risks associated with stem cell research, advocating for policies that support scientific advancement while safeguarding patient rights and ethical standards. Their influence can lead to more informed regulations that reflect societal values and the needs of those affected by various medical conditions.

In the context of stem cell research, advocacy groups also serve as a crucial bridge between the scientific community and the public. By communicating complex scientific concepts in accessible language, they help demystify the research process and address common misconceptions. This transparency is essential for fostering trust and ensuring that the public remains engaged in discussions about stem cell research. Furthermore, these groups often mobilise grassroots campaigns to gather support for specific legislative initiatives, demonstrating the power of collective action in shaping public policy.

Comparative analyses of international stem cell research laws reveal that the presence of strong advocacy groups often correlates with more progressive regulatory frameworks. Countries with active advocacy organisations tend to have more robust discussions around ethical considerations and patient rights. This influence can drive governments to adopt regulations that not only facilitate research but also protect individuals from potential exploitation. As such, advocacy groups play a critical role in promoting an ethical approach to stem cell research that is aligned with public sentiment and scientific integrity.

Additionally, advocacy groups are instrumental in ensuring that funding for stem cell research aligns with ethical standards. By collaborating with governmental bodies and private sector stakeholders, they can influence funding policies that prioritise ethical compliance and transparency. This can lead to more equitable access to research opportunities and ensure that advancements in stem cell technology benefit a wider range of patients. Their efforts in this arena underscore the importance of ethical governance in scientific funding and the role of advocacy in maintaining accountability within the research community.

In summary, the role of advocacy groups in stem cell research regulations is multifaceted and vital. They not only advocate for ethical practices and patient rights but also facilitate communication between the scientific community and the public. Their influence can lead to more informed policies that reflect societal values and promote responsible research. As the landscape of stem cell research continues to evolve, the contributions of these groups will remain essential in navigating the ethical complexities that arise in this dynamic field.

Case Studies of Public Influence on Policy Changes

The influence of public opinion on policy changes regarding stem cell research has been profound and multifaceted. In various countries, public sentiment has acted as a catalyst for legislative reforms, shaping the regulatory landscape in significant ways. For instance, in the United States, widespread advocacy for stem cell research led to increased federal funding and the establishment of guidelines that govern the ethical use of stem cells. This demonstrates how collective voices can drive policymakers to revisit existing regulations and consider public welfare as a priority.

One notable case study is the 2001 decision by then-President George W. Bush, who limited federal funding for embryonic stem cell research to existing lines. This decision sparked a nationwide debate, mobilising patient advocacy groups, scientists, and ethicists to rally for more inclusive funding policies. The ensuing public discourse highlighted the ethical dilemmas surrounding stem cell research, ultimately leading to policy shifts under subsequent administrations that expanded funding and support for a broader range of research initiatives.

Internationally, the impact of public opinion can also be observed in countries such as South Korea and the UK. In South Korea, the 2004 stem cell research scandal prompted a public outcry that led to stricter regulatory frameworks. This event underlined the importance of transparency and ethical compliance in stem cell research, as the public demanded accountability from researchers and regulatory bodies. Similarly, the UK's robust public engagement strategies surrounding stem cell research have fostered a more informed citizenry, resulting in regulations that reflect societal values and ethical considerations.

The role of pharmaceutical companies in shaping stem cell regulations cannot be overlooked. These entities often influence public opinion through funding research and advocacy efforts. Their vested interests can lead to lobbying for more permissive regulations, which may not always align with ethical considerations. The dynamics between public sentiment, corporate influence, and governmental action illustrate the complexity of creating balanced and fair regulations that prioritise patient rights and ethical governance.

In conclusion, case studies of public influence on policy changes in stem cell research reveal a dynamic interplay between societal values, ethical considerations, and regulatory frameworks. As public awareness and advocacy continue to evolve, they will undoubtedly shape the future of stem cell research legislation. Policymakers must remain attuned to public sentiment to ensure that regulations not only foster scientific advancement but also uphold ethical standards and respect patient rights.

Stem Cell Research Funding and Regulatory Compliance

Sources of Funding for Stem Cell Research

The funding landscape for stem cell research is multifaceted, encompassing various sources that significantly influence the direction and scope of scientific investigation in this field. Governmental bodies often serve as primary financiers, allocating taxpayer money to advance biomedical research initiatives. These funds are typically earmarked for projects that demonstrate potential for significant breakthroughs in medical treatment, particularly in regenerative medicine. However, the conditions surrounding these grants can impose strict regulatory compliance, affecting how research is conducted and reported.

In addition to government funding, private sector investment plays a crucial role in supporting stem cell research. Pharmaceutical companies and biotechnology firms are increasingly interested in the potential applications of stem cell technologies, often directing substantial resources towards promising projects. These investments are usually driven by the prospect of financial returns, which can create a complex relationship between profit motives and ethical considerations in research. The involvement of private entities may also lead to pressures that influence research priorities, often prioritising commercially viable outcomes over ethical scrutiny.

Non-profit organisations and philanthropic contributions represent another vital source of funding for stem cell research. These entities frequently support research initiatives that align with specific health missions or advocate for underserved medical conditions. Their funding can provide a more flexible approach, allowing researchers to explore innovative ideas without the constraints often associated with governmental funding. However, the reliance on such funding sources raises questions about the potential biases in research agendas and how they may affect the integrity of scientific inquiry.

Internationally, the disparity in funding availability for stem cell research can shape the regulatory landscape significantly. Countries with robust funding mechanisms often have more progressive research environments, while those with limited resources may struggle to keep pace. This disparity can lead to a competitive edge for nations that prioritise and invest in stem cell research, raising ethical considerations about global equity in biomedical advancements. The varying levels of support and regulation across different jurisdictions can lead to a patchwork of research standards and practices, complicating international collaboration.

As the field of stem cell research evolves, the interplay of funding sources continues to raise critical ethical questions. The balance between driving innovation and maintaining rigorous ethical standards is a persistent challenge for researchers, policymakers, and funding bodies alike. Understanding the sources of funding and their implications is essential for navigating the complex moral landscape of stem cell research regulations, ensuring that progress in this vital area of medicine is both scientifically sound and ethically grounded.

Compliance with Regulatory Frameworks

Compliance with regulatory frameworks is essential in ensuring that stem cell research is conducted ethically and responsibly. Various international, national, and local regulations govern the use of stem cells, reflecting differing societal values and ethical considerations surrounding this field. Health care personnel, ethicists, and biomedical researchers must navigate these complex regulations to ensure compliance while promoting scientific advancement. Understanding these frameworks not only aids in ethical research practices but also protects the rights of patients involved in clinical trials.

The ethical considerations in stem cell research regulations are manifold, as they often balance the potential benefits of research against moral objections. Internationally, different countries have adopted varying approaches to stem cell research, influenced by cultural, religious, and ethical beliefs. For instance, some countries have established comprehensive regulatory frameworks that allow for extensive research, while others impose strict limitations or bans on certain types of stem cell research. This comparative analysis highlights the importance of context in shaping regulatory policies and the need for ongoing dialogue among stakeholders to address ethical dilemmas.

Public opinion plays a significant role in shaping stem cell regulation policies, as societal attitudes can influence legislative decisions. Advocacy groups, patients, and the public often have strong views on stem cell research, which can lead to calls for more stringent regulations or, conversely, for more liberal access to research opportunities. Engaging with public opinion n is crucial for policymakers, as it ensures that regulations reflect societal values and concerns while fostering an environment conducive to scientific innovation.

The role of governmental bodies in shaping stem cell research legislation cannot be overstated. Regulatory agencies are tasked with establishing guidelines that ensure safety, efficacy, and compliance in stem cell research. These bodies also collaborate with ethical review boards to oversee clinical trials, ensuring that patient rights are respected throughout the research process. Moreover, the influence of pharmaceutical companies can complicate this landscape, as their interests may not always align with ethical research practices or patient welfare.

Finally, innovations in stem cell technology present unique regulatory challenges. As new techniques and applications emerge, regulatory frameworks must adapt to address these developments adequately. This requires a proactive approach from both regulatory bodies and researchers to ensure that emerging technologies are governed by sound ethical principles. Historical evolution of stem cell research regulations serves as a reminder of the need for flexibility and responsiveness in regulatory practices, ensuring that they not only protect individuals but also promote scientific progress in this dynamic field.

Consequences of Non-Compliance

Non-compliance with stem cell research regulations can have dire consequences for biomedical researchers and healthcare personnel alike. When institutions disregard established guidelines, the integrity of research is compromised, potentially leading to unethical practices and harmful outcomes for patients. The repercussions extend beyond individual researchers, impacting the reputation of the institutions involved, which can face public backlash and loss of funding. Non-compliance can also result in legal ramifications, including fines and restrictions on future research activities, thereby stifling scientific progress in a field that holds vast potential for medical advancements.

Furthermore, the ethical considerations surrounding stem cell research are paramount, and non-compliance undermines the foundational principles of biomedical ethics. Researchers have an obligation to ensure that their work adheres to ethical standards, particularly in light of public concerns regarding the moral implications of stem cell use. Violating these ethical norms can lead to a distrust of scientific research among the public, which may subsequently influence policy decisions and funding allocations. The erosion of public trust can have lasting effects on the future of stem cell research and its potential benefits to society.

The comparative analysis of international stem cell research laws reveals that non-compliance can isolate researchers from the global scientific community. Many countries have established stringent regulations to govern stem cell research, reflecting their cultural, ethical, and legal perspectives. When researchers fail to comply with these regulations, they risk being excluded from international collaborations, which are crucial for advancing knowledge and innovation in the field. This isolation can hinder the sharing of vital research findings and best practices, ultimately slowing the pace of scientific discovery.

Additionally, the influence of pharmaceutical companies on stem cell research regulations cannot be overlooked. Non-compliance can create an environment where unethical partnerships flourish, leading to the prioritisation of profit over patient welfare. This scenario not only jeopardises the integrity of the research but also poses significant risks to patient rights. Regulatory bodies must enforce compliance to ensure that research is conducted responsibly and that the interests of patients are safeguarded. Without proper oversight, the potential for exploitation of vulnerable populations in clinical trials increases, leading to ethical violations that could have been prevented.

In conclusion, the consequences of non-compliance in stem cell research are multifaceted and far-reaching. From legal penalties to ethical breaches, the implications affect researchers, institutions, and the broader societal trust in biomedical advancements. It is imperative for all stakeholders involved in stem cell research to adhere to regulations, not only to protect the integrity of their work but also to uphold the ethical standards that guide scientific inquiry. The future of stem cell research relies on a collective commitment to compliance and ethical governance.

Role of Governmental Bodies in Shaping Stem Cell Research Legislation

Key Governmental Agencies and Their Functions

In the realm of stem cell research, several key governmental agencies play pivotal roles in shaping regulations and policies that govern the field. In the United States, for instance, the National Institutes of Health (NIH) is central to funding biomedical research, including stem cell studies. The NIH not only provides financial support but also sets ethical guidelines that researchers must adhere to when conducting their studies. This oversight is crucial in ensuring that research is conducted responsibly and ethically, reflecting the moral considerations that underpin stem cell research.

Another significant agency is the Food and Drug Administration (FDA), which is tasked with regulating clinical trials involving stem cell therapies. The FDA ensures that any stem cell-based treatments entering the market meet stringent safety and efficacy standards. This agency's role is particularly important as it assesses the potential risks and benefits of new therapies, ensuring that patients are not exposed to unproven treatments. The FDA's comprehensive review process is an essential safeguard in the advancing field of regenerative medicine.

Internationally, various governmental bodies contribute to the regulation of stem cell research in their respective countries. For example, in the European

Union, the European Medicines Agency (EMA) plays a critical role in evaluating and approving stem cell therapies. Each country often has its own regulatory framework, which can lead to significant variations in how stem cell research is conducted and funded. This comparative analysis highlights the complexities involved in international stem cell research laws, as differing regulations can impact collaboration and innovation across borders.

Public opinion also significantly influences governmental agencies and their regulatory approaches to stem cell research. As ethical considerations become increasingly prominent in public discourse, agencies must navigate the delicate balance between scientific advancement and societal values. This dynamic interaction can lead to changes in policy and funding priorities, reflecting the evolving perceptions surrounding the ethical implications of stem cell research.

Lastly, it is essential to recognise the role of pharmaceutical companies in shaping stem cell research regulations. These entities often drive innovation but can also exert influence over regulatory frameworks through lobbying and funding initiatives. Understanding this relationship is vital for healthcare personnel, ethicists, and researchers who are navigating the intricate landscape of stem cell research, ensuring that patient rights and ethical considerations remain at the forefront of this rapidly evolving field.

Interactions Between Agencies and Researchers

The interactions between regulatory agencies and researchers in the field of stem cell research play a crucial role in shaping ethical practices and innovative advancements. Regulatory bodies, such as the Food and Drug Administration

(FDA) in the United States and the European Medicines Agency (EMA) in Europe, establish guidelines that researchers must adhere to ensure patient safety and ethical integrity. These agencies not only evaluate clinical trial applications but also monitor ongoing research to ensure compliance with established laws and regulations. The dynamic between these bodies and researchers can influence the pace at which new therapies are developed and brought to market.

Researchers often find themselves navigating a complex landscape of regulations that can vary significantly from one jurisdiction to another. This comparative analysis of international stem cell research laws reveals that while some countries adopt more permissive approaches, others impose stringent restrictions. Such disparities can hinder collaborative efforts and slow down global progress in stem cell therapies. Consequently, researchers must remain informed about the regulatory environment in which they operate, adapting their methodologies to meet both ethical standards and legal requirements.

Public opinion plays a pivotal role in shaping stem cell regulation policies. As societal values and ethical considerations evolve, they can directly impact government decisions regarding funding and regulation. Agencies tasked with overseeing stem cell research must consider public sentiment to maintain trust and support for scientific endeavours. Engaging with the community through public forums and consultations can help bridge the gap between researchers and the public, ensuring that regulatory policies reflect societal values and concerns.

The influence of pharmaceutical companies on stem cell research regulations cannot be overlooked. These entities often have significant resources to lobby for favourable regulations that align with their business interests. While such influence can drive innovation and funding, it also raises ethical questions about the prioritisation of profit over patient welfare. Regulatory agencies must balance the interests of these companies with the need for rigorous oversight and accountability in stem cell research practices.

Finally, the role of governmental bodies in shaping stem cell research legislation is vital for fostering an environment conducive to innovation while safeguarding ethical standards. As stem cell technologies continue to advance, regulators must adapt their frameworks to address emerging challenges. This ongoing dialogue between agencies and researchers is essential for developing policies that not only promote scientific progress but also protect patient rights and ensure ethical governance in stem cell research.

Legislative Advocacy and Change

Legislative advocacy plays a critical role in shaping the landscape of stem cell research regulations. Health care personnel, ethicists, and biomedical researchers must engage in continuous dialogue with policymakers to advocate for ethical guidelines that protect patient rights while fostering innovation. The complexity of stem cell research necessitates a nuanced understanding of both scientific advancements and the moral implications involved. By working collaboratively, these stakeholders can influence legislative frameworks that govern stem cell research and ensure they are both effective and ethically sound.

The ethical considerations in stem cell research regulations cannot be overstated. As new technologies emerge, they often outpace existing laws, creating a gap that can lead to ethical dilemmas. Advocacy efforts should focus on promoting regulations that are adaptable to scientific progress while safeguarding the welfare of patients involved in clinical trials. This balance is precarious, requiring ongoing education and engagement with the public to cultivate a broader understanding of the issues at hand.

Internationally, there is a diverse array of stem cell research laws that reflect varying cultural attitudes towards biomedical ethics. A comparative analysis of these regulations reveals significant differences in how countries prioritise ethical considerations versus scientific advancement. Legislative advocacy should aim to harmonise these approaches, fostering international collaboration while respecting local values. Understanding these differences is crucial for researchers who operate in a global context and seek to navigate the complexities of international regulations.

Public opinion significantly influences stem cell regulation policies. Advocacy efforts must therefore incorporate strategies to educate and engage the public, addressing misconceptions and highlighting the potential benefits of stem cell research. By fostering a well-informed public discourse, health care personnel and researchers can help shape policies that reflect societal values and ethical standards. This public engagement is essential for ensuring that regulations are not only scientifically rigorous but also socially acceptable.

Finally, the role of governmental bodies in shaping stem cell research legislation is pivotal. These entities must balance the interests of various stakeholders, including pharmaceutical companies, patient advocacy groups, and the scientific community. The influence of these companies can complicate the regulatory landscape, necessitating transparent discussions about funding and compliance. Effective advocacy will require building alliances with these entities to ensure that regulations promote both ethical research practices and innovation in stem cell technology, paving the way for future advancements in health care.

The Influence of Pharmaceutical Companies on Stem Cell Research Regulations

Industry Funding and Research Direction

The intersection of industry funding and research direction in stem cell research has become a critical area of focus within the broader discourse on ethical governance. As private and public entities invest heavily in this field, the motivations behind funding decisions often shape the research priorities. Such funding can drive innovation and expedite scientific advancements; however, it also raises ethical concerns regarding the potential for bias and the influence of profit-driven interests on research outcomes. Understanding these dynamics is essential for healthcare personnel and ethicists alike as they navigate the complex landscape of stem cell regulations.

Pharmaceutical companies, in particular, play a significant role in funding stem cell research, bringing both resources and expertise to the table. However, their involvement is not without controversy, as it can lead to conflicts of interest. Regulatory compliance becomes paramount in ensuring that research conducted under such funding adheres to ethical standards. Oversight committees must be vigilant in scrutinising funding sources and their implications for research integrity, thereby safeguarding patient rights and promoting transparent governance.

The historical evolution of stem cell research regulations often reflects the changing landscape of industry funding. In many jurisdictions, initial regulatory frameworks were developed in response to public concern over ethical issues, particularly the use of embryonic stem cells. As funding from industry stakeholders increased, so too did the pressure to adapt regulations that would facilitate advancements in technology while addressing ethical considerations. A comparative analysis of international laws reveals differing approaches to balancing these competing interests, highlighting the need for an ongoing dialogue among stakeholders.

Public opinion significantly influences the direction of stem cell research regulations, often swaying governmental bodies to act in accordance with societal values. Health care personnel and researchers must remain attuned to these shifts, as they can directly affect funding opportunities and regulatory frameworks. Engaging with the public through education and outreach can help demystify stem cell research and foster a more informed dialogue, ultimately leading to more ethically sound policies that reflect the collective values of society.

In conclusion, the interplay between industry funding and research direction in stem cell research presents both opportunities and challenges. Stakeholders must remain vigilant in ensuring that ethical considerations are at the forefront of decision-making processes. By fostering a collaborative environment among researchers, ethicists, and regulatory bodies, the field can continue to innovate while upholding the highest standards of ethical governance, ultimately benefiting patients and society at large.

Ethical Implications of Corporate Influence

The ethical implications of corporate influence in stem cell research are profound and multifaceted. As pharmaceutical companies increasingly invest in this promising field, their interests can shape the direction of research, often prioritising profit over patient welfare and scientific integrity. This dynamic raise critical questions about the extent to which corporate interests should dictate research agendas, particularly when the potential for medical breakthroughs intersects with ethical considerations surrounding human dignity and the sanctity of life.

Corporate funding can significantly impact the regulatory landscape of stem cell research. With substantial financial resources, companies may lobby for favourable regulations that expedite clinical trials or relax existing guidelines. This influence could lead to a regulatory environment that prioritises speed and profit over rigorous ethical scrutiny, potentially compromising patient safety and informed consent. The challenge lies in balancing the need for innovation with the imperative to uphold ethical standards that protect participants in research.

Moreover, the comparative analysis of international stem cell research laws reveals varying degrees of corporate influence across different jurisdictions. In some countries, strong regulations limit corporate involvement, thereby safeguarding ethical practices. In contrast, others may adopt a more permissive approach, allowing corporate interests to flourish unchecked. Such disparities not only affect the quality of research but also impact public trust in the scientific community, as perceptions of corporate greed can undermine confidence in the integrity of stem cell research.

Public opinion plays a crucial role in shaping stem cell regulation policies, often influenced by ethical concerns about corporate involvement. As stakeholders, patients and the general public have legitimate worries about how corporate interests might affect their rights and the governance of research. It is essential for policymakers to engage with the public, fostering transparency and dialogue to address these concerns and ensure that ethical considerations remain at the forefront of regulatory decisions.

Ultimately, the role of governmental bodies in shaping stem cell research legislation is pivotal in mitigating the ethical risks associated with corporate influence. By establishing robust regulatory frameworks that prioritise ethical principles, governments can help ensure that innovations in stem cell technology are developed responsibly. This approach not only safeguards patient rights but also promotes a research environment where ethical considerations are harmoniously integrated with scientific advancement, ensuring that the pursuit of knowledge does not come at the expense of moral integrity.

Regulatory Responses to Industry Practices

The regulatory responses to industry practices in the realm of stem cell research have evolved significantly over the past few decades. As advancements in stem cell technology have surged, so too have the ethical dilemmas associated with them. Governments and regulatory bodies worldwide have recognised the necessity of establishing frameworks to govern these practices, aiming to ensure safety, efficacy, and ethical compliance. These regulations vary widely across different jurisdictions, reflecting local cultural values, political landscapes, and public sentiments about stem cell research.

In many countries, the response to stem cell research has been shaped by historical context and public opinion. For instance, nations like the United States have seen a contentious debate surrounding federal funding for embryonic stem cell research, influenced by ethical concerns regarding the beginning of life. This public discourse has prompted governmental bodies to enact policies that either restrict or promote research based on societal values. In contrast, countries such as Sweden and the UK have adopted more permissive approaches, facilitating research while simultaneously instituting strict ethical guidelines to protect human rights and dignity.

The role of pharmaceutical companies cannot be understated in the regulatory landscape of stem cell research. These entities often wield significant influence over research agendas and funding, which can lead to conflicts of interest. Their involvement raises questions about the prioritisation of profits over patient welfare and ethical considerations. As such, regulatory frameworks must address these potential conflicts to ensure that stem cell research remains focused on advancing human health rather than merely serving commercial interests.

Regulatory frameworks for stem cell clinical trials are particularly crucial, as they directly impact patient safety and the integrity of scientific research. In many jurisdictions, there is a requirement for rigorous oversight to ensure that trials adhere to ethical standards and regulatory compliance. These frameworks often include provisions for informed consent, monitoring of adverse events, and transparency in reporting results. Such measures are essential not only for safeguarding participants but also for fostering public trust in stem cell research.

Lastly, the innovations in stem cell technology present ongoing regulatory challenges that require adaptive and forward-thinking approaches. As new techniques and therapies emerge, regulatory bodies must remain vigilant in assessing their implications for ethics and patient rights. The historical evolution of stem cell research regulations serves as a guide for navigating these challenges, illustrating the need for a robust and responsive regulatory environment that can accommodate the rapid pace of scientific advancement while upholding the highest ethical standards.

Regulatory Frameworks for Stem Cell Clinical Trials

Overview of Clinical Trial Regulations

The landscape of clinical trial regulations is complex and multifaceted, particularly when it comes to stem cell research. Regulatory bodies across various countries have established frameworks to ensure that clinical trials are conducted ethically and safely. These regulations aim to protect participants while facilitating scientific advancement. The intricacies of these regulations reflect the diverse ethical considerations that underlie stem cell research, highlighting the need for rigorous oversight in this rapidly evolving field.

One of the primary challenges in stem cell research regulations is the balance between innovation and safety. As new stem cell technologies emerge, regulatory frameworks must adapt to address the unique risks and ethical dilemmas they present. The role of governmental bodies is crucial, as they shape legislation that governs research practices. Additionally, public opinion plays a significant role in influencing regulatory policies, with societal values impacting the acceptance and funding of stem cell research initiatives.

Internationally, there is a notable variation in stem cell research laws, with some countries embracing more permissive approaches while others impose stringent restrictions. This comparative analysis reveals not only the cultural and ethical contexts of different nations but also the potential implications for global collaboration in research. Understanding these differences is essential for researchers and ethicists alike, as they navigate the regulatory landscape and seek to harmonise standards across borders.

Furthermore, the influence of pharmaceutical companies on stem cell research regulations cannot be overlooked. These companies often drive innovation and funding but may also prioritise profit over ethical considerations. This dynamic raise important questions about patient rights and the governance of stem cell research. Ensuring that regulations are in place to protect participants while fostering innovation is a delicate balance that requires ongoing dialogue among stakeholders.

In conclusion, the historical evolution of stem cell research regulations illustrates the ongoing struggle to harmonise scientific progress with ethical imperatives. As the field continues to advance, it is imperative for health care personnel, ethicists, and researchers to remain vigilant and engaged in the regulatory process. By doing so, they can contribute to a framework that not only protects patient rights but also encourages responsible innovation in stem cell technology.

Ethical Review Processes

Ethical review processes are crucial in the landscape of stem cell research, ensuring that studies meet rigorous ethical standards before they proceed. These processes involve comprehensive assessments by ethics committees, which evaluate the potential risks and benefits associated with research proposals. By scrutinising the ethical implications of stem cell research, these committees play a vital role in protecting both participants and the integrity of scientific inquiry. This layer of oversight is particularly important given the complex moral questions surrounding the use of human embryos and stem cells.

One significant aspect of ethical review processes is the comparative analysis of international regulations governing stem cell research. Different countries adopt varying approaches based on cultural, legal, and ethical perspectives. Some nations impose stringent restrictions, while others adopt a more permissive stance, reflecting broader societal attitudes towards biomedical innovation. Understanding these differences is essential for researchers who operate in a global environment and seek compliance with local laws while maintaining high ethical standards.

Moreover, the impact of public opinion cannot be underestimated in shaping ethical review processes. As societal views on stem cell research evolve, they influence legislative changes and the frameworks within which ethical reviews are conducted. Public discourse often highlights the need for transparency and accountability in research practices, pushing for greater involvement of community voices in ethical deliberations. This dynamic interplay between public sentiment and regulatory compliance underscores the necessity for ongoing dialogue between scientists, ethicists, and the public.

The role of governmental bodies in shaping stem cell research legislation also intersects with ethical review processes. These agencies not only establish regulatory frameworks but also provide guidance on ethical considerations that must be acknowledged during the review process. By fostering collaboration between researchers and regulatory authorities, governments can ensure that ethical standards keep pace with scientific advancements, thereby promoting responsible research practices that align with societal values.

Lastly, the influence of pharmaceutical companies on stem cell research regulations is an area of growing concern. As private entities invest heavily in stem cell innovations, their interests can potentially shape ethical review processes, raising questions about conflicts of interest and the prioritisation of profit over patient welfare. It is essential for oversight committees to remain vigilant, ensuring that ethical considerations remain at the forefront of decision-making in stem cell research, even amidst the pressures of commercialisation.

Case Studies of Notable Clinical Trials

The landscape of stem cell research is marked by numerous clinical trials that serve as critical case studies in understanding both the advancements and ethical dilemmas inherent in this field. One notable trial is the use of embryonic stem cells to treat spinal cord injuries, which has raised significant ethical concerns regarding the source of these cells. Such trials not only push the boundaries of scientific discovery but also force stakeholders to confront moral questions regarding patient rights and the implications of using embryonic cells. This case exemplifies the tension between innovative research and the ethical frameworks that govern it, highlighting the need for robust regulatory oversight.

Another significant clinical trial involved the application of induced pluripotent stem cells (iPSCs) to develop therapies for age-related macular degeneration. This research demonstrated the potential to create patient-specific cells, thereby mitigating the risk of immune rejection. However, it also sparked debates about the regulatory challenges associated with iPSCs, including concerns over long-term effects and the necessity for comprehensive regulatory compliance. The success of this trial underscores the importance of creating adaptive regulatory frameworks that can keep pace with rapid technological advancements in the sector.

Internationally, the comparison of stem cell research laws offers insightful case studies. Countries such as Sweden and the United Kingdom have established clear and comprehensive regulations that facilitate research while ensuring ethical standards are maintained. In contrast, nations with more restrictive laws often see a brain drain, where talented researchers relocate to more permissive environments. These contrasting scenarios illustrate how public opinion and governmental policies can shape the landscape of stem cell research, influencing funding opportunities and the overall advancement of the field.

The involvement of pharmaceutical companies in stem cell research also presents a complex case study. Their substantial financial investment can drive innovation and expedite the development of new therapies. However, ethical concerns arise regarding the potential influence of profit motives on research integrity and regulatory compliance. The balancing act between fostering innovation and ensuring ethical governance is crucial for maintaining public trust and advancing the field responsibly.

Lastly, the historical evolution of stem cell research regulations provides a rich backdrop to current discussions. From initial hesitations surrounding the use of human embryos to today's more nuanced approach that embraces both ethical considerations and scientific progress, this evolution reflects changing societal values. Case studies from the past highlight the importance of adaptable regulatory frameworks that respond to emerging technologies and societal concerns, ensuring that patient rights remain at the forefront of stem cell research governance.

Patient Rights and Stem Cell Research Governance

Rights of Participants in Research

Participants in research, particularly in the context of stem cell studies, possess fundamental rights that must be acknowledged and protected. These rights are rooted in the principles of autonomy, informed consent, and the necessity for transparency in all research practices. Health care personnel and researchers must ensure that participants are fully aware of the nature of the research, the potential risks involved, and their right to withdraw at any time without any repercussions. Upholding these rights is not merely a legal obligation but a moral imperative that fosters trust between participants and researchers.

Informed consent is a cornerstone of ethical research practices, particularly in sensitive areas like stem cell research. Participants should be provided with comprehensive information about the research protocol, including the purpose, procedures, potential benefits, and risks associated with the study. This information must be presented in a clear and understandable manner, allowing participants to make an educated decision about their involvement. The dynamic nature of stem cell research, with its evolving technologies and methodologies, necessitates ongoing communication and re-consent, ensuring that participants remain informed throughout their engagement in the research.

The rights of participants extend beyond informed consent to include the right to privacy and confidentiality. Researchers are responsible for safeguarding the personal information of participants and ensuring that any data collected is anonymised whenever possible. In the context of stem cell research, where genetic material may be involved, the implications of privacy breaches can be profound. Therefore, ethical oversight committees must rigorously evaluate research proposals to ensure that participant rights regarding privacy are adequately addressed and protected.

Furthermore, participants in stem cell research have the right to access information regarding the outcomes of the research they contributed to. This transparency not only empowers participants but also helps to reinforce public trust in the research process. By providing feedback and results, researchers can demonstrate accountability and encourage future participation in scientific studies. Health care personnel and oversight committees must develop mechanisms to facilitate this feedback loop, ensuring that participants feel valued and informed about the impact of their contributions.

Finally, the evolving landscape of stem cell research regulations necessitates an ongoing dialogue about participant rights. As new technologies and methodologies emerge, the ethical considerations surrounding participant involvement must be constantly reassessed. Engaging stakeholders, including participants, health care personnel, and ethicists, in this dialogue is essential for developing robust regulatory frameworks that uphold the rights of individuals involved in research. By prioritising participant rights, the research community can foster an ethical environment that encourages innovation while respecting the dignity and autonomy of those who contribute to scientific advancement.

Governance Structures and Oversight

The governance structures surrounding stem cell research are multifaceted, reflecting the complexity of ethical, legal, and scientific dimensions involved. Different countries adopt varied approaches to oversight, with some implementing stringent regulations while others maintain a more permissive environment. This divergence often stems from cultural values, historical contexts, and public attitudes toward biotechnology. Consequently, understanding these governance frameworks is crucial for stakeholders involved in stem cell research, as they navigate the moral landscape shaped by regulatory compliance and ethical considerations.

Oversight committees play a pivotal role in ensuring that stem cell research adheres to established ethical norms and legal requirements. These committees, often comprising ethicists, scientists, and legal experts, evaluate research proposals to assess potential risks and benefits. Their decisions are influenced not only by scientific merit but also by societal values surrounding human dignity and the moral status of stem cells. As a result, the function of these committees is not merely bureaucratic; they serve as guardians of public trust in scientific research.

The impact of public opinion on stem cell regulation policies cannot be underestimated. In many cases, legislative frameworks have been shaped by societal debates surrounding the moral implications of stem cell research. Advocacy groups, both for and against stem cell research, mobilise public sentiment to influence policymakers, highlighting the fluid relationship between public perceptions and regulatory practices. This dynamic underscore the importance of transparent communication between researchers and the public to foster informed dialogue about ethical issues.

Governmental bodies are instrumental in shaping stem cell research legislation, with their policies often reflecting the political climate and prevailing ethical considerations. These entities must balance the promotion of scientific innovation with the protection of patient rights and ethical standards. Additionally, the influence of pharmaceutical companies can complicate this landscape, as their interests may not always align with public welfare. Regulatory frameworks must therefore be designed to mitigate potential conflicts of interest while ensuring that advancements in stem cell technology are safely and ethically pursued.

Lastly, the historical evolution of stem cell research regulations reveals a trajectory of increasing sophistication in governance structures. As scientific knowledge expands and new technologies emerge, regulatory frameworks must adapt to address novel ethical challenges. Innovations in stem cell technology, such as gene editing and tissue engineering, present unique regulatory hurdles that require ongoing dialogue among stakeholders. Ensuring that governance structures remain responsive to these changes is vital for fostering a responsible and ethically sound environment for stem cell research.

Advocacy for Patient-Centric Approaches

The concept of patient-centric approaches in stem cell research advocacy is gaining significant traction among healthcare personnel and ethicists alike. This paradigm shift emphasises the importance of aligning research objectives with the needs and preferences of patients. By prioritising patient voices, researchers can ensure that ethical considerations are not merely theoretical but are grounded in the real-world experiences of those affected by these advancements. This approach not only enhances the moral legitimacy of research but also fosters trust between patients and researchers, which is vital for the successful implementation of stem cell therapies.

Furthermore, the regulatory landscape surrounding stem cell research is evolving to reflect this patient-centric ethos. Various international frameworks are beginning to incorporate patient rights and perspectives into their guidelines, recognising that patients are not just subjects of research but active participants in the process. These regulations aim to protect patients while promoting innovation, ensuring that the benefits of stem cell research are accessible and equitable. The challenge remains for regulatory bodies to balance these interests effectively, considering the complexities of scientific advancement and ethical obligations.

Another critical aspect of advocacy for patient-centric approaches is the role of public opinion in shaping stem cell research policies. As societal values and perceptions shift, they significantly influence the legislative environment surrounding stem cell research. Advocacy groups play a pivotal role in educating the public and policymakers about the potential benefits and risks associated with stem cell therapies. This grassroots engagement can lead to more informed decisions, ultimately resulting in regulations that better reflect the desires and concerns of the community.

Moreover, the influence of pharmaceutical companies on stem cell research regulations cannot be overlooked in this discussion. While these entities can provide essential funding and resources to advance research, their interests may not always align with those of patients. Advocacy for patient-centric approaches necessitates a vigilant awareness of the potential conflicts of interest that arise when profit motives intertwine with research ethics. Ensuring that patient welfare remains the priority requires robust oversight and transparency in how these relationships are managed within the regulatory frameworks.

In conclusion, the advocacy for patient-centric approaches in stem cell research is a multifaceted endeavour that requires collaboration among healthcare professionals, ethicists, and regulatory bodies. As the field continues to evolve, it is imperative to keep the patient at the forefront of discussions surrounding ethical considerations and legislative frameworks. By fostering an environment where patient needs are prioritised, the potential for stem cell research to transform healthcare can be fully realised, leading to innovations that are not only scientifically groundbreaking but also ethically sound and socially responsible.

Innovations in Stem Cell Technology and Their Regulatory Challenges

Emerging Technologies in Stem Cell Research

Emerging technologies in stem cell research are reshaping the landscape of biomedical science and raising important ethical considerations. Techniques such as induced pluripotent stem cells (iPSCs) and gene editing technologies like

CRISPR have revolutionised the ability to derive and manipulate stem cells. These innovations offer the promise of personalised medicine, but they also introduce complex regulatory challenges that necessitate careful oversight and ethical scrutiny. As the capabilities of stem cell research expand, so too does the need for comprehensive regulations that address both scientific potential and moral implications.

The rapid advancement of stem cell technologies has prompted a comparative analysis of international laws governing this field. Different countries have adopted varied approaches to stem cell research, reflecting diverse cultural attitudes toward ethics and science. Some nations have embraced permissive frameworks that encourage innovation, while others impose stringent restrictions that limit research possibilities. This divergence highlights the ongoing debate about the balance between fostering scientific advancement and protecting human rights, particularly in the context of patient consent and the use of embryonic stem cells.

Public opinion plays a crucial role in shaping stem cell regulation policies. As societal values evolve, so too do the expectations placed on researchers and policymakers. The influence of public sentiment can lead to increased funding for research initiatives, but it can also result in backlash against perceived ethical violations. Engaging with communities to understand their perspectives on stem cell research is essential for developing regulations that reflect societal norms and ethical standards, ensuring that research is conducted transparently and responsibly.

Governmental bodies are pivotal in establishing the regulatory frameworks that guide stem cell clinical trials. Agencies such as the Food and Drug Administration (FDA) in the United States and the European Medicines Agency (EMA) in Europe set forth guidelines that researchers must follow to ensure safety and efficacy. However, the fast-paced nature of technological advancements in stem cell research often outstrips existing regulations, leading to calls for more adaptive and responsive legislative frameworks. Policymakers must remain vigilant and proactive in addressing the gaps that may arise as new technologies emerge.

Finally, the role of pharmaceutical companies in influencing stem cell research regulations cannot be overlooked. These entities often drive funding and innovation in the field, but their interests can sometimes conflict with ethical considerations. As they engage in partnerships with research institutions, questions arise regarding the prioritisation of profit over patient welfare. Regulatory bodies must navigate this complex landscape, working to ensure that ethical standards are upheld while also fostering an environment conducive to scientific progress and public health benefits.

Regulatory Adaptations to New Innovations

As innovations in stem cell technology emerge, regulatory frameworks must adapt to address the unique challenges posed by these advancements. The rapid pace of scientific discovery often outstrips existing regulations, which can lead to gaps in oversight that may compromise ethical standards. Regulatory bodies are increasingly recognising the need for flexible approaches that allow for the incorporation of new technologies while ensuring patient safety and ethical compliance. This adaptability is crucial in maintaining public trust and facilitating responsible research practices.

Ethical considerations are at the forefront of discussions regarding the regulation of stem cell research. The balance between encouraging innovation and protecting human rights is delicate and requires ongoing dialogue among stakeholders. Ethical frameworks must evolve alongside scientific advancements to ensure that the rights of patients and research subjects are safeguarded. This includes addressing concerns related to informed consent, the commodification of human tissue, and the long-term implications of stem cell therapies.

A comparative analysis of international stem cell research laws reveals significant variations in regulatory approaches, influenced by cultural, ethical, and political factors. Some countries adopt permissive stances towards stem cell research, fostering innovation, while others impose stringent restrictions based on moral grounds. These differences can complicate international collaborations and may impact the global landscape of biomedical research. Understanding these regulatory environments is essential for researchers and policymakers working in the field.

Public opinion plays a pivotal role in shaping stem cell regulation policies. As societal attitudes towards stem cell research evolve, they can significantly influence legislative decisions. Policymakers must engage with the public to gauge perceptions and address concerns, ensuring that regulations reflect societal values while promoting scientific progress. This engagement is vital in fostering a collaborative environment where ethical considerations are prioritised alongside technological advancements.

Finally, the influence of pharmaceutical companies on stem cell research regulations cannot be overlooked. As these companies invest in stem cell technologies, their interests may impact regulatory frameworks and funding priorities. It is essential for regulatory bodies to maintain independence and transparency in their decision-making processes to avoid conflicts of interest. By fostering a regulatory landscape that encourages innovation while adhering to ethical standards, the future of stem cell research can be navigated responsibly and effectively.

Future Challenges in Regulation

The landscape of stem cell research regulation is fraught with challenges that will shape its future trajectory. As advancements in stem cell technology continue to emerge, regulatory frameworks must evolve to keep pace with the scientific innovations. This includes addressing the ethical implications associated with new methodologies and ensuring that regulations remain relevant in light of public opinion and international law. Regulatory bodies face the daunting task of balancing the need for stringent oversight with the necessity of fostering an environment conducive to scientific progress.

One significant challenge lies in the comparative analysis of international stem cell research laws. Different countries adopt varying stances on stem cell research, influenced by cultural, ethical, and political factors. This disparity creates complications for multinational research initiatives and raises questions about the harmonisation of regulations. As researchers collaborate across borders, a unified approach to regulation becomes imperative to prevent ethical breaches and to promote a coherent framework that respects patient rights and scientific integrity.

Public opinion plays a crucial role in shaping stem cell regulation policies. As societal attitudes towards stem cell research evolve, so too must the governance structures that support it. Engaging with the public to understand their concerns and expectations can help regulatory bodies to create more responsive and transparent policies. This interaction is vital, as it not only influences funding avenues but also impacts the legitimacy of research practices in the eyes of the community.

The influence of pharmaceutical companies on stem cell research regulations presents another complex challenge. The potential for profit in stem cell therapies can lead to conflicts of interest that may compromise ethical standards. Regulatory agencies must navigate these relationships carefully, ensuring that the pursuit of innovation does not undermine the principles of patient safety and ethical governance. This requires a robust framework that holds companies accountable while also encouraging responsible research and development.

Finally, the historical evolution of stem cell research regulations provides a critical context for understanding current challenges. The lessons learned from past controversies, such as those surrounding embryonic stem cell research, inform contemporary regulatory practices. As the field advances, stakeholders must remain vigilant, adapting regulations to address emerging ethical dilemmas and ensuring that patient rights are safeguarded. The future of stem cell research regulation hinges on collaborative efforts among health care personnel, ethicists, and policymakers, striving for a balanced approach that prioritises both innovation and ethical integrity.

Historical Evolution of Stem Cell Research Regulations

Key Historical Events Shaping Regulation

The regulation of stem cell research has been profoundly shaped by key historical events that highlight both the ethical dilemmas and scientific advancements associated with this field. One pivotal event was the discovery of embryonic stem cells in the 1980s, which opened new avenues for medical research but also ignited heated debates about the moral status of human embryos. This period marked the beginning of a complex dialogue between scientists, ethicists, and policymakers, leading to the first regulatory frameworks aimed at overseeing stem cell research practices. The establishment of these regulations was crucial in addressing public concerns while fostering scientific innovation.

In the late 1990s, events such as the cloning of Dolly the sheep further escalated discussions surrounding stem cell research regulations. Cloning raised significant ethical questions regarding the manipulation of life and the potential for human cloning, prompting governments worldwide to reassess their legal and ethical stances. As a result, many countries introduced stringent regulations to prevent misuse of stem cell technologies, reflecting a growing public demand for accountability in scientific research. These regulations varied greatly across nations, illustrating the complex interplay between cultural values and scientific advancement.

The early 2000s saw the rise of patient advocacy groups, which played a crucial role in influencing public opinion and, consequently, regulatory policies. These organisations highlighted the potential benefits of stem cell research for treating debilitating conditions, urging policymakers to consider the therapeutic possibilities rather than solely focusing on ethical concerns. As public support for stem cell research grew, particularly in the United States, funding for research initiatives increased, leading to a more robust regulatory environment that aimed to balance ethical considerations with the need for scientific progress.

Internationally, the regulatory landscape for stem cell research has evolved in response to both scientific advancements and public sentiment. Comparative analyses of various countries' laws reveal significant disparities in how stem cell research is approached. For example, while some countries have embraced permissive regulations that encourage innovation, others maintain strict prohibitions, reflecting differing cultural attitudes towards biotechnology. This divergence highlights the necessity for a cohesive international dialogue to harmonise regulatory frameworks and ensure ethical compliance in stem cell research.

In recent years, the emergence of new stem cell technologies, including induced pluripotent stem cells (iPSCs), has introduced additional regulatory challenges. These innovations promise to revolutionise regenerative medicine, yet they also complicate existing regulatory frameworks. As governmental bodies continue to adapt to these advancements, the influence of pharmaceutical companies has become increasingly evident, often shaping the direction of stem cell research regulations through lobbying and funding efforts. The ongoing evolution of stem cell research regulations will require a careful balance between fostering innovation, protecting patient rights, and addressing ethical concerns in this rapidly advancing field.

Evolution of Ethical Standards

The evolution of ethical standards in stem cell research has been shaped by a myriad of factors, including scientific advancements, societal values, and regulatory frameworks. From the early days of embryonic stem cell research, where ethical considerations were largely absent, to the contemporary era where guidelines are meticulously delineated, the journey has been complex. Initial explorations into stem cell technology were often characterised by a lack of consensus on ethical implications, reflecting a burgeoning field that was outpacing ethical discourse. As the scientific community began to recognise the potential for both breakthroughs and ethical dilemmas, the call for structured ethical standards grew louder.

In response to the rapid advancements in stem cell research, various international bodies began to establish ethical guidelines aimed at ensuring responsible conduct. The introduction of frameworks such as the Declaration of Helsinki and the Belmont Report marked significant milestones, asserting the importance of informed consent, beneficence, and justice in biomedical research.

These principles laid the groundwork for more specific regulations governing stem cell research, highlighting the need to balance scientific inquiry with ethical obligations. As nations grappled with their respective ethical stances, the global landscape became increasingly diverse, prompting a comparative analysis of different regulatory approaches.

Public opinion has played a crucial role in shaping stem cell research regulations, as societal attitudes towards the moral implications of stem cell use vary widely. In some countries, public support has led to more permissive regulations, while in others, ethical concerns have resulted in stringent restrictions. The interplay between public sentiment and regulatory frameworks has often forced policymakers to navigate a delicate balance, ensuring that regulations reflect both scientific potential and ethical accountability. This dynamic underscore the importance of engaging the public in discussions about stem cell research, as their views can significantly influence legislative outcomes.

Furthermore, the impact of funding on stem cell research regulation cannot be overlooked. Governmental bodies, philanthropic organisations, and private enterprises all contribute to the financial landscape of biomedical research, and their priorities often dictate the direction of ethical standards. The role of pharmaceutical companies, in particular, has raised questions about the influence of profit motives on regulatory compliance and ethical governance. As these entities push for accelerated research and development, it is essential to scrutinise how their interests align with patient rights and the broader societal good.

In conclusion, the evolution of ethical standards in stem cell research reflects an ongoing dialogue between science, ethics, and public policy. As innovations in stem cell technology continue to emerge, regulatory challenges will persist, necessitating a robust framework that can adapt to new developments. The historical context of these standards informs current practices and highlights the importance of vigilance in upholding ethical principles in the face of rapid scientific progress. The future of stem cell research will depend on our ability to navigate these complexities while ensuring that ethical considerations remain at the forefront of scientific inquiry.

Future Directions in Regulation

As the field of stem cell research rapidly advances, the future directions in regulation must adapt to the evolving ethical landscape. Regulatory frameworks need to be dynamic, accommodating innovations while ensuring patient safety and ethical standards. Governments and international bodies have a pivotal role in shaping these regulations, necessitating robust dialogue among stakeholders, including researchers, ethicists, and healthcare professionals. This collaborative approach will foster a regulatory environment that is both flexible and protective of human rights.

Ethical considerations in stem cell research regulations remain at the forefront of legislative dialogues. The need to balance scientific progress with moral implications is crucial. Ethical frameworks should not only guide research practices but also address public concerns regarding the use of human embryos and the potential commodification of human life. As societal values shift, regulations must reflect these changes while maintaining a commitment to ethical integrity.

Comparative analyses of international stem cell research laws reveal significant discrepancies in regulatory approaches. Some countries embrace permissive regulations, fostering innovation, while others impose stringent restrictions that may hinder research progress. Understanding these variations is essential for developing harmonised global guidelines that respect cultural differences while promoting ethical research practices across borders.

The impact of public opinion on stem cell regulation policies cannot be underestimated. As societal awareness and understanding of stem cell research grow, so too does the influence of public sentiment on legislative decisions. Engaging the public in discussions about stem cell research can lead to more informed policies that reflect community values and concerns, ultimately shaping the direction of future regulations.

Pharmaceutical companies also play a critical role in shaping stem cell research regulations. Their involvement can drive funding and innovation, yet it raises questions about the potential for conflicts of interest. Establishing clear guidelines for corporate involvement in research is essential to ensure that regulatory compliance prioritises patient rights and ethical standards above profit motives. As innovations in stem cell technology continue to emerge, regulatory bodies must remain vigilant and responsive to the challenges these advancements present.

Conclusion and Future Prospects

Summary of Key Findings

The exploration of stem cell research regulations has unveiled a complex landscape characterised by diverse ethical considerations and legal frameworks across the globe. This summary of key findings highlights the significant attempts made internationally to establish regulatory measures that govern stem cell research. Countries have adopted varying approaches, influenced by cultural, ethical, and scientific priorities, which reflect the rich tapestry of values that underpin their respective health care systems. These differences underscore the necessity for a comparative analysis to inform best practices in regulatory compliance and ethical governance.

Ethical considerations emerge as a pivotal theme within the discourse on stem cell research regulations. The moral implications of stem cell use, particularly regarding human embryonic stem cells, have provoked vigorous debates among ethicists, researchers, and the public. This dialogue has led to the development of ethical guidelines that seek to balance scientific advancement with respect for human dignity and rights. Stakeholders must navigate these ethical waters carefully, as the outcomes will significantly shape future research directions and public trust in biomedical innovations.

Public opinion plays a critical role in the formulation of stem cell regulation policies. Findings indicate that societal attitudes towards stem cell research can significantly influence legislative actions and funding allocations. Public support or opposition often reflects broader societal values and ethical concerns, which policymakers must address to ensure that regulations resonate with the community's expectations. This interplay between public sentiment and regulatory frameworks is essential for fostering a conducive environment for responsible scientific exploration.

The influence of pharmaceutical companies on stem cell research regulations cannot be overlooked. These entities often provide substantial funding for research initiatives, which may inadvertently affect regulatory practices and governance. The findings suggest that while such financial contributions can propel scientific advancements, they also raise questions about the integrity of research and the potential for conflicts of interest. A balanced approach is needed to ensure that corporate interests do not overshadow ethical considerations and patient rights in the realm of stem cell research.

Lastly, the historical evolution of stem cell research regulations reveals a trajectory that is continuously shaped by innovations in stem cell technology. As advancements occur, regulatory frameworks must adapt to address emerging challenges associated with new methodologies and applications. The findings emphasise the importance of maintaining a dynamic regulatory environment that fosters innovation while safeguarding ethical standards and patient welfare. This delicate balance will be crucial as the field progresses and faces new ethical dilemmas and regulatory hurdles.

Recommendations for Policy Makers

In shaping effective stem cell research policies, it is crucial for policymakers to engage in extensive dialogue with healthcare personnel, ethicists, and biomedical research scientists. Such collaborative discussions can illuminate the ethical dilemmas that arise in stem cell research, ensuring that regulations reflect a balance between innovation and moral responsibility. Policymakers should prioritise transparency in the regulatory process to foster trust among stakeholders and the public, thereby enhancing the legitimacy of the regulatory framework.

Another vital recommendation is to conduct a comparative analysis of international stem cell research laws. Understanding how different countries navigate the ethical and regulatory challenges of stem cell research can provide valuable insights. Policymakers can learn from both the successes and failures of these various approaches, enabling them to craft more informed and adaptive policies that resonate with the values of their own societies.

Public opinion plays a significant role in shaping stem cell regulation policies. Policymakers should implement mechanisms for ongoing public engagement to gauge societal attitudes toward stem cell research and its implications. By considering public sentiment, policymakers can ensure that regulations are not only scientifically sound but also socially accepted. This can lead to more robust funding opportunities and support for research initiatives that align with the expectations of the community.

Furthermore, it is essential for governmental bodies to establish clear guidelines regarding the influence of pharmaceutical companies on stem cell research regulations. Transparency in funding sources and potential conflicts of interest must be addressed to cultivate an environment of ethical compliance.

Policymakers should strive to create regulatory frameworks that not only promote innovation in stem cell technology but also safeguard patient rights and ensure accountability in research practices.

Lastly, as technological advancements in stem cell research continue to evolve, policymakers must remain adaptable and proactive. This includes revisiting and revising existing regulations to accommodate new scientific discoveries and methodologies. By fostering an environment that encourages innovation while enforcing strict regulatory compliance, policymakers can ensure that stem cell research continues to contribute positively to healthcare outcomes without compromising ethical standards.

Future Trends in Stem Cell Research Regulations

The landscape of stem cell research regulations is continuously evolving, shaped by technological advancements and societal perceptions. As stem cell therapies become more mainstream, regulatory frameworks are being re-evaluated to ensure they can accommodate innovative approaches while maintaining ethical standards. This adaptation is crucial as it not only affects the development of new treatments but also influences public trust in biomedical research. By examining emerging trends, stakeholders can better navigate the complexities of regulation in this dynamic field.

Ethical considerations remain at the forefront of stem cell research regulations. With advancements in technology such as induced pluripotent stem cells (iPSCs), new ethical dilemmas arise regarding consent, sourcing of materials, and the potential for genetic modifications. These issues prompt regulatory bodies to reassess existing laws and guidelines to ensure they align with contemporary ethical standards. A proactive approach to ethics in regulation will be essential in fostering responsible research practices that respect patient rights and societal values.

Internationally, the divergence in stem cell research laws presents both challenges and opportunities for harmonisation. Countries vary significantly in their regulatory approaches, from stringent prohibitions to permissive frameworks. This comparative analysis highlights the need for a cohesive strategy that balances innovation with ethical oversight. As global collaboration in biomedical research increases, aligning regulations can facilitate advancements while safeguarding ethical considerations across borders.

Public opinion plays a significant role in shaping stem cell regulation policies. As societal views shift, influenced by media coverage and advocacy groups, regulatory bodies must remain responsive to public concerns and aspirations. Engaging with the community can help demystify stem cell research and foster a more informed dialogue about its potential benefits and risks. This engagement is vital for building public trust and ensuring that regulations reflect societal values and expectations.

Finally, the influence of pharmaceutical companies on stem cell research regulations cannot be overlooked. As key players in the development and funding of new therapies, these companies often advocate for regulatory changes that support innovation. However, this relationship raises questions about the balance between promoting research and ensuring ethical compliance. A transparent regulatory framework that considers the interests of all stakeholders, including patients, researchers, and industry, is essential for fostering a responsible and sustainable environment for stem cell research.

Pause for Thought

- Stem cell research is a pivotal area in modern biomedical science, offering promising avenues for regenerative medicine and therapeutic interventions giving opportunities for treating diseases such as Parkinson's disease, diabetes and spinal cord injuries. However, the essential guard rails to these opportunities are complex ethical considerations.

- Stem cell research is influenced by the ethical considerations which is shaped by the cultural, social, and political landscape. In some regions, there are stringent regulations which limit research to certain types of stem cells while others adopt a more permissive approach, encouraging innovation and explanations.

- The intersection of government policy and the scientific inquiry requires continuous dialogue between regulating agencies and the scientific community to adapt to new discoveries and societal needs. This collaboration is vital for regulatory oversight that both supports research and protect patient rights.

- Ethical regulations are designed to protect human dignity, ensure safety, and foster public trust in scientific endeavours. Without such ethical oversight the potential for exploitation of vulnerable populations and the misuse of research findings could increase significantly. The importance of ethical regulations is underscored by the complex moral questions that surround stem cell research, thus necessitating a careful balance between scientific advancement and ethical responsibility.

- Comparative analysis of international stem cell research laws reveal significant disparities in regulatory approaches. Some nations like the United Kingdom have developed robust frameworks that facilitate research whilst imposing strict ethical standards whereas others maintain more lenient regulations. This divergence often results from cultural attitudes towards science and ethics, with public opinion playing a crucial role.

- The influence of public opinion on stem cell regulatory policies have come from a variety of bodies, advocacy groups, patient organisation, and the media have all contributed to shaping perceptions about the benefits and risk associated with stem cell research. Thus, regulatory bodies are often compelled to be guided by public sentiments when drafting legislation.

- The evolving landscape of stem cell technology presents ongoing regulatory challenges that must be addressed. Innovations are outpacing existing regulatory framework, creating potential gaps in oversight. Governmental bodies alongside pharmaceutical companies, play a crucial role in adopting to these changes by developing comprehensive regulatory strategies that protect patient rights while promoting scientific advancement.

- Legislative efforts often reflect a balancing act between scientific innovation and ethical considerations. In the United States, the national institute of health guidelines 2000 was a step towards formal regulation which established parameters for federal funding of embryonic stem cells research. This prompted discussions surrounding the moral implications of using human embryo, ultimately influencing public discourse and legislative frameworks across the globe.

- Countries like Sweden and the United Kingdom have adopted more permissive regulations, allowing for extensive research and clinical applications, while Germany enforce strict limitations. This analysis reveals how public opinion, is influenced by cultural and religious factors and their role in shaping national policies.

- The influence of governmental bodies such as the food and drug administration in the United States of America and the European medicines agency in Europe have established rigorous frameworks for clinical trials involving stem cells, ensuring patient safety and ethical compliance. Here the policies are refined by engaging with researchers and ethicist to refine policies that govern clinical applications.

Take Home Nuggets

- The implementation of regulations surrounding stem cell research present numerous challenges that can impede progress in this vital field. This is not made easy by the complexity and variability of existing laws across different jurisdictions. This inconsistency creates confusion among researchers and healthcare personnel who may have difficulty navigating the regulatory landscape.

- The moral status of stem cells is a pivotal topic in the realm of biomedical ethics particularly as it applies to stem cell research regulations. Integral to this ethical dilemma is the timing of the beginning of life and the manipulation of cellular materials that have the potential to develop into human beings.

- Various ethical frameworks, including utilitarianism, deontology and virtue ethics, provide different perspectives on the moral consideration owed to stem cells, complicating the regulatory landscape surrounding their use in research and therapy.

- Informed consent is a fundamental ethical principle in health care and biomedical research, underscoring the importance of autonomy for patients and research participants. The ethical considerations of autonomy in stem cell research are amplified by the diverse cultures, legal and social perspectives that exists globally.

- A key take away relating to regulatory oversight is that in countries like Canada and Australia, government oversight committees have been instrumental in creating robust frameworks that prioritise patient rights and ethical considerations. These committees often provide crucial oversight on clinical trials, ensuring that stem cell research aligns with ethical standards and public expectations. This governance not only safeguards patient rights but also bolsters public trust in the scientific community.

- The influence of public opinion on policy changes regarding stem cells research has been profound and multifaceted. In various countries public sentiment has acted as a catalyst for legislative reforms, shaping the regulatory landscape in significant ways. In the United States widespread advocacy for stem cell research led to increased federal funding and the establishment of guidelines that govern the ethical use of stem cells.

- Internationally, the impact of public opinion can also be observed in countries such as South Korea, the 2004 stem cell research scandal prompted a public outcry that led to stricter regulatory frameworks. This event underlined the importance of transparency and ethical compliance in stem cell research, as the public demanded accountability from researchers and regulatory bodies. Similarly, the United Kingdom's robust public engagement strategies surrounding stem cell research have fostered a more informed citizenry resulting in regulations that reflect societal values and ethical considerations.

- Scientific investigation into stem cell research is multifaceted and encompasses various sources that significantly influence the direction and scope of the scientific investigation. Governmental bodies which often serve as primary financiers, allocate taxpayers money to advance biomedical research initiatives. There funds are typically earmarked for projects that demonstrate potential for significant break through in medical treatment. The conditions surrounding these grants can impose strict regulatory compliance affecting how research is conducted and reported.

- Non-compliance with stem cell research regulations can have dire consequences for biomedical researchers and health care personnel alike. When institutions disregard established guidelines, the integrity of research is compromised, potentially leading to unethical practices and harmful outcomes for patients. The repercussions extend beyond individual researchers impacting the reputation of the institutions involved, which can face public backlash and loss of funding. Non-compliance can also result in legal ramifications including fines and restrictions on future research activities.

- The interactions between regulatory agencies and researchers in the field of stem cell research play a crucial role in shaping ethical practices and innovative advancements. Regulatory bodies such as the food and drug administration in the United States and the European medical agency (EMA) in Europe establish guidelines that researchers must adhere to ensure patient safety and ethical integrity. These agencies not only evaluate clinical trial applications but also monitor ongoing research to ensure compliance with established laws and regulations.

Chapter 6
The Concept of Personhood in Stem Cell Research

Definition and Historical Context

The concept of personhood is pivotal in the discourse surrounding stem cell research, as it raises profound ethical, legal, and philosophical questions. At its core, personhood refers to the status of an entity as a person, which carries with it a host of rights and moral considerations. Historically, this concept has evolved significantly, influenced by cultural, religious, and scientific developments. Understanding the historical context of personhood is essential for grasping its implications in contemporary biomedical practices, especially in stem cell research, where the origins of stem cells often intersect with debates about when life and personhood begin.

In the early 20th century, the definition of personhood was largely tied to biological and developmental milestones. This perspective was shaped by advancements in embryology and a growing understanding of human development. However, as stem cell research emerged in the latter half of the century, particularly with the advent of embryonic stem cells, traditional definitions began to be challenged. The scientific ability to manipulate and cultivate stem cells from very early embryos posed new questions about the moral status of these entities, which some argue should be afforded personhood rights from the moment of fertilisation.

Cultural perspectives also play a significant role in shaping definitions of personhood, as different societies and religions offer varying interpretations. In some cultures, personhood is conferred at conception, while in others, it may be associated with viability outside the womb or certain cognitive capacities. These differing views create a complex landscape that affects public opinion and policy decisions regarding stem cell research. Furthermore, the impact of religion cannot be overlooked, as many religious traditions influence beliefs about the sanctity of life and the moral implications of stem cell usage, often leading to polarised debates in the public sphere.

The ethical implications of personhood definitions extend to funding and governance in stem cell research. Concepts of personhood can significantly influence the allocation of resources, as funding bodies may be swayed by the prevailing moral and ethical frameworks that define personhood in their respective jurisdictions. Moreover, these definitions can affect regulatory approaches, with some countries adopting stringent laws that reflect conservative interpretations of personhood, while others embrace more liberal stances that permit broader research in regenerative medicine.

Finally, the intersection of disability rights and personhood in stem cell discourse presents an additional layer of complexity. Advocates for individuals with disabilities argue that personhood should not be contingent upon the absence of disability or the potential for certain capabilities. This perspective challenges traditional notions of what it means to be a person and calls for a more inclusive understanding that embraces diversity in human experience. As the field of stem cell research continues to advance, ongoing philosophical debates will likely shape both public perception and policymaking, underscoring the necessity for a nuanced examination of personhood in this vital area of biomedical ethics.

The Biological Basis for Personhood

The concept of personhood is fundamental when discussing the ethical dimensions of stem cell research. It serves as a philosophical foundation upon which various arguments for and against stem cell therapies are built. Understanding what constitutes a person biologically can lead to significant implications for the treatment of diseases and the development of regenerative medicine. This discussion often centres around the definitions of life and the stages of human development, which are contentious topics among scientists, ethicists, and the public alike.

Biologically, personhood can be examined through the lens of developmental biology, where the characteristics that define human life emerge. This includes discussions about the zygote, embryo, and foetus, and at what point they may acquire personhood status. The implications of these definitions extend into legal frameworks, affecting how stem cell research is regulated, and influencing funding opportunities. As such, the biological basis for personhood is not just an academic inquiry but one that has real-world consequences for the advancement of medical science and ethical practice.

Cultural perspectives also play a crucial role in shaping the understanding of personhood within the context of stem cell research. Different societies have varying beliefs regarding the onset of personhood, often influenced by religious views and moral philosophies. These perspectives can create a divide in public opinion and impact policy-making processes, making it essential for healthcare professionals and researchers to engage with these cultural narratives. Recognising the diverse opinions on personhood can foster a more inclusive dialogue about the ethical use of stem cells in medicine.

The intersection of disability rights and personhood adds another layer of complexity to the discourse. Many advocates argue that the definitions of personhood should include considerations of quality of life and the potential for suffering, particularly in the context of disabilities. This perspective challenges the traditional views of personhood, necessitating a more nuanced approach to stem cell therapies aimed at treating or preventing disabilities. Engaging with these concepts is vital for stem cell oversight bodies to ensure that policies reflect a comprehensive understanding of personhood that respects all individuals' rights.

In summary, the biological basis for personhood is a multifaceted topic that intertwines scientific inquiry with ethical, cultural, and political dimensions. The ongoing debates surrounding personhood in relation to stem cell research highlight the need for healthcare personnel and biomedical scientists to be well-informed about these issues. By understanding the implications of personhood definitions, stakeholders can better navigate the ethical challenges posed by stem cell therapies and contribute to a more informed public discourse.

Key Philosophical Theories

The concept of personhood in stem cell research is a profound philosophical inquiry that influences ethical, legal, and social discussions surrounding this field. Different philosophical theories outline what constitutes personhood, ranging from biological criteria to psychological characteristics. For instance, some theories suggest that personhood begins at conception, while others argue that it is linked to cognitive abilities or the capacity for self-awareness. This divergence in thought complicates the ethical landscape of stem cell research, particularly when considering the rights and moral status of embryos and stem cells.

Ethical implications of personhood are particularly significant in the context of stem cell therapy. The debate centres on whether embryos should be afforded the same moral considerations as living persons. This raises questions about the acceptability of using embryonic stem cells for research and therapy, especially if the potential benefits to patients are substantial. Moreover, healthcare personnel and biomedical scientists must navigate these ethical waters carefully, as their decisions can have far-reaching consequences on patient care and societal norms surrounding life and death.

Legal definitions of personhood also play a crucial role in shaping the regulatory framework for stem cell research. Various jurisdictions have adopted differing definitions, which impacts the legality of certain research practices. In some areas, legal personhood is granted at conception, while in others, it may not be recognised until viability outside the womb. These legal distinctions not only affect the funding and conduct of stem cell research but also influence public perception and policymaking in biotechnology.

Cultural perspectives on personhood further complicate the discourse on stem cell usage. Diverse belief systems and traditions shape how different societies view the beginning of life and the moral implications of manipulating human cells.

For example, religious perspectives often dictate the stance individuals and communities take on the use of embryonic stem cells, leading to significant variations in acceptance and support for research initiatives. Understanding these cultural dimensions is vital for stakeholders engaged in stem cell research and therapy.

Finally, philosophical debates surrounding personhood intersect with broader societal issues, including disability rights. The discussion often includes the rights of individuals with disabilities and how these intersect with the perceived status of embryos or stem cells. As arguments for and against personhood evolve, they inform funding priorities for stem cell research and influence how policies are crafted, reflecting the complex and multifaceted nature of this ongoing dialogue in regenerative medicine.

Ethical Implications of Personhood in Stem Cell Therapy

Moral Status of Embryos

The moral status of embryos is a complex and contentious issue within the realm of stem cell research, particularly as it pertains to the concept of personhood. This debate encompasses various ethical implications, particularly concerning the classification of embryos as potential persons or mere biological entities. In examining the moral consideration afforded to embryos, it is essential to navigate the philosophical arguments that assert personhood begins at conception versus those that posit it emerges at later developmental stages. This distinction has profound implications for the ethical frameworks guiding stem cell research and therapy.

Legal definitions of personhood significantly influence the moral status assigned to embryos in various jurisdictions. In some countries, laws may recognise embryos as persons with rights, while in others, they are not afforded such status until certain milestones of development are reached. This disparity reflects the cultural perspectives surrounding personhood, where societal values and religious beliefs play pivotal roles in shaping legal definitions. Understanding these legal contexts is crucial for healthcare personnel and biomedical scientists as they navigate the ethical landscape of stem cell research.

Cultural perspectives on personhood also highlight the diversity of opinions regarding the use of embryonic stem cells. In some cultures, the sanctity of life is paramount, leading to a strong opposition against any research involving embryos. In contrast, other cultures may prioritise the potential benefits of stem cell therapies for treating debilitating conditions. These varying viewpoints underscore the importance of engaging with different cultural narratives and the role they play in influencing public perceptions and policymaking in biotechnology.

Philosophical debates surrounding personhood and embryonic stem cells further complicate the moral landscape. The discourse often centres on questions of identity, autonomy, and moral agency. Proponents of embryonic stem cell research argue that the potential to alleviate suffering through scientific advancements outweighs the moral considerations associated with the embryo's status. Conversely, opponents assert that recognising the embryo's moral worth is essential to uphold ethical standards in medicine and research. This ongoing dialogue is critical in shaping the ethical frameworks that govern stem cell research practices.

Finally, the intersection of personhood concepts with disability rights adds another layer of complexity to the conversation. The discourse surrounding personhood must consider the implications for individuals with disabilities and how these definitions may affect funding and access to stem cell therapies. As policymaking continues to evolve in the field of biotechnology, understanding the nuanced implications of personhood, particularly in relation to vulnerable populations, will be essential for ensuring equitable and ethical advancements in regenerative medicine.

Ethical Considerations in Stem Cell Applications

The ethical considerations surrounding stem cell applications are deeply intertwined with the complex concept of personhood. This notion poses significant implications for how we define life, individuality, and moral status within the context of stem cell research and therapy. The varying interpretations of personhood can dramatically influence both public opinion and policymaking, particularly in relation to the use of embryonic stem cells. As health care personnel and biomedical scientists navigate these challenging waters, it is essential to engage with the diverse perspectives that shape our understanding of what it means to be a person in this scientific domain.

Legal definitions of personhood play a crucial role in regulating stem cell research. These definitions vary widely across jurisdictions, reflecting differing cultural and philosophical beliefs. In some regions, personhood may be ascribed at conception, while others may adopt a more fluid approach, recognising personhood at later developmental stages. Such legal frameworks not only impact the permissibility of various stem cell applications but also influence funding opportunities and research directions. As oversight bodies consider these definitions, they must balance scientific innovation with ethical responsibility.

Cultural perspectives on personhood further complicate the discourse surrounding stem cell usage. In many societies, religious beliefs significantly shape views on the sanctity of life and the moral implications of manipulating human cells. For instance, certain religious doctrines may oppose embryonic research altogether, while others might advocate for its potential to alleviate suffering. This cultural landscape necessitates that biomedical professionals remain sensitive to the beliefs of the communities they serve, ensuring that their practices align with broader societal values while advancing scientific progress.

Philosophical debates about personhood also fuel the ongoing dialogue within stem cell ethics. Questions about what constitutes personhood—be it consciousness, capacity for relationships, or biological markers—are critical to understanding the moral status of embryos and stem cells. These discussions not only inform ethical guidelines but also impact public perceptions and acceptance of regenerative medicine. Engaging with these philosophical inquiries allows health care professionals and researchers to navigate the ethical complexities inherent in their work effectively.

Finally, the intersection of disability rights and personhood in stem cell discourse raises important ethical questions about inclusivity and the value of diverse human experiences. As advancements in regenerative medicine hold the promise of curing or alleviating disabilities, it is vital to consider how personhood definitions may marginalise certain individuals or communities. Fostering an inclusive dialogue that respects the dignity of all persons, regardless of ability, is essential in shaping a future where stem cell applications are ethically sound and socially responsible.

Balancing Benefits and Risks

The discussion surrounding stem cell research often revolves around the delicate balance between the potential benefits and the associated risks. As healthcare personnel and biomedical scientists navigate this complex landscape, it is crucial to consider not only the scientific advancements but also the ethical implications tied to the concept of personhood. This balance requires careful consideration of the moral status attributed to stem cells, as well as the potential for innovative therapies that could transform patient care and improve quality of life.

The ethical implications of personhood in stem cell therapy present a multifaceted challenge. On one hand, the promise of regenerative medicine offers hope for treating previously incurable conditions, raising questions about the moral weight of the entities involved in research. On the other hand, the various definitions of personhood can lead to significant ethical dilemmas, as differing perspectives may either support or oppose certain research practices, thereby affecting the direction of scientific inquiry and funding.

Legal definitions of personhood play a critical role in shaping the regulatory landscape for stem cell research. Legislation varies widely across different jurisdictions, with some countries affording embryos a high degree of moral consideration, while others adopt a more permissive stance towards research. Understanding these legal frameworks is essential for oversight bodies and researchers alike, as they navigate the ethical terrain and seek to align their practices with both scientific goals and societal values.

Cultural perspectives on personhood also influence public perceptions and policy-making in the realm of biotechnology. In many societies, religious beliefs significantly shape attitudes towards stem cell research, leading to diverse interpretations of when life begins and the moral implications of manipulating embryonic cells. Engaging with these cultural narratives is vital for fostering dialogue and consensus, as it can help bridge the divide between scientific advancement and ethical considerations in healthcare.

Ultimately, the intersection of personhood concepts and disability rights adds another layer of complexity to the discourse surrounding stem cell research. Advocates for individuals with disabilities often argue for a more inclusive understanding of personhood that recognises the value of all lives, regardless of their biological status. This nuanced perspective can inform policymaking and funding decisions, ensuring that the benefits of stem cell research are accessible to all, while also considering the ethical ramifications of how personhood is defined and applied in practice.

Legal Definitions of Personhood in Relation to Stem Cell Research

Overview of Legal Frameworks

The legal frameworks surrounding stem cell research and the concept of personhood are complex and multifaceted. These frameworks are shaped by various ethical, cultural, and philosophical considerations that influence how personhood is defined and understood. In many jurisdictions, the legal definitions of personhood vary significantly, reflecting differing societal values and beliefs about when life begins and what constitutes moral consideration. This diversity in legal perspectives poses challenges for researchers and healthcare professionals navigating the regulatory landscape of stem cell therapies.

In the context of stem cell research, the ethical implications of personhood are particularly significant. Stakeholders must grapple with the moral status of embryos and the ethical considerations of utilising stem cells derived from them. The discourse often involves weighing the potential benefits of stem cell therapies against the rights of what some consider potential persons. As such, the legal frameworks must not only address scientific and medical concerns but also engage with ethical arguments that arise from competing views on personhood.

Cultural perspectives on personhood significantly influence the legal landscape of stem cell research. Different cultures may hold varying beliefs regarding the moral status of embryos and the ethicality of stem cell research. For instance, some cultures may view embryonic stem cells as equivalent to human life, while others may not. These cultural beliefs can affect public opinion and, consequently, the legislative processes that govern stem cell research, leading to disparities in how laws are enacted and enforced across different regions.

Philosophical debates surrounding personhood also play a crucial role in shaping the legal frameworks for stem cell research. Questions about what it means to be a person and the criteria that confer personhood are central to these discussions. Philosophers have proposed various definitions of personhood, ranging from biological criteria to psychological characteristics. These debates often inform legal definitions and can influence policymakers as they craft legislation that seeks to balance scientific advancement with ethical considerations.

Finally, the intersection of religion and personhood in stem cell ethics cannot be overlooked. Religious beliefs often shape individuals' and societies' views on the sanctity of life and the moral implications of using stem cells in research. This intersection can lead to varied interpretations of personhood, which directly impacts funding for stem cell research and public perceptions of regenerative medicine. As society continues to grapple with these complex issues, the legal frameworks governing stem cell research will likely evolve in response to ongoing ethical, cultural, and philosophical discourses.

Variations in National Legislation

The concept of personhood in the realm of stem cell research is significantly influenced by variations in national legislation. Different countries approach the definition and implications of personhood in diverse ways, which consequently shapes their legal frameworks regarding stem cell research and therapy. For instance, some nations may confer personhood status from the moment of conception, thereby imposing strict regulations on the use of embryonic stem cells. In contrast, others may adopt a more permissive stance, allowing broader research opportunities that seek to balance ethical considerations with scientific advancements.

Ethical implications stemming from these legislative variations are profound, as they influence not only the legal landscape but also public perception and acceptance of stem cell therapies. Countries that recognise a higher degree of personhood may face resistance from both the public and medical communities when proposing new stem cell treatments. Conversely, nations with more liberal definitions may encourage innovation, attracting funding and fostering an environment conducive to scientific discovery. This dichotomy highlights the importance of understanding how ethical principles are interpreted within different legislative contexts.

Cultural perspectives play a critical role in shaping national legislation on personhood and stem cell usage. In societies where religious beliefs strongly inform moral viewpoints, there may be stringent restrictions on research involving embryonic stem cells or cloning. Countries with a secular approach, however, might be more open to exploring the potential of stem cell therapies, reflecting a prioritisation of scientific progress over religious considerations. This cultural backdrop not only affects legislation but also influences the debate surrounding personhood, ethics, and the rights of individuals with disabilities in the context of regenerative medicine.

Philosophical debates surrounding personhood are also central to the legal discourse on stem cell research. These debates often intersect with disability rights, as the definitions of personhood can have significant implications for individuals with disabilities and their access to innovative treatments. Legal definitions that exclude certain populations from the category of personhood may lead to ethical dilemmas regarding the allocation of resources and funding for stem cell research, raising questions about inclusivity and equity in healthcare.

Ultimately, the variations in national legislation regarding personhood and stem cell research underscore the complex interplay between ethics, law, culture, and philosophy. As health care personnel, biomedical scientists, and oversight bodies navigate this landscape, they must consider how differing legal definitions impact not only scientific progress but also the broader societal implications of stem cell therapies. Understanding these variations is crucial for fostering informed dialogue and responsible policymaking in the field of biotechnology.

Case Studies of Legal Challenges

The exploration of personhood in stem cell research has led to numerous legal challenges across various jurisdictions. In the United States, significant cases such as Roe v. Wade have established a precedent for the rights of embryos, leading to ongoing debates about when personhood begins. These legal battles often hinge on the interpretation of the law concerning the rights of the unborn and the implications for stem cell research funding. As healthcare personnel and biomedical scientists navigate this landscape, understanding these cases is crucial for addressing the ethical and legal dimensions of their work.

In Europe, the legal definitions of personhood vary significantly, impacting the regulatory environment for stem cell research. For instance, the European Union's Charter of Fundamental Rights does not explicitly recognise the embryo as a person, allowing for broader research opportunities compared to countries where embryos are afforded full legal protection. Such differences underscore the importance of cultural perspectives in shaping the legal framework surrounding stem cell research. This interplay between legal definitions and cultural beliefs plays a vital role in determining how stem cell therapies are developed and implemented across different regions.

The influence of religious beliefs on personhood definitions cannot be overstated, particularly in jurisdictions where faith plays a pivotal role in legislative processes. In many cases, religious groups advocate for the recognition of embryos as persons, arguing that this status should protect them from research exploitation. This has led to significant pushback against funding for stem cell research in countries where religious views dominate public policy. Understanding these dynamics is essential for healthcare professionals and researchers who must navigate these complex moral landscapes while pursuing scientific advancement.

Moreover, the intersection of disability rights and personhood presents another layer of complexity in legal challenges surrounding stem cell research. Advocates for disability rights argue that the focus on personhood can inadvertently devalue individuals with disabilities, shifting the narrative towards a more exclusionary understanding of life and worth. This has spurred legal actions aimed at ensuring that stem cell research does not undermine the rights and dignity of disabled individuals, thus highlighting the need for inclusive discussions about personhood in the context of regenerative medicine.

Ultimately, the ongoing philosophical debates surrounding personhood and embryonic stem cells continue to shape the legal landscape of stem cell research. These discussions influence public perception and, consequently, policymaking in biotechnology. As healthcare personnel and oversight bodies engage with these complex issues, they must remain informed about the evolving legal definitions of personhood and their implications for research funding, ethical considerations, and societal values in the realm of stem cell therapy.

Cultural Perspectives on Personhood and Stem Cell Usage

Influence of Cultural Norms

Cultural norms play a pivotal role in shaping the discourse surrounding personhood, particularly in the context of stem cell research. Different societies hold varying beliefs about the beginning of life, which directly influence their ethical stance towards embryonic and adult stem cell usage. In cultures where life is viewed as beginning at conception, any manipulation of embryos can evoke strong moral objections, leading to policies that restrict research funding and advancements in regenerative medicine. Conversely, cultures with a more liberal interpretation of personhood may advocate for the potential benefits of stem cell therapies, prioritising scientific progress over traditional views of life.

The ethical implications of personhood are further complicated by the intersection of cultural perspectives and legal definitions. In some jurisdictions, personhood is legally recognised at various stages of development, impacting the regulatory landscape for stem cell research. This legal framework often reflects the dominant cultural attitudes, creating a complex web of ethical considerations that healthcare personnel and biomedical scientists must navigate. Understanding these cultural underpinnings is essential for professionals involved in stem cell research, as they directly influence both practice and policy.

Moreover, philosophical debates surrounding personhood often reflect broader cultural narratives, encompassing religious beliefs, societal values, and historical context. The role of religion cannot be overstated; it shapes individual and collective perceptions of personhood and has been a significant factor in the opposition to certain stem cell research practices. This influence is evident in public discourse and policymaking, as religious groups frequently mobilise to advocate for restrictive measures against embryonic research, citing the sanctity of life as a paramount concern.

Public perceptions of personhood also impact funding for stem cell research, as societal attitudes can dictate governmental and private investment. When personhood is viewed through a lens of potential medical advancement, funding may be more readily available; however, when ethical concerns overshadow scientific promise, researchers may face significant obstacles. This dynamic highlights the necessity for continued public education and dialogue regarding the benefits of stem cell therapies, particularly in areas where cultural resistance is strong.

Finally, the comparative analysis of personhood definitions across global legislative frameworks reveals a diverse landscape influenced by cultural norms. These differences not only affect the permissibility of stem cell research but also highlight the importance of inclusive discussions that consider the intersections of disability rights and personhood. As the field of regenerative medicine continues to evolve, an understanding of these cultural influences will be critical for healthcare personnel, biomedical scientists, and stem cell oversight bodies in fostering ethical and effective practices in research.

Case Studies from Different Cultures

The exploration of personhood in relation to stem cell research varies significantly across different cultures, reflecting diverse ethical, philosophical, and religious beliefs. In Japan, for instance, the cultural emphasis on harmony and collective well-being influences perceptions of personhood. Here, stem cell research is often viewed through the lens of societal benefit, where the potential to alleviate suffering is prioritised over the moral status of the embryo. This cultural perspective encourages a more utilitarian approach to the ethical dilemmas posed by stem cell therapies, allowing for broader acceptance of scientific advancements in regenerative medicine.

In contrast, many Latin American countries exhibit a strong alignment between personhood and religious beliefs, particularly within Catholic communities. The legal definitions of personhood in these regions often extend protection to embryos from the moment of conception. Consequently, stem cell research faces significant scrutiny and legal hurdles. The ethical implications of this perspective challenge healthcare personnel and policymakers to navigate a complex landscape where religious doctrine profoundly influences public opinion and legislative frameworks surrounding biotechnological advancements.

Furthermore, in the context of Western cultures, particularly in the United States and parts of Europe, the debates surrounding personhood are often polarised. These discussions encompass a wide range of philosophical arguments, from those advocating for embryonic stem cells based on the potential for life-saving therapies, to those who argue for the moral status of the embryo as a person. The intersection of these views significantly impacts funding opportunities for research, as public perception and legislative support are often swayed by the prevailing definitions of personhood.

Additionally, perspectives on personhood can also reflect an intersection with disability rights movements. In various cultures, the discourse surrounding disability and personhood challenges traditional views, prompting a re-evaluation of what it means to be a person. This evolving understanding can influence ethical considerations in stem cell research, particularly in how therapies are developed and accessed by individuals with disabilities. Engaging with this dimension is crucial for biomedical scientists and oversight bodies to ensure that innovations in stem cell therapy are inclusive and equitable.

Ultimately, the comparative analysis of personhood definitions across cultures provides invaluable insights into the ethical landscape of stem cell research. By examining case studies from different cultural contexts, healthcare personnel and policymakers can better understand the implications of their decisions on both scientific progress and societal values. This cultural sensitivity can foster a more nuanced dialogue about personhood and its ethical dimensions, paving the way for more informed and respectful approaches to stem cell research and therapy across the globe.

The Role of Public Discourse

Public discourse plays a vital role in shaping the ethical landscape surrounding stem cell research, particularly concerning the concept of personhood. As health care personnel and biomedical scientists engage in discussions about the implications of personhood, they contribute to a broader understanding of how these definitions influence research and therapy. The dialogue surrounding personhood is not merely academic; it has tangible effects on policy-making and public perception, making it essential for stakeholders to actively participate in these conversations.

The ethical implications of personhood in stem cell therapy are profound, often igniting fierce debates among various groups. Different cultural perspectives contribute to diverse definitions of personhood, influencing how individuals and communities perceive the moral status of embryos and stem cells. As such, public discourse becomes a platform where these varying perspectives can be articulated and examined, allowing for a more nuanced understanding of the ethical dimensions involved in stem cell research.

Legal definitions of personhood also play a crucial role in the discourse, as they directly impact regulatory frameworks governing stem cell research. Health care professionals and oversight bodies must navigate these legal landscapes, which can vary significantly across jurisdictions. Engaging in public discourse allows these stakeholders to advocate for legal definitions that align with ethical considerations and scientific advancements, ensuring that regulations support rather than hinder innovation in regenerative medicine.

Philosophical debates surrounding personhood, particularly in relation to embryonic stem cells, are further enriched by public engagement. As society grapples with questions of identity and moral worth, the role of religion and its influence on personhood beliefs cannot be overlooked. By participating in public discussions, stakeholders can highlight how these philosophical and religious perspectives inform policies and funding decisions related to stem cell research.

Ultimately, the intersection of personhood concepts with disability rights and public perceptions significantly influences the future of stem cell research. As the discourse evolves, it is crucial for health care personnel, scientists, and policymakers to remain engaged and informed. This ongoing dialogue not only shapes the ethical framework of stem cell research but also impacts funding, policymaking, and the general societal acceptance of regenerative medicine.

Philosophical Debates Surrounding Personhood and Embryonic Stem Cells

Major Philosophical Arguments

In the realm of stem cell research, the concept of personhood serves as a pivotal issue, prompting extensive philosophical debates. Major philosophical arguments centre around the definition of when personhood begins, which is often anchored in biological, psychological, and social dimensions. Some argue that personhood commences at conception, while others propose that it emerges at later developmental stages. This divergence in perspectives significantly influences ethical considerations and research practices in the field, particularly as it pertains to embryonic stem cells.

Ethical implications of personhood in stem cell therapy are profound, as they dictate the moral status of embryos and their use in research. Those who advocate for a strict definition of personhood from conception often oppose the utilisation of embryonic stem cells, viewing it as morally unacceptable. Conversely, proponents of a more expansive definition argue for the therapeutic potential of stem cells in alleviating suffering, highlighting the benefits that could arise from such research. This ethical dichotomy directly impacts the framework within which stem cell research operates, influencing both scientific inquiry and clinical application.

Legal definitions of personhood vary significantly across jurisdictions, which adds another layer of complexity to the conversation. In some countries, laws affirm personhood from conception, while others adopt a more permissive stance that allows for stem cell research under certain conditions. These legal frameworks not only reflect cultural attitudes towards personhood but also shape the regulatory environment for stem cell research. Understanding these legal variations is essential for health care personnel and biomedical scientists, as they navigate the ethical landscape of their work.

Cultural perspectives on personhood further complicate the discourse, as different societies hold diverse beliefs about the beginning of life and the moral implications of stem cell research. In many cultures, religious beliefs play a crucial role in shaping these views, influencing public opinion and policymaking. The intersection of religion and personhood can lead to significant disparities in how stem cell research is perceived and funded, impacting the availability of resources for scientific advancement in various contexts.

Lastly, the impact of personhood concepts on funding for stem cell research cannot be overlooked. As funding bodies assess the ethical ramifications of their investments, they often consider prevailing public perceptions and philosophical debates regarding personhood. This interplay between ethical discourse and financial support ultimately influences the trajectory of stem cell research and its potential contributions to regenerative medicine. Engaging in these philosophical arguments is vital for stakeholders in the field, as it not only shapes policy but also informs the ethical foundations of biomedical practice.

Theories of Identity and Consciousness

The theories of identity and consciousness play a pivotal role in shaping the discourse surrounding personhood, particularly in the context of stem cell research. These theories explore the essence of what it means to be a person, delving into the complexities of consciousness and self-awareness. In the realm of biomedical science, understanding these concepts is essential for addressing ethical implications that arise when considering the use of stem cells. By comprehending the nuances of identity, healthcare personnel and oversight bodies can better navigate the moral landscapes of stem cell therapy, ensuring that practices align with ethical standards and societal values.

Philosophical debates surrounding personhood and embryonic stem cells further complicate the narrative. Different philosophical frameworks offer varied definitions of personhood, each with its own implications for the ethical treatment of stem cells. Some argue that personhood begins at conception, while others suggest it emerges during later developmental stages. This divergence in thought influences not only ethical considerations but also legal definitions of personhood, impacting regulations and policies related to stem cell research. A thorough understanding of these philosophical underpinnings is crucial for professionals involved in stem cell oversight and research.

Cultural perspectives also significantly influence the conversation about personhood in stem cell usage. Diverse beliefs and values across cultures lead to varying interpretations of what constitutes a person and, consequently, the moral status of stem cells. Healthcare personnel must be cognisant of these cultural dimensions when engaging with patients and communities about stem cell therapies. Additionally, these perspectives can shape public perceptions and influence funding for stem cell research, as societal values often dictate the prioritisation of certain types of research over others.

Religion plays an instrumental role in shaping views on personhood and stem cell ethics. Many religious beliefs articulate specific views on the beginning of life, which can directly influence opinions on the ethical acceptability of stem cell research. For instance, certain faiths may oppose embryonic stem cell research based on their beliefs regarding the sanctity of life. Understanding these religious perspectives is vital for healthcare professionals and policymakers, as they navigate the complexities of public sentiment and ethical considerations in stem cell research.

Lastly, the intersection of disability rights and personhood in stem cell discourse highlights the need for inclusive discussions about identity and ethics. The implications of personhood concepts extend to how we view individuals with disabilities, raising important questions about equality and access to stem cell therapies. This dialogue is crucial for ensuring that all voices are heard in the policymaking process, ultimately fostering a more equitable approach to biotechnology and regenerative medicine. Addressing these multifaceted issues requires a collaborative effort among healthcare personnel, biomedical scientists, and oversight bodies to ensure that the ethical dimensions of personhood are respected and upheld in stem cell research.

Implications for Policy and Ethics

The ethical landscape surrounding stem cell research is complex and deeply intertwined with the concept of personhood. As healthcare personnel, biomedical scientists, and oversight bodies engage with this intricate subject, it becomes apparent that definitions of personhood significantly influence ethical considerations. The implications for policy are profound, as varying interpretations can lead to divergent approaches in regulating stem cell research and therapy. Understanding the philosophical underpinnings of personhood is essential for developing ethical frameworks that guide research practices and clinical applications.

Legal definitions of personhood vary widely across jurisdictions, impacting the governance of stem cell research. In some regions, embryos are granted full personhood status, while others consider them as potential life without legal recognition. This disparity creates challenges for researchers, who must navigate a patchwork of laws that can stifle innovation or, conversely, lead to ethical oversights. Policymakers must carefully evaluate these legal definitions to create harmonised regulations that uphold both scientific advancement and ethical integrity in stem cell research.

Cultural perspectives on personhood also play a critical role in shaping public perceptions of stem cell usage. Different societies may hold varied beliefs about the moral status of embryos, influenced by historical, religious, and social contexts. These cultural attitudes can sway public opinion, impacting funding decisions and the prioritisation of research agendas. It is crucial for scientists and policymakers to engage with these cultural narratives to foster a more inclusive dialogue around stem cell ethics that respects diverse viewpoints while advancing scientific knowledge.

The interplay between personhood and funding for stem cell research cannot be overlooked. Funding bodies often align their support with prevailing ethical views, which are themselves shaped by public perception and cultural attitudes. This can create a cycle where ethical considerations dictate financial resources, potentially limiting the scope of research that can be pursued. As such, it is essential for stakeholders to advocate for balanced funding mechanisms that support innovative research while considering the ethical implications of personhood.

Finally, the influence of personhood arguments on policymaking in biotechnology is significant. Policymakers must grapple with the philosophical debates surrounding the moral and ethical status of embryos when crafting legislation. These discussions often extend into the realm of disability rights, where personhood definitions can affect the rights and dignity of individuals with disabilities. As society moves forward, it is imperative that the implications of personhood are thoughtfully integrated into the policy framework to ensure that ethical considerations remain at the forefront of stem cell research and therapy.

The Role of Religion in Shaping Views on Personhood in Stem Cell Ethics

Overview of Key Religious Perspectives

The concept of personhood is a pivotal topic within the realm of stem cell research, influencing various ethical and legal discussions. Different religious perspectives provide foundational insights into how personhood is defined, impacting policies and practices in biomedical science. For many faith traditions, personhood is associated with the belief that life begins at conception, thereby attributing moral value and rights to embryos. This belief frequently shapes the ethical framework within which stem cell therapies are considered, particularly when the source of stem cells involves the destruction of embryos.

In the Christian tradition, particularly within Catholic doctrine, the belief is that human life commences at the moment of fertilisation. This perspective leads to a strong opposition against embryonic stem cell research, as it is seen as violating the sanctity of life. Conversely, some Protestant denominations may adopt a more nuanced approach, allowing for the use of stem cells derived from embryos that are no longer viable or intended for implantation. This variability highlights the need for healthcare personnel to understand the diverse religious beliefs that inform their patients' views and decisions regarding stem cell therapies.

Judaism also offers a significant viewpoint on personhood, where interpretations may vary between Orthodox, Conservative, and Reform branches. Generally, Jewish law emphasises the value of life and the potential of the embryo but may allow for stem cell research under certain conditions, particularly when it aligns with the preservation of life. Such perspectives illustrate the complexities involved in the ethical debates surrounding stem cell research, where religious beliefs can both support and challenge scientific advancement.

Islamic teachings further complicate the discourse on personhood and stem cell research. The Islamic view often holds that the soul is infused into the embryo at a certain stage, which varies among scholars; thus, this influences the permissibility of using embryonic stem cells. The intersection of religious ethics and biomedical science necessitates a collaborative approach, where healthcare providers engage with patients' beliefs to navigate the ethical landscape of stem cell research effectively.

Ultimately, the role of religion in shaping views on personhood in stem cell ethics cannot be understated. As healthcare personnel and biomedical scientists engage in research and therapeutic applications, understanding these religious perspectives is crucial. The ongoing dialogue between science, ethics, and faith will continue to influence public perceptions and policymaking in biotechnology, highlighting the importance of respect and sensitivity towards diverse beliefs in this evolving field.

Influence of Religious Beliefs on Policy

The intersection of religious beliefs and policymaking in the realm of stem cell research is a complex and often contentious issue. Religious doctrines profoundly shape the understanding of personhood, which in turn influences legislative frameworks and health care practices. Various faith traditions offer differing interpretations of when life begins, which significantly impacts how stem cell research is viewed and regulated. For health care personnel and biomedical scientists, navigating these beliefs is crucial to ensuring ethical compliance and fostering respectful dialogues with diverse patient populations.

In many cultures, religious beliefs serve as a moral compass, guiding opinions on the ethical implications of personhood in stem cell therapy. For instance, certain groups may advocate for the sanctity of life from conception, arguing against the use of embryonic stem cells. This perspective often leads to calls for stringent regulations or outright bans on specific research practices. Conversely, other religious perspectives may emphasise the potential for healing and the moral obligation to alleviate suffering through scientific advancements, thereby supporting a more permissive stance towards stem cell research.

Legal definitions of personhood are heavily influenced by religious thought, which complicates the creation of uniform policies across different jurisdictions. In some countries, laws reflect the religious majority's beliefs, resulting in restrictive measures on stem cell research. In contrast, secular legal frameworks may adopt a more liberal approach, allowing for a broader scope of research opportunities. This disparity in legal definitions raises critical questions about the rights of embryos and foetuses, positioning religious beliefs at the forefront of policy debates.

Public perceptions of personhood in relation to regenerative medicine are often shaped by religious narratives, which can either support or hinder funding for stem cell research. When faith-based organisations advocate for research initiatives, they can mobilise substantial resources and public support. However, opposition from religious groups can lead to financial and legislative obstacles, impacting the progress of scientific inquiry. Thus, understanding the religious landscape is essential for stakeholders involved in stem cell research to secure necessary funding and navigate potential roadblocks effectively.

The philosophical debates surrounding personhood and the role of religion in shaping these views are critical in informing policymaking in biotechnology. As discussions evolve, it becomes increasingly important for health care professionals and policymakers to engage with diverse religious perspectives to foster an inclusive approach to personhood. By doing so, they can ensure that policies reflect a comprehensive understanding of ethical dimensions in stem cell research, ultimately contributing to a more nuanced dialogue that respects both scientific advancement and individual belief systems.

Interfaith Dialogues on Stem Cell Issues

Interfaith dialogues on stem cell issues provide a crucial platform for discussing the ethical implications of personhood in stem cell research. Different religious traditions offer diverse perspectives on the beginning of life and the moral status of embryos. For instance, while some faiths may regard embryos as persons from conception, others might adopt a more nuanced view, allowing for the exploration of stem cell therapies under certain ethical guidelines. This diversity of beliefs necessitates respectful dialogue among healthcare personnel, biomedical scientists, and oversight bodies to navigate these complex issues effectively.

The intersection of religion and ethics in stem cell research highlights the need for a clear understanding of how personhood is defined across various cultures. In many traditions, the concept of personhood is often intertwined with spiritual beliefs, which influences how individuals and communities perceive the use of stem cells. Engaging with these cultural perspectives can foster a more comprehensive approach to policymaking, ensuring that legislation surrounding stem cell research reflects a balance between scientific advancement and ethical considerations rooted in diverse beliefs.

Philosophical debates surrounding the concept of personhood further complicate discussions in stem cell ethics. Scholars and ethicists often challenge the parameters of what constitutes a person, raising questions about the moral implications of using embryonic stem cells for research and therapy. These debates can shape public perceptions significantly, as they influence how society views the potential of regenerative medicine. Engaging in interfaith dialogues can help clarify these philosophical positions, allowing for a more informed public discourse.

Legal definitions of personhood in relation to stem cell research vary widely across jurisdictions and have significant implications for funding and regulation. Different countries have adopted various stances on the ethical boundaries of stem cell research, often reflecting the dominant cultural and religious beliefs of their populations. By fostering interfaith discussions, stakeholders can better understand these legal landscapes and work towards creating policies that respect both scientific inquiry and ethical standards.

Ultimately, the role of interfaith dialogue in addressing stem cell issues cannot be underestimated. By bringing together diverse perspectives, these conversations can lead to more inclusive and ethically sound approaches to stem cell research. As healthcare personnel, biomedical scientists, and oversight bodies engage in this dialogue, they can contribute to the development of frameworks that respect personhood while promoting scientific innovation in regenerative medicine.

The Impact of Personhood Concepts on Funding for Stem Cell Research

Funding Landscape and Personhood

The funding landscape for stem cell research is markedly influenced by the evolving concept of personhood. As ethical debates continue to shape the discourse surrounding stem cells, particularly embryonic stem cells, funding bodies are increasingly scrutinising the implications of personhood on their financial support. Institutions and organisations that allocate funding often grapple with the ethical dilemmas posed by the potential classification of embryos as persons, which can significantly alter the trajectory and feasibility of research projects. Consequently, researchers must navigate these complex ethical landscapes to secure necessary funding while adhering to regulatory requirements and institutional policies.

The ethical implications of personhood extend beyond the mere allocation of resources; they also affect the public perception of stem cell therapies. As various cultural perspectives inform the understanding of personhood, researchers and healthcare professionals must engage in dialogue that addresses these nuances. The diverse beliefs surrounding the beginning of life and the moral status of embryos can lead to varying levels of acceptance or resistance to funding stem cell research. This cultural context is crucial, as it shapes stakeholder expectations and influences the priorities of funding agencies.

Legal definitions of personhood also play a significant role in the funding landscape for stem cell research. In various jurisdictions, laws that define when personhood begins can either facilitate or hinder research efforts. For instance, in regions where embryos are granted full personhood status, funding may be more restrictive, limiting the scope of permissible research. Alternatively, in areas with more liberal definitions, researchers may find greater financial support. Understanding these legal frameworks is essential for researchers, as they must align their proposals with the prevailing legal and ethical standards to secure funding.

Philosophical debates surrounding personhood further complicate the landscape of stem cell research funding. Differing philosophical views on what constitutes personhood can lead to conflicting positions on funding allocation. Some argue for a more inclusive definition that encompasses embryos, while others advocate for a more restrictive approach that prioritises the potential for human life. These philosophical disputes not only impact individual funding decisions but also influence broader policymaking within the realm of biotechnology and regenerative medicine.

Finally, the intersection of personhood concepts with public perceptions and disability rights is a critical area for consideration in the funding landscape. As the discourse evolves, advocates for disability rights remind us that personhood should encompass a broader understanding of human dignity and potential. This intersection challenges traditional narratives and calls for a re-evaluation of how funding bodies approach stem cell research. As public perceptions shift, funding agencies may need to adapt their strategies to reflect a more inclusive understanding of personhood, ensuring that all voices are heard in the ongoing ethical debates surrounding stem cell research.

Ethical Funding Practices

Ethical funding practices in stem cell research are crucial for ensuring that advancements in regenerative medicine align with societal values and ethical standards. Funding sources can significantly influence the direction of research, often reflecting the underlying beliefs about personhood and the moral status of embryos. As health care personnel and biomedical scientists navigate these waters, it is essential to critically assess not only the financial implications but also the ethical ramifications of funding decisions.

The concept of personhood plays a pivotal role in shaping funding strategies for stem cell research. Divergent views on when personhood begins can result in disagreements over the appropriateness of using embryonic stem cells. Consequently, funding bodies may establish criteria that either support or restrict research based on their interpretation of personhood, which in turn affects the scope and progress of scientific inquiry in this field.

Legal definitions of personhood vary significantly across jurisdictions, impacting the regulatory landscape for stem cell research funding. In some regions, personhood laws may impose strict limitations on the use of embryos for research, deterring potential investors and institutions from supporting projects that could lead to significant breakthroughs in regenerative medicine. Understanding these legal frameworks is essential for stakeholders aiming to navigate the complexities of funding and research effectively.

Cultural perspectives on personhood also shape the ethical funding practices in stem cell research. Different communities hold unique beliefs and values that influence their views on the moral implications of stem cell usage. Funding organisations must consider these cultural contexts to foster public trust and ensure that their financial contributions align with the ethical expectations of the communities they serve.

Finally, the intersection of disability rights and personhood in stem cell discourse highlights the need for inclusive funding practices. By engaging with a diverse range of perspectives, funding bodies can promote research that not only advances scientific knowledge but also respects the dignity and rights of all individuals. This approach not only encourages ethical funding practices but also supports a more comprehensive understanding of personhood in the context of stem cell research.

Case Studies of Funding Outcomes

Case studies of funding outcomes in stem cell research reveal significant variations based on the perceptions of personhood and its ethical implications. In regions where a more permissive understanding of personhood exists, funding for innovative stem cell therapies tends to flourish. These environments often encourage collaboration between public and private sectors, leading to substantial investment in research and development. For instance, countries that recognise the potential of embryonic stem cells often see increased grants and financial support, resulting in breakthroughs that can enhance medical treatment options.

Conversely, in jurisdictions where personhood is strictly defined or where ethical concerns dominate the discourse, funding can be severely restricted. Regulatory bodies may impose stringent guidelines that limit the scope of research, creating an environment of uncertainty for investors and researchers alike. Such constraints can hinder the progress of promising stem cell therapies, leaving potential advancements in medical science unrealised. This dichotomy highlights the critical role that legal and ethical definitions of personhood play in shaping the funding landscape for stem cell research.

Cultural perspectives also significantly influence funding outcomes in stem cell research. In societies where religious beliefs strongly dictate views on personhood, funding may be directed away from certain types of research, particularly those involving embryonic stem cells. These cultural attitudes can lead to public resistance against funding initiatives that are perceived as ethically contentious. As a result, researchers must navigate a complex landscape of cultural sensitivities when seeking financial support for their projects.

The intersection of personhood concepts and funding is particularly evident in public perceptions of stem cell research. Campaigns aimed at educating the public about the potential benefits of stem cell therapies can positively influence funding decisions. When the public is informed and supportive, policymakers are more likely to allocate funds towards research that aligns with those views. Thus, the success of funding initiatives often hinges on the ability to engage effectively with the public and address their concerns regarding the ethical implications of stem cell research.

Lastly, the influence of personhood arguments extends to policymaking in biotechnology. Policymakers must balance ethical concerns with the potential for scientific advancement, often leading to compromises that can affect funding allocations. By analysing case studies where funding outcomes were directly influenced by personhood debates, stakeholders can better understand the intricate relationship between ethics, culture, and finance in stem cell research. This understanding is crucial for navigating the complexities of funding in a field that is continuously evolving.

Public Perceptions of Personhood in Relation to Regenerative Medicine

Surveys and Public Opinion Studies

Surveys and public opinion studies play a crucial role in understanding the evolving perceptions of personhood in the context of stem cell research. These studies gather insights from various segments of the population, including healthcare personnel, biomedical scientists, and the public. By examining these perspectives, researchers can identify the ethical implications that influence public sentiment and policymaking in this sensitive area of biotechnology. The findings often reveal significant variations based on demographic factors such as age, education, and cultural background, which can shape responses to the complex issues surrounding personhood.

In the realm of stem cell therapy, ethical implications are deeply intertwined with public opinions on personhood. Surveys often reflect a spectrum of beliefs, with some individuals advocating for the sanctity of life from conception, while others prioritise the potential benefits of regenerative medicine for those suffering from debilitating conditions. These differing viewpoints highlight the moral dilemmas faced by researchers and policymakers alike, as they navigate the challenging landscape of ethical decision-making in stem cell research. Public opinion can sway funding priorities and influence the direction of scientific inquiry, making it imperative to understand the underlying beliefs that drive these opinions.

Legal definitions of personhood, as they relate to stem cell research, are also shaped by public perception. Surveys can illuminate how different segments of society interpret laws regarding the status of embryos and stem cells. The legal framework surrounding personhood varies across jurisdictions, and public opinion can play a pivotal role in shaping these laws. As debates continue over the status of embryonic stem cells and their ethical implications, understanding public sentiment through surveys can provide critical insights for lawmakers and advocates working to align legal definitions with societal values.

Cultural perspectives significantly influence public opinions on personhood in the context of stem cell usage. Surveys often reveal how cultural beliefs, including religious views, affect attitudes toward stem cell research and therapy. For instance, in societies with strong religious convictions regarding the beginning of life, there may be heightened opposition to embryonic stem cell research. Conversely, cultures that emphasise scientific progress and potential medical advancements may exhibit more favourable views. By analysing these cultural dimensions, stakeholders can better navigate the complex interplay between ethics, law, and public opinion in stem cell discourse.

Finally, the role of public opinion studies extends to the intersection of disability rights and personhood discussions in stem cell discourse. Surveys can gauge how perceptions of personhood influence the rights of individuals with disabilities, particularly in relation to the potential for stem cell therapies. Understanding these dynamics is essential for fostering inclusive discussions that respect the dignity of all individuals, regardless of their condition. As public opinion continues to evolve, it remains a critical factor in shaping the future landscape of stem cell research and its ethical implications.

Media Influence on Perceptions

The media plays a pivotal role in shaping public perceptions surrounding the concept of personhood, particularly within the context of stem cell research. Coverage of scientific advancements often frames the narrative, influencing how individuals and communities understand the ethical implications of personhood in relation to stem cell therapy. The portrayal of stem cells in news reports, documentaries, and social media can either demystify or sensationalise the subject, thereby impacting public opinion and, ultimately, policy-making decisions. As health care personnel and biomedical scientists engage with these narratives, they must critically evaluate how media representations can skew perceptions and influence ethical discussions.

Strategies for Public Engagement

Public engagement is vital in navigating the complex ethical dimensions of personhood within stem cell research. Health care personnel, biomedical scientists, and oversight bodies must actively involve the public to bridge gaps in understanding and address concerns surrounding the implications of personhood. Strategies for public engagement should prioritise transparency, providing clear information about the scientific processes and ethical considerations involved in stem cell research. This transparency fosters trust and encourages informed discussions among diverse community stakeholders.

Educational initiatives play a crucial role in shaping public perceptions of personhood and stem cell therapy. By organising workshops, seminars, and public forums, professionals can facilitate dialogue that highlights the ethical, cultural, and philosophical debates surrounding personhood. These initiatives should aim to create an inclusive environment where individuals from various backgrounds can express their views and engage in meaningful conversations about the implications of stem cell research, including its potential to address disability rights and enhance regenerative medicine.

Collaborative partnerships with community organisations and advocacy groups are essential for effective public engagement. These partnerships can help amplify diverse voices and ensure that the perspectives of underrepresented populations are considered in discussions about personhood and stem cell ethics. By working together, health care personnel and biomedical scientists can better understand the cultural and religious influences that shape public opinions, leading to more nuanced and respectful dialogues.

Utilising digital platforms is another effective strategy for enhancing public engagement. Social media, webinars, and online forums provide accessible avenues for disseminating information and facilitating discussions on the ethical dimensions of personhood in stem cell research. By leveraging these tools, professionals can reach a broader audience, engage with varying viewpoints, and respond to questions and concerns in real-time, thereby fostering a more informed and participatory public discourse.

Lastly, it is crucial to monitor and evaluate the impact of public engagement strategies. Collecting feedback and assessing the effectiveness of outreach efforts will help identify areas for improvement and ensure that the dialogue surrounding personhood in stem cell research remains relevant and responsive to public needs. Continuous engagement not only enhances understanding but also contributes to the development of policies that reflect the diverse values and beliefs of society, ultimately shaping a more ethical framework for stem cell research.

The Influence of Personhood Arguments on Policymaking in Biotechnology

Policy Development Processes

Policy development processes in the realm of stem cell research are crucial in navigating the complex ethical landscape surrounding personhood. The concept of personhood raises significant questions about when life begins and who qualifies for rights and protections. This complexity necessitates a robust policy framework that balances scientific advancement with ethical considerations. Stakeholders, including healthcare personnel and biomedical scientists, must engage in ongoing dialogue to ensure that policies reflect a comprehensive understanding of personhood and its implications for stem cell therapy.

In shaping policies, it is essential to consider the legal definitions of personhood as they relate to stem cell research. Different jurisdictions may interpret personhood differently, affecting the permissibility of certain research practices. Policymakers must navigate these varying definitions while considering the ethical implications of their decisions. This legal landscape can directly influence funding availability, as financial support often hinges on the alignment of research with prevailing legal interpretations of personhood.

Cultural perspectives play a significant role in the policy development process, influencing public perceptions and acceptance of stem cell research. Various cultures may have distinct beliefs regarding personhood and its implications for embryonic stem cells, which can affect societal attitudes towards regenerative medicine. Policymakers need to be attuned to these cultural sensitivities to create policies that resonate with the communities they serve, ensuring wider acceptance and support for stem cell initiatives.

Philosophical debates surrounding personhood provide a critical backdrop for policy formulation. Engaging with these debates allows policymakers to consider the moral implications of their decisions, particularly regarding the intersection of disability rights and personhood in stem cell discourse. By addressing these philosophical questions, policies can be developed that not only advance scientific knowledge but also uphold ethical standards in relation to all individuals impacted by stem cell research.

Finally, the influence of religious perspectives on personhood cannot be overlooked in the policy-making process. Religious beliefs often shape individuals' views on the moral status of embryonic stem cells, which can lead to varied opinions on the acceptability of certain research practices. Policymakers must navigate these diverse beliefs while striving to create inclusive policies that reflect a respectful understanding of different viewpoints on personhood, ultimately fostering an environment conducive to ethical and responsible stem cell research.

Case Studies of Legislative Changes

Legislative changes regarding the concept of personhood in stem cell research have varied significantly across different jurisdictions, reflecting a complex interplay of ethical, cultural, and legal considerations. In the United States, for instance, the debate over personhood gained traction with various state-level initiatives aimed at defining embryos and foetuses as persons. These legislative measures not only influence the scope of biomedical research but also affect funding allocations and institutional policies, creating a ripple effect throughout the healthcare and scientific communities.

In contrast, countries like the United Kingdom have adopted a more regulated approach to stem cell research, with the Human Fertilisation and Embryology Act providing a framework that balances scientific advancement with ethical considerations. The UK legislation explicitly permits research on embryos up to 14 days old, reflecting a compromise that acknowledges the potential of stem cell therapies while also recognising the moral complexities involved. This legislative stance not only facilitates innovation but also shapes public perception by demonstrating a commitment to ethical oversight in the realm of biotechnology.

Cultural perspectives play a crucial role in shaping legislative changes related to personhood, as seen in the comparative analysis of global practices. For example, in many predominantly Catholic countries, strong religious beliefs influence policies that restrict stem cell research based on the idea of personhood. These cultural attitudes can lead to stringent laws that limit scientific exploration, demonstrating how deeply held beliefs can conflict with medical advancements and the potential benefits of regenerative medicine.

Philosophical debates surrounding the definition of personhood further complicate the legislative landscape. The varying interpretations of when life begins impact not only legal definitions but also ethical discussions in stem cell therapy. For instance, some argue that personhood begins at conception, which would categorically prohibit certain types of stem cell research, while others suggest a more nuanced approach that considers viability and consciousness. Such philosophical discourse is essential for policymakers as they navigate the ethical implications of their decisions.

Ultimately, the intersection of disability rights and personhood in stem cell discourse raises additional questions about who is afforded rights and protections within legislative frameworks. By examining case studies of legislative changes, one can observe how definitions of personhood can either support or hinder advancements in stem cell research, particularly for individuals with disabilities. These case studies illustrate the profound impact that legislative definitions of personhood have on the future of biotechnology and the ethical landscape of healthcare.

Advocacy and Lobbying Efforts

Advocacy and lobbying efforts play a crucial role in shaping the landscape of stem cell research, particularly in the context of personhood. These efforts are often driven by various stakeholders, including health care professionals, biomedical scientists, and ethicists, who seek to influence public perception and policy regarding the ethical implications of personhood in stem cell therapy. By fostering dialogue and engagement among diverse groups, advocacy initiatives can help clarify the complexities surrounding personhood, thereby aiding in the establishment of coherent legal frameworks and ethical guidelines.

One significant aspect of advocacy involves raising awareness about the diverse cultural perspectives on personhood and its implications for stem cell usage. Different societies may hold varying views on when personhood begins, which can significantly impact research funding and regulatory policies. Advocacy groups often work to highlight these cultural differences, promoting a more inclusive dialogue that can lead to more equitable policies and practices in stem cell research and therapy.

Moreover, the philosophical debates surrounding personhood and embryonic stem cells are central to lobbying efforts. Advocates engage with policymakers and the public to discuss the moral and ethical considerations that underpin personhood definitions. By framing these debates in relatable terms, they aim to influence legislative actions and funding decisions, ensuring that ethical considerations are not overshadowed by scientific advancements.

Religious perspectives also play a pivotal role in advocacy and lobbying efforts, as they can significantly shape views on personhood in the context of stem cell ethics. Religious organisations often mobilise their communities to advocate for specific definitions of personhood that align with their beliefs, thereby impacting the broader discourse on stem cell research. Understanding these influences is essential for health care personnel and policymakers alike, as it can aid in navigating the complex ethical terrain of this field.

Lastly, the intersection of disability rights and personhood discourse is an emerging area of focus in advocacy efforts. As stem cell research progresses, there is a pressing need to consider how concepts of personhood affect individuals with disabilities. Advocacy groups are increasingly highlighting the importance of inclusive definitions of personhood that recognise the value of all individuals, regardless of their physical or cognitive abilities, thereby influencing policymaking and funding in biotechnology.

Comparative Analysis of Personhood Definitions in Global Stem Cell Legislation

Regional Variations and Trends

The discourse surrounding personhood in stem cell research is characterised by notable regional variations that reflect differing cultural, legal, and ethical frameworks. In the United States, the debate often leans towards individual rights and the autonomy of scientific inquiry, which has led to a relatively permissive stance on stem cell research. In contrast, countries in Europe may adopt a more cautious approach, influenced by a collective commitment to ethical standards that prioritise potential life and human dignity, resulting in stricter regulations surrounding the use of embryonic stem cells.

Cultural perspectives play a critical role in shaping these regional trends. In many Asian countries, traditional beliefs concerning the sanctity of life often intertwine with modern scientific practices, creating a complex landscape where stem cell research is both embraced for its potential and scrutinised for its ethical implications. This cultural lens can significantly affect public perception and the willingness of governments to fund and support stem cell initiatives, highlighting the importance of understanding local attitudes towards personhood.

Legal definitions of personhood vary significantly across jurisdictions, influencing the operational landscape for stem cell research. In some regions, legal frameworks explicitly define embryos as persons, thereby restricting research activities and funding opportunities. Conversely, in areas where personhood is not legally recognised until birth, researchers may experience greater freedom in their work, although they must navigate the ethical implications of such definitions.

Philosophical debates surrounding personhood also manifest regionally, with varying degrees of influence from religious perspectives. For instance, in predominantly religious countries, arguments against embryonic stem cell research may be more prevalent, as religious doctrines often emphasise the moral status of embryos. This can lead to significant public opposition, affecting policymaking and the overall landscape of stem cell research in those areas.

Ultimately, the intersection of personhood concepts with disability rights further complicates the discourse, particularly in regions where advocacy for individuals with disabilities is strong. This intersection raises important questions about inclusivity and the ethical frameworks that govern stem cell research, prompting ongoing debates that reflect regional values and priorities. As such, understanding these regional variations is vital for healthcare personnel, biomedical scientists, and oversight bodies engaged in the field of stem cell research, as it shapes the ethical and practical frameworks within which they operate.

Implications for International Collaboration

The implications for international collaboration in the context of stem cell research are profound, especially when considering the varying definitions and interpretations of personhood across different cultures and legal frameworks. As research in this field continues to advance, it becomes crucial for countries to engage in open dialogues that bridge these diverse perspectives. Such collaboration can facilitate a more unified approach to ethical standards and practices in stem cell research, ultimately leading to improved outcomes in regenerative medicine.

One significant aspect is the ethical implications of personhood in stem cell therapy, which often differ widely from one nation to another. These differences can influence funding allocation and the prioritisation of research projects. By fostering international partnerships, stakeholders can better navigate these complexities, ensuring that ethical considerations surrounding personhood do not hinder scientific progress. This cooperative spirit can help align research goals with the ethical expectations of various societies.

Legal definitions of personhood also play a critical role in shaping collaborative efforts. Variations in legislation can create barriers to research and the sharing of resources. By engaging in international dialogue, countries can work towards creating harmonised legal frameworks that respect cultural sensitivities while promoting scientific advancement. This alignment can help mitigate conflicts that arise from differing legal interpretations, enabling smoother international collaborations.

Cultural perspectives on personhood are pivotal in understanding how different societies approach stem cell usage. Engaging with these perspectives allows for a more inclusive dialogue that respects the beliefs and values of various communities. This understanding can enhance international collaborations by fostering mutual respect and cooperation among researchers, ethicists, and policymakers, ultimately leading to more culturally sensitive approaches to stem cell research.

Finally, the influence of personhood arguments on policy-making in biotechnology cannot be understated. As countries navigate the ethical landscape of stem cell research, collaborative efforts can lead to the development of policies that reflect a more comprehensive understanding of personhood. By pooling resources and sharing insights, international stakeholders can create a more coherent global framework that addresses the ethical, legal, and cultural dimensions of personhood in stem cell research.

Future Directions for Harmonisation

The future directions for harmonisation in the realm of personhood within stem cell research present a complex yet crucial landscape. As global perspectives on personhood vary widely, it is imperative that health care personnel, biomedical scientists, and stem cell oversight bodies engage in a concerted effort to reconcile these diverse views. This involves not only legal frameworks but also ethical considerations that impact the development and application of stem cell therapies. A unified approach is essential to ensure that ethical standards are upheld while fostering innovation in regenerative medicine.

Legal definitions of personhood across different jurisdictions significantly influence stem cell research initiatives. As countries grapple with the implications of these definitions, harmonisation becomes a necessity to facilitate international collaboration and funding. Establishing a common ground on the legal status of stem cells can help streamline research processes and enhance public trust in scientific advancements. This legal clarity would also alleviate the concerns of funding bodies, thereby promoting a more robust investment in stem cell research.

Cultural perspectives play a pivotal role in shaping the discourse around personhood and stem cell usage. Different cultural backgrounds can lead to varying interpretations of what constitutes personhood, impacting public perceptions and ethical considerations. Future discussions must encompass these cultural nuances to promote a more inclusive narrative that respects diverse beliefs while advocating for scientific progress. This cultural engagement is vital for the acceptance and integration of stem cell therapies within various societies.

Philosophical debates surrounding personhood, particularly in relation to embryonic stem cells, continue to challenge researchers and ethicists alike. Addressing these debates in a constructive manner can pave the way for a more nuanced understanding of personhood that transcends binary classifications. Future harmonisation efforts should encourage interdisciplinary dialogues that incorporate philosophical, ethical, and scientific perspectives to enrich the discourse surrounding stem cell research and its implications.

Finally, the role of religion in shaping views on personhood cannot be overlooked. Religious beliefs profoundly influence ethical stances and public attitudes towards stem cell research. By recognising and respecting these influences, stakeholders can foster a more harmonious approach to personhood in the context of biomedical advancements. Engaging with religious leaders and communities will be pivotal in shaping policies that reflect a comprehensive understanding of personhood, thus ensuring ethical integrity in stem cell research.

The Intersection of Disability Rights and Personhood in Stem Cell Discourse

Disability Rights Perspectives

The intersection of disability rights and personhood within the context of stem cell research invites a critical examination of ethical principles and legal definitions. In many societies, personhood has traditionally been understood through a narrow lens that often excludes individuals with disabilities. This raises significant ethical dilemmas as stem cell therapy continues to evolve and expand, potentially offering new treatments for various conditions, including those that affect disabled individuals. Therefore, it is crucial to consider how these perspectives shape the broader discourse on personhood in stem cell research.

Ethical Dilemmas in Stem Cell Research

The exploration of ethical dilemmas in stem cell research is profoundly intertwined with the evolving concept of personhood. This notion raises critical questions regarding when life begins and the moral status of embryos used in research. Health care personnel and biomedical scientists must grapple with these ethical implications, as they navigate the fine line between scientific advancement and the respect for potential life. The varying definitions of personhood significantly impact not only the ethical landscape but also the legal frameworks governing stem cell research.

Legal definitions of personhood vary widely across jurisdictions, influencing the permissibility of stem cell research and therapy. In some countries, embryos are afforded full legal rights, which restricts research opportunities. In contrast, other regions adopt a more lenient stance, allowing for extensive exploration in regenerative medicine. These legal distinctions underscore the necessity for oversight bodies to continuously evaluate and adapt policies that align with both scientific progress and ethical standards.

Cultural perspectives on personhood also play a pivotal role in shaping public opinion and policymaking in biotechnology. Different societies possess diverse beliefs rooted in tradition, religion, and ethics, which influence how stem cell research is perceived and accepted. For instance, in cultures that view the embryo as a person from conception, there may be stronger opposition to stem cell therapies that involve embryo destruction. Therefore, understanding these cultural contexts is vital for health care professionals and policymakers alike.

Philosophical debates surrounding personhood further complicate the discourse on embryonic stem cells. Ethical theories, such as utilitarianism and deontological ethics, offer contrasting views on the moral significance of embryos. These debates not only inform individual beliefs but also shape institutional policies and funding decisions for stem cell research. As such, the intersection of ethics and philosophy remains a critical area for ongoing discussion among biomedical scientists and oversight bodies.

Lastly, the implications of personhood concepts extend to disability rights and the broader societal understanding of what it means to be human. The dialogue surrounding personhood in stem cell ethics must include voices from diverse backgrounds, including those with disabilities, to ensure that all perspectives are recognised. This inclusive approach can enrich the ethical considerations of stem cell research and promote a more comprehensive understanding of its potential impacts on society at large.

Advocating for Inclusive Policies

In the evolving landscape of stem cell research, advocating for inclusive policies is paramount. Health care personnel, biomedical scientists, and oversight bodies must recognise the ethical implications entwined with the concept of personhood. These policies should be designed not only to protect potential life but also to consider the diverse perspectives surrounding personhood, informed by cultural, legal, and philosophical debates. This holistic approach ensures that the dialogue surrounding stem cell therapy remains comprehensive and inclusive, thereby fostering a more equitable healthcare environment.

Legal definitions of personhood vary significantly across jurisdictions, impacting the regulatory framework governing stem cell research. Advocates for inclusive policies must engage with these legal complexities to promote regulations that respect both the potential of stem cell therapies and the rights of individuals involved. This requires a collaborative effort among stakeholders to influence legislation that accommodates the myriad of beliefs regarding personhood, especially as they relate to embryonic stem cells and their potential uses in regenerative medicine.

Cultural perspectives play a crucial role in shaping the discourse on personhood and stem cell usage. Different communities may hold varying beliefs regarding the moral status of embryos and the implications of stem cell research. By advocating for inclusive policies, stakeholders can facilitate a dialogue that respects these cultural differences while striving to establish common ground. This inclusivity can enhance public understanding and acceptance of stem cell therapies, which is essential for advancing the field.

Philosophical debates surrounding personhood significantly influence public perceptions and, consequently, funding for stem cell research. The advocacy for inclusive policies must address these philosophical questions, ensuring that funding mechanisms are aligned with a broader understanding of personhood. By doing so, stakeholders can advocate for resources that support diverse research initiatives while challenging narrow definitions that may restrict scientific progress.

Finally, the intersection of disability rights and personhood in stem cell discourse cannot be overlooked. Advocating for inclusive policies means recognising the voices of individuals with disabilities who have a stake in the outcomes of stem cell research. By integrating their perspectives into the policymaking process, the community can promote a more nuanced understanding of personhood that values all lives, ultimately leading to more ethical and inclusive practices in biotechnology.

Pause for Thought

- The concept of personhood is pivotal in the stem cell research discussion, as it raises ethical, legal and philosophical questions.

- Personhood refers to the status of an entity as a person which carries with it a hosts of rights and moral considerations, the concept has been shaped by the cultural, religious and scientific developments.

- The concept of personhood has changed over the years. In the early 20th century, the definition of personhood was largely tied to biological and developmental milestones. This was shaped by advances in embryology and a growing understanding of human development. With time traditional definitions began to be challenged. The scientific ability to manipulate and cultivate stem cells from very early embryos posed questions about the moral status of these entities which some argue should be afforded personhood status.

- Different societies and religions offer varying interpretations of personhood. In some cultures, personhood is conferred at conception, while in others, it may be associated with viability outside the womb or certain properties.

- The ethical implications of personhood influences funding and governance in stem cell research. The concepts of personhood can influence the allocation of resources as funding bodies may be swayed by the prevailing moral and ethical frameworks that define personhood in respective jurisdictions.

- The biological basis of personhood has real-world implications for the advancement of medical science and ethical practice.

- The intersection of personhood concepts with disability rights is a complex conversation. This must consider the implications for individuals with disability and how these definitions may affect funding and access to stem cell therapies. Understanding the implications of personhood, in relation to vulnerable population is essential for ensuring equitable and ethical advancements in regenerative medicine.

- The exploration of personhood in stem cell research has led to numerous legal challenges across various jurisdictions. In the United States of America, Roe versus Wade have established a precedent for the right of embryos leading to ongoing debates about when person begins. These legal battles often revolve around the law concerning the rights of the unborn and the implication for stem cell research findings.

- The European union's charter of fundamental rights does not explicitly recognize the embryo as a person, allowing for broader research opportunities compared to countries where embryo are afforded full legal protection.

- In Japan, the cultural emphasis is a harmony and collective well-being which influences perceptions of personhood. Here, stem cell research is often considered from the basis of societal benefit where the potential to alleviate suffering is prioritized over the moral status of the embryo.

Take Home Nuggets

- Theories of identity and consciousness play a pivotal role in shaping the discussion around personhood as it relates to stem cell research.

- Different religious perspectives provide foundational insights into how personhood is defined, thus impacting policies and practices in biomedical science. For many faith traditions, personhood is associated with the belief that life begins at conception, thereby attributing moral value and rights to embryos.

- The intersection of religious ethics and biomedical science necessitates a collaborative approach where healthcare providers engage with patients' belief to navigate the ethical landscape of stem cell research effectively. The ongoing dialogue between science, ethics and faith will continue to influence public perceptions and policy making in biotechnology, highlighting the importance of respect and sensitivity towards diverse beliefs in this evolving field.

- Interfaith dialogue on stem cell issues provides a crucial platform for discussing the ethical implications of personhood in stem cell research. Diversity of beliefs necessitates respectful dialogue among healthcare personnel, biomedical scientist and oversight bodies to navigate these complex issues effectively.

- Debates challenging the parameters of what constitutes a person, raises questions about the moral implications of using embryonic stem cells for research and therapy. These debates shape public perceptions significantly, as they influence how society views the potential of regenerative medicine. Interfaith dialogue can help clarify these philosophical positions, allowing for a more informed public discourse.

- The moral dilemma faced by researchers and policy makers is nestled between the concept of personhood versus the greater societal good.

- The concept of personhood raises significant questions about when life begins and who qualifies for rights and protection. A robust framework that balances scientific advancement with ethical considerations is therefore necessary.

- Legislative changes regarding the concept of personhood in stem cell research have varied significantly across different jurisdictions, reflecting a complex interplay of ethical, cultural, and legal consideration.in the

United States of America, defining the embryo and foetus as persons allowed for debate over personhood to proliferate.

- In the United Kingdom, there is a regulated approach to stem cell research with the human fertilisation and embryology authority providing a framework that balances scientific advancement with ethical considerations. The United Kingdom legislation explicitly permits research on embryos up to 14 days old. This reflects a compromise that acknowledges the potential of stem cell therapies while also recognising the moral complexities involved.

- As research in stem cells continues to develop, it is crucial for countries to engage in open dialogue that bridge these diverse perspectives.

Chapter 7
Importance of Regulatory Standards

Regulatory standards play a crucial role in ensuring the safety and efficacy of stem cell research. By establishing clear guidelines, these standards act as guard rails that help researchers navigate the complex ethical landscape inherent in this field. Compliance with regulatory frameworks not only protects the rights of participants but also enhances the credibility of research outcomes, ultimately fostering public trust in scientific advancements. In a rapidly evolving area like stem cell research, adherence to these standards is essential for maintaining integrity and accountability.

Ethical frameworks underpinning regulatory standards are vital for guiding researchers in making informed decisions. They provide a foundation for assessing the moral implications of stem cell research, helping to balance scientific inquiry with respect for human dignity. These frameworks encourage researchers to engage with oversight bodies and advocate for practices that align with ethical considerations. By embedding ethics into the regulatory process, researchers can ensure that their work contributes positively to society while minimising potential harm.

Regulatory compliance in stem cell laboratories involves strict adherence to guidelines that govern laboratory practices and research protocols. This compliance is not merely a bureaucratic exercise; it represents a commitment to the highest standards of scientific integrity and participant safety. Laboratories must implement best practices for obtaining informed consent, ensuring that participants are fully aware of the implications of their involvement in research. Such practices are integral to fostering transparency and building trust among participants and the wider community.

Advocacy groups play a significant role in shaping the landscape of stem cell research by promoting awareness and adherence to regulatory standards. These organisations often serve as a bridge between the scientific community and the public, facilitating dialogue on ethical concerns and regulatory practices. Their contributions can influence policy changes and enhance the overall framework within which stem cell research operates. By actively participating in discussions around regulation, advocacy groups help ensure that the voices of patients and the public are heard in shaping research agendas.

Effective risk assessment and management are paramount in conducting stem cell trials, necessitating rigorous regulatory oversight. Researchers must evaluate potential risks to participants and develop strategies to mitigate these risks while pursuing scientific objectives. Education and training programmes for stem cell researchers are essential for ensuring that they are well-versed in both regulatory compliance and ethical considerations. Such initiatives not only enhance the capabilities of researchers but also contribute to a culture of responsibility that prioritises participant welfare and scientific integrity.

Guard Rails for Stem Cell Research

Defining Guard Rails

In the realm of stem cell research, defining guard rails is essential to ensure that scientific inquiry proceeds ethically and responsibly. These guard rails serve as the framework within which researchers operate, establishing clear boundaries that protect both participants and the integrity of the research. By delineating acceptable practices, these guidelines assist in navigating the complex ethical landscape inherent in stem cell studies, where the potential for significant medical advancements must be balanced against the risks involved.

One of the primary aspects of guard rails is the establishment of ethical frameworks that govern consent procedures. Informed consent is not merely a formality; it is a fundamental component of respect for autonomy and the rights of the participants. Best practices in this area necessitate that researchers communicate risks, benefits, and the nature of the research in a manner that is comprehensible to participants. This ensures that individuals are truly informed and can make decisions aligned with their values and preferences.

Regulatory compliance is another crucial element of guard rails in stem cell laboratories. Adherence to established regulations not only safeguards participants but also enhances the credibility of the research being conducted. Regulatory bodies provide oversight that helps to maintain rigorous standards in the handling and use of stem cells, ensuring that laboratories operate within legal and ethical parameters. This compliance builds public trust, which is vital for the continued advancement of stem cell research.

The role of advocacy groups cannot be understated when discussing guard rails. These organisations often act as intermediaries between the scientific community and the public, advocating for ethical practices and providing education on the implications of stem cell research. Their input is invaluable in shaping policies and ensuring that diverse perspectives are considered in the formulation of guidelines. Through collaboration, advocacy groups help fortify the guard rails that protect both researchers and participants.

Finally, risk assessment and management strategies must be integrated into the guard rails framework. By identifying potential risks associated with stem cell trials, researchers can implement measures to mitigate these risks effectively. Additionally, education and training programmes for stem cell researchers are essential in fostering an understanding of ethical practices and regulatory requirements. By equipping researchers with the knowledge and skills necessary to navigate the complexities of stem cell research, these programmes reinforce the importance of maintaining robust guard rails throughout the research process.

Historical Context of Regulations

The historical context of regulations surrounding stem cell research is pivotal in understanding the current landscape of compliance and ethical standards in laboratories. From the early discoveries in the field of regenerative medicine to the present day, various events have shaped the regulations that govern this complex area of science. Notably, the isolation of stem cells in the late 20th century sparked intense debates about the ethical implications and the need for regulatory frameworks to ensure responsible research practices.

In the early stages, many countries lacked specific regulations addressing stem cell research, leading to a patchwork of guidelines that varied significantly across regions. As public interest grew, so did concerns about the ethical treatment of human subjects and the potential for exploitation. This prompted the establishment of oversight bodies that aimed to create a cohesive regulatory environment, which would safeguard both researchers and participants while promoting scientific advancement.

The introduction of ethical frameworks was a significant milestone in the evolution of regulations. These frameworks sought to balance the pursuit of scientific knowledge with the moral responsibilities owed to individuals. Key principles emerged, including the necessity for informed consent, respect for autonomy, and the minimisation of harm. Such ethical considerations became fundamental in shaping best practices within laboratories, ensuring that research protocols align with societal values and expectations.

Advocacy groups have played a crucial role in the regulatory landscape of stem cell research. Their efforts have not only raised public awareness but also influenced policymaking by voicing the concerns of various stakeholders, including patients, researchers, and ethicists. By engaging in dialogue with regulatory bodies, these groups have contributed to a more informed and responsive regulatory environment, which is essential for the advancement of stem cell science.

Finally, risk assessment and management have become integral components of regulatory compliance in stem cell laboratories. As the field continues to evolve, ongoing education and training programmes for researchers are essential in ensuring that they are equipped with the knowledge to navigate the complex regulatory landscape. By fostering a culture of compliance and ethical awareness, the stem cell research community can better manage the risks associated with innovative therapies, ultimately leading to safer and more effective outcomes for patients.

Key International Guidelines

The landscape of stem cell research is governed by a variety of international guidelines that ensure ethical standards and regulatory compliance. These frameworks are crucial for health care personnel and biomedical scientists as they navigate the complex terrain of stem cell applications. Key international bodies, such as the World Health Organization and the International Society for Stem Cell Research, have established comprehensive guidelines that address both the scientific and ethical considerations inherent in stem cell research. These guidelines serve as guard rails, providing direction and clarity in an evolving field that holds immense potential for medical advancements.

Ethical frameworks play a pivotal role in shaping the conduct of stem cell research. They outline the moral principles that researchers must adhere to, including respect for human dignity and the necessity of informed consent. Best practices for obtaining consent are particularly vital, ensuring that participants in stem cell trials are fully aware of the risks and benefits involved. This ethical diligence not only protects the rights of individuals but also fosters trust between researchers and the community, which is essential for the advancement of scientific knowledge.

Regulatory compliance in stem cell laboratories is not merely a legal obligation but a cornerstone of responsible research. Adhering to international guidelines helps laboratories maintain high standards of safety and efficacy. These regulations encompass a wide range of practices, from laboratory management to the ethical sourcing of stem cells. Compliance is monitored by oversight bodies that conduct regular audits and evaluations, ensuring that research activities align with both ethical expectations and scientific integrity.

The role of advocacy groups cannot be understated in the realm of stem cell research. These organisations act as intermediaries between the scientific community and the public, promoting awareness and understanding of stem cell therapies. They also advocate for policies that support responsible research practices and funding for stem cell studies. By fostering dialogue and collaboration, advocacy groups enhance the regulatory landscape, ensuring that the voices of stakeholders are heard and considered in the ongoing discourse surrounding stem cell research.

Finally, risk assessment and management in stem cell trials are essential components that contribute to the overall success and safety of research initiatives. A thorough risk analysis allows researchers to identify potential hazards and implement strategies to mitigate them. Furthermore, education and training programmes for stem cell researchers are crucial in equipping them with the knowledge and skills necessary to conduct ethically and scientifically sound research. Such initiatives not only enhance the competency of researchers but also elevate the standards of the field.

Ethical Frameworks for Stem Cell Research

Ethical Principles in Research

Ethical principles are foundational to the integrity of research, particularly in sensitive fields like stem cell research. Researchers must adhere to frameworks that ensure respect for human dignity, welfare, and rights. These principles guide the development of regulations and compliance measures that govern laboratories, ensuring that research is conducted responsibly and ethically. This is vital not only for the legitimacy of scientific inquiry but also for maintaining public trust in scientific advancements.

Consent is a critical component of ethical research practices. Best practices dictate that participants must be fully informed about the nature of the research, potential risks, and benefits before agreeing to participate. This process involves clear communication and the provision of comprehensive information to ensure that consent is truly informed. Researchers must continually assess their consent procedures, adapting them to reflect the evolving ethical standards and the expectations of participants.

In the realm of stem cell research, advocacy groups play a pivotal role in shaping ethical standards and regulatory compliance. These organisations often act as intermediaries, providing a voice for patients and the public while ensuring that research aligns with societal values. Their involvement can facilitate dialogue between researchers, regulatory bodies, and the community, fostering a collaborative environment that prioritises ethical considerations and public interest in research outcomes.

Risk assessment and management are also essential aspects of ethical research practices. Researchers are tasked with evaluating potential risks to participants and the broader community, implementing strategies to mitigate these risks. This proactive approach not only safeguards individuals involved in trials but also enhances the credibility of the research process. Comprehensive risk management plans are crucial for compliance with regulatory standards and for the ethical conduct of research.

Education and training programmes for stem cell researchers must incorporate ethical principles prominently. These programmes should equip researchers with the knowledge and skills necessary to navigate the complex ethical landscape of their work. Continuous education on ethical issues, informed consent, and risk management is vital for fostering a culture of compliance and care within stem cell laboratories. By investing in training, institutions can ensure that their personnel uphold the highest ethical standards, ultimately benefiting both research integrity and patient welfare.

Informed Consent and Autonomy

Informed consent is a foundational principle in biomedical research, particularly in the context of stem cell laboratories. It ensures that participants are fully aware of the nature of the research, the potential risks and benefits, and their rights as participants. This process not only respects the autonomy of individuals but also fosters trust between researchers and participants, which is vital for the integrity of scientific inquiry. Health care personnel must be well-versed in obtaining informed consent, as this is not merely a legal requirement but an ethical obligation that underpins the research framework.

Autonomy in the context of stem cell research refers to the capacity of individuals to make informed choices about their participation in research studies. This is especially critical given the complexities and uncertainties surrounding stem cell therapies. Researchers and regulatory bodies must ensure that participants are not only informed but also empowered to make decisions that align with their values and beliefs. Education and training programmes play a crucial role in equipping health care personnel and researchers with the skills needed to facilitate this autonomy effectively.

The ethical frameworks guiding stem cell research emphasise the importance of informed consent as a safeguard against coercion and exploitation. These frameworks provide guidelines for researchers to follow, ensuring that consent is obtained in a manner that is transparent and respectful. Advocacy groups also play a significant role in promoting ethical standards and protecting the rights of participants. Their involvement helps to raise awareness about the importance of informed consent and encourages adherence to best practices in the field.

Risk assessment and management are integral to the informed consent process. Participants must be made aware of any potential risks associated with their involvement in stem cell research. This includes both physical risks and the implications of participating in trials. By providing comprehensive information about these risks, researchers can help participants make informed decisions, thereby reinforcing their autonomy. Furthermore, clear communication about potential outcomes helps to build a strong foundation of trust between participants and researchers.

In conclusion, informed consent and autonomy are critical components of ethical stem cell research. Compliance with regulatory standards and best practices ensures that participants are respected and their rights protected. As the field of stem cell research continues to evolve, ongoing education and collaboration among health care personnel, biomedical scientists, and oversight bodies will be essential in maintaining high ethical standards. By prioritising informed consent, the integrity of research and the welfare of participants can be upheld, ultimately advancing the field in a responsible manner.

Balancing Innovation and Ethics

In the rapidly evolving field of stem cell research, the interplay between innovation and ethics is a pressing concern for healthcare personnel, biomedical scientists, and regulatory bodies alike. As advancements in technology open new avenues for treatment and research, it becomes imperative to establish guard rails that ensure these innovations do not compromise ethical standards. The challenge lies in fostering an environment where scientific progress is balanced with a commitment to ethical practices, safeguarding the rights and welfare of participants involved in stem cell studies.

Ethical frameworks are essential in guiding researchers through the complex landscape of stem cell research. These frameworks provide a structure within which ethical considerations can be assessed, ensuring that all aspects of the research process align with societal values and expectations. The development of comprehensive guidelines that address consent procedures, risk assessment, and participant management is crucial. Such frameworks not only enhance the credibility of research but also build public trust, which is vital for the continued support of stem cell studies.

Regulatory compliance in stem cell laboratories serves as a cornerstone for maintaining ethical standards in research. Adhering to established regulations not only protects participants but also ensures that the research conducted is both scientifically valid and ethically sound. Oversight bodies play a significant role in enforcing these regulations, and their collaboration with researchers can lead to best practices that promote transparency and accountability in all aspects of stem cell research. This partnership is fundamental to navigating the ethical complexities that arise as science advances.

The role of advocacy groups in stem cell research cannot be understated, as they often serve as a bridge between the scientific community and the public. These groups advocate for ethical considerations and help to raise awareness about the potential benefits and risks associated with stem cell therapies. Their influence is essential in shaping public policy and ensuring that the voices of patients and families are heard in the regulatory process. By fostering dialogue between researchers, regulators, and the community, advocacy groups contribute to a more informed and ethically conscious research environment.

Finally, risk assessment and management in stem cell trials is a critical component of ethical research practice. Identifying potential risks and implementing strategies to mitigate them ensures that participant safety remains a priority. Education and training programmes for stem cell researchers are vital in promoting a culture of ethical awareness and responsibility. By equipping researchers with the necessary knowledge and tools, we can cultivate an environment where innovation thrives alongside ethical integrity, ultimately leading to the responsible advancement of stem cell research.

Regulatory Compliance in Stem Cell Laboratories

Overview of Regulatory Bodies

Regulatory bodies play a crucial role in overseeing stem cell research, ensuring that ethical standards and compliance measures are adhered to. These organisations are tasked with establishing guidelines that protect the rights and welfare of research participants, while also promoting scientific integrity. The collaboration between various regulatory agencies helps create a robust framework that not only supports innovation but also mitigates potential risks associated with stem cell research.

In the UK, the Human Fertilisation and Embryology Authority (HFEA) is one of the primary regulatory bodies responsible for overseeing activities involving human embryos and stem cells. This agency sets strict guidelines for research protocols, focusing on ethical considerations and safety requirements. By enforcing compliance with these standards, the HFEA ensures that stem cell laboratories operate within a framework that prioritises both scientific advancement and public trust.

Internationally, organisations such as the World Health Organisation (WHO) and the International Society for Stem Cell Research (ISSCR) provide essential guidance on ethical frameworks for stem cell research. These bodies promote best practices and encourage countries to adopt regulations that align with global standards. By fostering international collaboration, these organisations help address issues of ethical disparities and enhance the quality of stem cell research worldwide.

Advocacy groups also play a significant role in the regulatory landscape of stem cell research. They serve as a bridge between the scientific community, policymakers, and the public, advocating for transparency and ethical practices. These groups work tirelessly to educate stakeholders about the importance of informed consent and patient rights, ensuring that research participants are fully aware of the implications of their involvement in stem cell trials.

Finally, risk assessment and management are integral components of compliance in stem cell laboratories. Regulatory bodies require thorough evaluations of potential risks associated with stem cell research activities. Training programmes for researchers are essential in equipping them with the knowledge and skills necessary to conduct ethical and compliant research. By prioritising education and awareness, regulatory bodies ensure that stem cell research is conducted responsibly and ethically, fostering public confidence in scientific progress.

Compliance Frameworks

Compliance frameworks in stem cell laboratories are essential for ensuring that research adheres to ethical and regulatory standards. These frameworks provide a structured approach to managing the complexities of stem cell research, which often involves sensitive ethical considerations regarding human subjects. By establishing clear guidelines, compliance frameworks serve as guard rails that help researchers navigate the legal landscape while promoting responsible scientific inquiry.

The ethical frameworks underlying compliance in stem cell research are particularly crucial as they guide the conduct of researchers and the treatment of human subjects. These frameworks help ensure that consent processes are transparent and that participants are fully informed about the risks and benefits of their involvement. Furthermore, they promote respect for the autonomy of individuals participating in research, thus fostering trust between researchers and the communities they serve.

Regulatory compliance in stem cell laboratories encompasses various aspects, including adherence to local, national, and international regulations. Laboratories must implement best practices for quality assurance and risk management to mitigate potential ethical breaches. This includes regular audits, training programmes for staff, and the establishment of incident reporting mechanisms to ensure that any deviations from established protocols are promptly addressed.

Advocacy groups play a vital role in stem cell research by serving as intermediaries between the scientific community, policymakers, and the public. These organisations often work to influence regulatory frameworks, ensuring that the voices of patients, researchers, and ethical committees are considered in the development of compliance standards. By promoting dialogue and transparency, advocacy groups help to shape a research environment that prioritises ethical considerations alongside scientific advancement.

Finally, effective education and training programmes for stem cell researchers are integral to fostering a culture of compliance within laboratories. These programmes should cover not only the technical aspects of stem cell research but also the ethical implications and regulatory requirements. By equipping researchers with the necessary knowledge and skills, we can ensure that they are better prepared to navigate the complexities of compliance, ultimately leading to safer and more responsible research outcomes.

Auditing and Inspections

Auditing and inspections are fundamental components of ensuring compliance within stem cell laboratories. These processes help to confirm that laboratories adhere to established regulatory standards and ethical frameworks, thereby safeguarding the integrity of research and the welfare of participants. Regular audits not only assess adherence to protocols but also identify areas for improvement, fostering a culture of continuous enhancement in research practices.

The role of oversight bodies in conducting these audits cannot be overstated. They provide an external perspective, ensuring that laboratories are not only compliant with the regulations but also ethical in their approach to research. This oversight is crucial in maintaining public trust in stem cell research, as it assures stakeholders that scientific inquiry is conducted responsibly and transparently.

Additionally, inspections serve as a means of risk assessment and management in stem cell trials. By evaluating laboratory practices and protocols, inspectors can identify potential risks that may affect research outcomes or participant safety. This proactive approach aids in the development of best practices, which are essential for minimising risks and enhancing the overall quality of research conducted in the field.

Education and training programmes for stem cell researchers also play a vital role in the auditing and inspection process. These programmes equip personnel with the necessary knowledge and skills to understand regulatory compliance and ethical considerations. By fostering a well-informed workforce, laboratories can ensure that their staff are capable of meeting the rigorous standards set forth by oversight bodies, thereby improving the likelihood of successful audits and inspections.

Finally, the involvement of advocacy groups in the auditing process adds another layer of accountability. These organisations can provide valuable insights into public concerns and ethical considerations, helping to shape the auditing criteria and inspection processes. Engaging advocacy groups ensures that the voices of stakeholders are heard, promoting a balanced approach to compliance that prioritises both scientific progress and ethical responsibility.

Best Practices for Consent in Stem Cell Research

Importance of Informed Consent

Informed consent is a cornerstone of ethical practice in stem cell research, ensuring that participants are fully aware of the implications of their involvement. It involves providing potential subjects with comprehensive information regarding the study, including its purpose, procedures, risks, and benefits. This process not only respects the autonomy of individuals but also fosters trust between researchers and participants, which is vital for the integrity of scientific inquiry.

The importance of informed consent extends beyond mere compliance with regulations; it embodies the ethical commitment to respect and protect the rights of research participants. In the context of stem cell laboratories, where the complexities of scientific advancements can often overwhelm participants, clarity and transparency are paramount. Researchers must ensure that the consent process is conducted in a manner that is understandable to individuals from diverse backgrounds, thereby enhancing their ability to make informed decisions.

Best practices for obtaining informed consent in stem cell research involve not only verbal communication but also the provision of written materials that outline the study's details. It is essential for healthcare personnel and biomedical scientists to be trained in effective communication strategies that cater to varying levels of health literacy. By employing simple language and avoiding jargon, researchers can significantly improve participants' comprehension and comfort levels regarding their involvement.

Advocacy groups play a crucial role in shaping informed consent practices within stem cell research. These organisations often work to educate the public about the potential of stem cell therapies and the importance of ethical standards in research. Their involvement can enhance public trust, facilitate dialogue between researchers and communities, and ultimately lead to more robust consent processes that truly reflect the values and concerns of society.

In conclusion, the significance of informed consent in stem cell research cannot be overstated. It is not merely a regulatory requirement but a fundamental ethical obligation that underpins the relationship between researchers and participants. By adhering to best practices and engaging with advocacy groups, stem cell laboratories can ensure that their research is conducted with the highest standards of ethical integrity, ultimately contributing to the advancement of medical science while safeguarding the rights of individuals involved.

Elements of Effective Consent Processes

In the context of stem cell research, effective consent processes are crucial for ensuring ethical compliance and safeguarding participants' rights. A well-structured consent process goes beyond merely obtaining a signature; it necessitates a clear understanding of the research purpose, procedures, and potential risks involved. Health care personnel and biomedical scientists must communicate these elements transparently to foster trust and encourage informed participation. This dialogue not only aligns with ethical frameworks but also adheres to regulatory compliance requirements in stem cell laboratories.

Moreover, the role of advocacy groups cannot be understated in the consent process. These organisations often serve as intermediaries, helping to educate potential participants about the implications of their involvement in research. They advocate for best practices in consent, ensuring that the voices of patients and participants are represented. Engaging advocacy groups in the consent process helps to bridge gaps in understanding and addresses concerns related to risk assessment and management in stem cell trials.

Another key aspect of an effective consent process is the incorporation of educational and training programmes for researchers. Such initiatives equip stem cell researchers with the necessary skills to communicate complex information in an accessible manner. Training should focus on the nuances of consent, including how to address participants' questions and concerns comprehensively. This empowers researchers to create a supportive environment that respects participants' autonomy while also facilitating informed decision-making.

Regularly reviewing and updating consent materials is also essential to maintain relevance and clarity. As research practices evolve and new findings emerge, consent information must reflect these changes. Health care personnel should be proactive in revising consent documentation, incorporating feedback from participants to improve comprehension. This commitment to continuous improvement not only enhances the quality of the consent process but also reinforces the ethical foundations of stem cell research.

In conclusion, the elements of effective consent processes in stem cell research are multi-faceted and require collaboration among various stakeholders. By prioritising transparency, engaging advocacy groups, implementing robust training programmes, and committing to ongoing revisions, the research community can uphold the highest standards of ethical compliance. This holistic approach not only protects participants but also advances the integrity of stem cell research.

Challenges in Consent in Diverse Populations

The process of obtaining consent for participation in stem cell research presents unique challenges, particularly in diverse populations. These challenges arise from varying cultural perceptions of medical research and differing levels of understanding regarding the implications of stem cell therapies. In many communities, historical mistrust towards medical institutions can complicate the consent process. Health care personnel must navigate these complexities while ensuring that participants are fully informed and capable of making autonomous decisions.

Ethical frameworks play a crucial role in guiding consent practices within diverse populations. It is imperative that researchers are trained to recognise the cultural nuances that may influence a participant's willingness to consent. This includes understanding language barriers and providing materials that are accessible to individuals from various backgrounds. By tailoring consent processes to accommodate these differences, researchers can foster a more inclusive environment that respects the rights and beliefs of all participants.

Regulatory compliance is another significant aspect of consent in stem cell laboratories. Oversight bodies must ensure that consent protocols adhere to established ethical standards while also considering the specific needs of diverse populations. This necessitates ongoing dialogue between researchers, regulatory agencies, and community advocates. By involving advocacy groups in the development of consent strategies, researchers can better align their practices with the values and expectations of the communities they serve.

Best practices for obtaining consent must also evolve to meet the needs of diverse populations. This includes employing culturally competent communication strategies and utilising community engagement to build trust. Training programmes for stem cell researchers should emphasise the importance of these practices, equipping them with the skills to effectively engage with participants from various cultural backgrounds. By prioritising informed consent, researchers can enhance the integrity of their studies and promote ethical research practices.

Finally, risk assessment and management in stem cell trials should incorporate perspectives from diverse populations. This includes recognising potential risks that may be perceived differently across cultures. Researchers must be diligent in addressing these concerns during the consent process, ensuring that participants feel safe and respected. Education and training programmes must reflect this commitment to inclusivity, thereby empowering researchers to conduct ethically sound studies that honour the diversity of the populations they engage with.

The Role of Advocacy Groups in Stem Cell Research

Introduction to Advocacy in Stem Cell Research

Advocacy in stem cell research plays a crucial role in shaping the landscape of scientific inquiry and regulatory compliance. For healthcare personnel, biomedical scientists, and oversight bodies, understanding the nuances of advocacy is essential for navigating the complex ethical frameworks that govern this field. Advocacy groups not only raise awareness about the potential benefits of stem cell research but also ensure that ethical considerations are at the forefront of scientific advancement. This dual focus on promotion and ethics is vital for building public trust and fostering a collaborative environment between researchers and the community.

The ethical frameworks guiding stem cell research are multi-faceted, involving considerations of consent, risk assessment, and the societal implications of scientific progress. Health care personnel must be well-versed in these frameworks to advocate effectively for patient rights and safety. Best practices for obtaining informed consent are particularly important, as they empower participants in research while safeguarding their autonomy. Advocacy groups often provide resources and training to help researchers implement these best practices, thereby enhancing the quality of research and compliance with regulatory standards.

Regulatory compliance in stem cell laboratories is another critical area where advocacy plays a significant role. Advocacy groups work alongside regulatory bodies to ensure that laboratories adhere to established guidelines, thereby minimising risks associated with stem cell trials. These groups often engage in dialogue with policymakers to influence regulations that govern research practices. By advocating for robust compliance measures, they help protect both researchers and participants, ensuring that scientific exploration occurs within ethical and legal boundaries.

Risk assessment and management are key components of stem cell trials, and effective advocacy can enhance these processes. Advocacy groups can facilitate discussions about potential risks, guiding researchers in their efforts to mitigate them. By promoting transparency and open communication, these groups help foster a culture of safety and responsibility in stem cell research. This collaborative approach not only aids researchers in developing safer protocols but also reassures the public about the integrity of ongoing research.

Finally, education and training programmes for stem cell researchers are essential for instilling a strong ethical foundation in the next generation of scientists. Advocacy groups play a pivotal role in the development of these programmes by providing expertise and resources. By equipping researchers with the knowledge, they need to navigate ethical dilemmas and regulatory requirements, advocacy initiatives contribute to a more informed and responsible scientific community. This focus on education ultimately supports the advancement of stem cell research while prioritising ethical considerations and public confidence.

Collaborations Between Advocacy Groups and Researchers

Collaborations between advocacy groups and researchers are vital for the advancement of stem cell research, particularly within the context of regulatory compliance and ethical frameworks. Advocacy groups play a crucial role in representing patient interests and ensuring that the voices of those affected by various conditions are heard in scientific discussions. By partnering with researchers, these groups can help to bridge the gap between scientific inquiry and patient needs, fostering a more inclusive research environment that prioritises ethical considerations and adheres to regulatory standards.

The partnership between advocacy organisations and researchers enhances the development of robust ethical frameworks for stem cell research. Advocacy groups bring valuable insights into the societal implications of research, helping scientists to understand the ethical landscape surrounding their work. This collaboration can lead to the establishment of guidelines that not only comply with regulations but also resonate with public sentiments and moral obligations, thereby promoting transparency and trust in the research process.

Moreover, advocacy groups can assist in the creation of best practices for obtaining informed consent in stem cell research. By working together, researchers and advocacy organisations can develop educational materials that clearly communicate the risks and benefits of participation in research trials. This collaboration ensures that prospective participants are well-informed and that their consent is truly informed, which is essential for maintaining ethical integrity in research.

Risk assessment and management in stem cell trials also benefit significantly from the collaboration between advocacy groups and researchers. Advocacy organisations often have access to patient experiences and concerns, which can inform researchers about potential risks that may not be immediately apparent. By integrating these insights into the design and implementation of trials, researchers can better anticipate and mitigate risks, ultimately leading to safer and more effective clinical outcomes.

Education and training programmes for stem cell researchers are another area where advocacy groups can provide crucial support. By collaborating on educational initiatives, advocacy organisations can help ensure that researchers are not only knowledgeable about the scientific aspects of stem cell research but also about the ethical implications and societal expectations surrounding their work. This holistic approach to training fosters a generation of researchers who are not only skilled in their field but also committed to upholding the highest standards of ethical practice and regulatory compliance.

Impact of Advocacy on Policy and Public Opinion

Advocacy plays a pivotal role in shaping policy and influencing public opinion, particularly in the realm of stem cell research. By bringing together stakeholders, including scientists, healthcare professionals, and patients, advocacy groups create a platform for dialogue that raises awareness of the ethical and regulatory issues surrounding stem cell technologies. These organisations not only provide critical information but also mobilise public support, thereby creating an environment conducive to policy change and improved regulatory frameworks.

One significant impact of advocacy is the establishment of ethical frameworks that guide stem cell research. Advocacy groups often collaborate with regulatory bodies to define standards that prioritise patient safety and ethical considerations. By championing transparency and accountability, these organisations help to foster trust among the public and ensure that research practices align with societal values and expectations.

Moreover, advocacy efforts contribute to the development and implementation of best practices for consent in stem cell research. This is crucial in safeguarding participants' rights and ensuring that they are fully informed about the risks and benefits of their involvement. Advocacy groups work to educate both researchers and participants about the importance of informed consent, ultimately enhancing the ethical standards of research practices within the stem cell community.

In the context of risk assessment and management in stem cell trials, advocacy plays a vital role in promoting safe research practices. By highlighting successful case studies and sharing insights from past experiences, advocacy organisations can guide researchers in navigating potential challenges. This proactive approach not only mitigates risks but also reinforces the credibility of stem cell research in the eyes of regulatory bodies and the public.

Lastly, advocacy groups are instrumental in the education and training of stem cell researchers. They organise workshops, seminars, and training programmes that equip researchers with the knowledge and skills necessary to operate within the regulatory landscape. By fostering a culture of continuous learning and compliance, these groups ensure that the next generation of stem cell researchers is well-prepared to contribute to this rapidly evolving field while adhering to ethical and regulatory standards.

Risk Assessment and Management in Stem Cell Trials

Identifying Risks in Stem Cell Research

Identifying risks in stem cell research is essential for ensuring the safety and efficacy of scientific advancements in this field. The complex nature of stem cell biology presents unique challenges that require diligent assessment and proactive management. Health care personnel and biomedical scientists must work collaboratively to establish guard rails that not only protect participants but also promote ethical standards throughout the research process.

Ethical frameworks play a crucial role in identifying potential risks associated with stem cell research. These frameworks guide researchers in making informed decisions, ensuring that the dignity and rights of individuals involved are respected. Oversight bodies are responsible for evaluating research proposals to ensure compliance with ethical guidelines, which helps mitigate risks related to informed consent and the potential misuse of stem cells.

Regulatory compliance in stem cell laboratories is paramount for the integrity of research. Adherence to established regulations not only safeguards participants but also enhances the credibility of research findings. Best practices for obtaining consent must be strictly followed, ensuring that participants are fully aware of the risks and benefits associated with their involvement in clinical trials. This transparency is vital in fostering trust between researchers and participants.

Risk assessment and management strategies are essential components of stem cell trials. By systematically identifying potential hazards, researchers can implement measures to minimise risks. This proactive approach not only protects participants but also contributes to the overall success of scientific endeavours in the field of regenerative medicine.

Education and training programmes for stem cell researchers are critical in promoting a culture of safety and compliance. Continuous professional development ensures that personnel are equipped with the latest knowledge and skills necessary to navigate the complexities of stem cell research. Advocacy groups also play a significant role by raising awareness and supporting initiatives aimed at identifying and managing risks, ultimately leading to safer and more effective research outcomes.

Developing Risk Management Strategies

Developing robust risk management strategies is essential for ensuring the integrity and safety of stem cell research. This involves identifying potential risks associated with various stages of research, from laboratory practices to clinical trials. Health care personnel and biomedical scientists must work collaboratively to assess these risks and implement measures that mitigate them. By establishing a culture of compliance and care, organisations can foster an environment where ethical considerations are prioritised alongside scientific advancement.

A critical aspect of risk management in stem cell laboratories is the implementation of guard rails to navigate the complex regulatory landscape. Oversight bodies play a pivotal role in setting these frameworks, ensuring that research adheres to established ethical standards. This not only protects the rights of participants but also enhances public trust in stem cell research. By aligning with best practices, laboratories can develop protocols that are both compliant and ethically sound.

Moreover, effective consent processes are integral to risk management strategies. Researchers must ensure that participants are fully informed about the risks and benefits of their involvement in studies. This requires ongoing education and training programmes that equip researchers with the tools to communicate these concepts clearly. By prioritising informed consent, laboratories can reduce the potential for ethical breaches and enhance participant engagement in research initiatives.

Advocacy groups also play a vital role in shaping risk management strategies within the realm of stem cell research. Their contributions help to highlight public concerns and ethical dilemmas, guiding researchers and oversight bodies in their decision-making processes. Engaging with these groups fosters a collaborative approach to risk assessment, ensuring that diverse perspectives are considered in the development of research policies. This engagement ultimately leads to more comprehensive and ethically responsible research practices.

Finally, continuous risk assessment and management are necessary throughout the lifespan of stem cell trials. Regular evaluations allow for the identification of new risks and the adaptation of strategies accordingly. By cultivating a proactive approach to risk management, laboratories can not only comply with regulations but also advance the field of stem cell research in a manner that prioritises ethical standards and patient welfare. This commitment to safety and ethics will help to build a sustainable future for stem cell therapies.

Case Studies of Risk Management

In the realm of stem cell research, effective risk management is crucial to ensure compliance with regulatory standards and ethical frameworks. Case studies from various laboratories illustrate how proactive measures have been implemented to identify and mitigate potential risks. For instance, a prominent stem cell research facility adopted a comprehensive risk assessment protocol that involved regular audits and stakeholder consultations. This initiative not only enhanced their compliance with regulations but also fostered a culture of transparency and accountability within the laboratory environment.

Another notable case study involved a partnership between a stem cell laboratory and an oversight body. Together, they established a framework for best practices in obtaining informed consent from research participants. By prioritising participant education and engagement, this collaboration improved the quality of consent processes and reduced the likelihood of ethical breaches. The positive outcomes from this partnership underscore the importance of involving advocacy groups in the development of consent strategies, highlighting their role in safeguarding participant rights and interests.

Moreover, a specific trial on stem cell therapies for degenerative diseases faced significant regulatory challenges. The research team implemented an adaptive management approach, allowing for continuous monitoring and adjustment of their protocols based on interim findings. This flexibility not only ensured compliance with evolving regulatory requirements but also allowed the team to manage risks more effectively, ultimately leading to successful trial outcomes. Such adaptive strategies are essential in navigating the complexities of stem cell research.

In another case, a laboratory focused on the ethical implications of donor selection in stem cell research showcased the need for robust ethical frameworks. Through a series of workshops and training programmes, researchers were educated on the ethical considerations surrounding donor consent and the potential impacts on diverse populations. This emphasis on education ensured that all staff were equipped to handle ethical dilemmas, promoting a culture of ethical awareness and responsibility.

Lastly, the role of advocacy groups cannot be overstated in facilitating dialogue between researchers, regulatory bodies, and the public. A case study highlighting this collaboration demonstrated how advocacy groups helped to bridge communication gaps, ensuring that community concerns were addressed in the research process. This engagement not only enhanced public trust but also reinforced the necessity of incorporating diverse perspectives in risk management strategies, ultimately contributing to more robust regulatory compliance in stem cell laboratories.

Education and Training Programmes for Stem Cell Researchers

Importance of Education and Training

Education and training are essential components in the field of stem cell research, serving as the foundation for ensuring compliance with regulatory standards and ethical frameworks. As the landscape of stem cell research evolves, healthcare personnel and biomedical scientists must be equipped with the latest knowledge and skills. This not only enhances their competency but also fosters a culture of responsibility and integrity in research practices. By prioritising education, we can cultivate a workforce that is well-informed about the complexities and implications of stem cell applications.

The importance of a structured training programme cannot be overstated, particularly in the context of regulatory compliance. Training helps researchers understand the various guard rails established for stem cell research, including ethical considerations and safety protocols. These programmes should cover best practices for obtaining informed consent, which is crucial for maintaining trust and transparency with research participants. A well-trained researcher is better equipped to navigate the intricate regulatory landscape, ensuring that all activities are conducted within legal and ethical boundaries.

Moreover, education and training serve to enhance risk assessment and management strategies in stem cell trials. Effective training enables researchers to identify potential risks early and develop mitigation strategies. This proactive approach not only safeguards participants but also protects the integrity of the research. By instilling a thorough understanding of risk management principles, training programmes can significantly reduce the likelihood of adverse events, thereby reinforcing public confidence in stem cell research.

Advocacy groups play a pivotal role in supporting educational initiatives within the stem cell research community. These organisations often provide resources and training opportunities that are tailored to the needs of researchers and healthcare professionals. By collaborating with advocacy groups, institutions can amplify their educational efforts, ensuring that the workforce remains informed about the latest developments and best practices in the field. This partnership is vital for fostering an environment of continuous learning and improvement.

In conclusion, the emphasis on education and training within stem cell laboratories cannot be overlooked. It is imperative for healthcare personnel, biomedical scientists, and oversight bodies to invest in comprehensive training programmes. Such initiatives not only promote compliance with regulatory standards but also enhance the ethical conduct of research. By prioritising education, we can ensure that stem cell research is conducted responsibly, ultimately benefiting both science and society at large.

Curriculum Development for Stem Cell Research

The development of a curriculum for stem cell research is crucial in establishing a robust foundation for future researchers. It must encompass various aspects, including ethical frameworks, regulatory compliance, and best practices for consent. This curriculum should cater to the diverse audience of healthcare personnel, biomedical scientists, and oversight bodies, ensuring that all stakeholders are equipped with the necessary knowledge and skills. By integrating these elements, the curriculum can foster a culture of compliance and care within stem cell laboratories.

An essential component of the curriculum is the inclusion of ethical frameworks that guide stem cell research. Training should emphasise the importance of ethical considerations, such as respect for donors and informed consent. This ensures that researchers understand the moral implications of their work and are committed to conducting research that aligns with societal values. Advocacy groups play a vital role in this aspect, as they can provide insights and support in developing ethical guidelines that resonate with the public and scientific community alike.

Regulatory compliance is another critical pillar of the curriculum, helping to navigate the complex landscape of stem cell research regulations. Participants should receive training on the various local, national, and international regulations governing stem cell research. Understanding these regulations is vital for ensuring that research is conducted ethically and legally, thus minimising risks associated with non-compliance. Additionally, this knowledge empowers researchers to advocate for more supportive regulatory environments.

Risk assessment and management strategies must also be integrated into the curriculum to prepare researchers for potential challenges in stem cell trials. Educating researchers on identifying, evaluating, and mitigating risks can enhance the safety and efficacy of their studies. Furthermore, practical workshops and case studies can provide hands-on experience in managing real-world scenarios, reinforcing the importance of thorough risk management in clinical research settings.

Lastly, education and training programmes should be designed to promote continuous professional development for stem cell researchers. This can include workshops, seminars, and online courses that keep researchers updated on the latest advancements in the field. By fostering a culture of lifelong learning, the curriculum can ensure that researchers remain at the forefront of stem cell research, ultimately benefiting patient care and scientific innovation.

Continuing Education and Professional Development

Continuing education and professional development are critical components in maintaining the standards of compliance and care within stem cell laboratories. As the field rapidly evolves, healthcare personnel and biomedical scientists must engage in lifelong learning to keep abreast of regulatory changes and advancements in stem cell research. This ongoing education not only enhances individual competencies but also ensures that laboratories adhere to the highest ethical frameworks and guard rails established by oversight bodies.

Training programmes should encompass a range of topics, including best practices for obtaining informed consent in stem cell research. Understanding the nuances of consent is vital, as it impacts the ethical integrity of research studies and the trust placed in scientific inquiry by the public. Workshops and seminars designed around these themes can equip professionals with the necessary knowledge and skills to navigate complex consent processes effectively.

Moreover, risk assessment and management in stem cell trials are pivotal areas that require continuous professional development. As researchers encounter new challenges, they must be prepared to identify potential risks and implement strategies to mitigate them. Regular training sessions focusing on risk management can foster a culture of safety and compliance, ultimately enhancing the quality of research outcomes.

The role of advocacy groups in stem cell research also warrants attention in continuing education initiatives. These organisations often provide valuable insights into patient perspectives and ethical considerations that may not be fully addressed in standard training. By collaborating with advocacy groups, stem cell laboratories can ensure that their practices align with community values and expectations, fostering greater acceptance and support for their work.

In conclusion, the commitment to continuing education and professional development within the field of stem cell research is essential for ensuring regulatory compliance and ethical integrity. By prioritising education, healthcare personnel and biomedical scientists can better navigate the complexities of stem cell research, ultimately leading to improved outcomes and enhanced public trust in the scientific community. It is imperative that training programmes evolve continually to meet the dynamic needs of the field and uphold the best practices in research.

Future Directions in Stem Cell Research Compliance

Emerging Trends and Technologies

The landscape of stem cell research is continually evolving, driven by advancements in technology and a growing understanding of ethical considerations. Emerging trends indicate a significant shift towards more precise and personalised approaches to treatment, leveraging innovations in gene editing and regenerative medicine. As these technologies develop, laboratories must adapt their compliance frameworks to ensure they align with regulatory standards while still fostering innovation. This balancing act will be crucial as research moves forward in a rapidly changing environment.

Ethical frameworks are also seeing transformation in new technologies. As stem cell research becomes increasingly complex, the need for robust ethical guidelines has never been more pressing. Stakeholders, including healthcare personnel, biomedical scientists, and oversight bodies, must engage in ongoing dialogue to establish frameworks that address the nuances of emerging methodologies. This collaboration will help ensure that ethical considerations remain at the forefront of research practices, particularly in relation to consent and the rights of donors.

Regulatory compliance in stem cell laboratories is essential for maintaining public trust and safety. As new technologies emerge, regulatory bodies are challenged to keep pace with scientific advancements. Laboratories must stay informed of changes in regulations and ensure they implement best practices to meet compliance requirements. This may involve adopting new protocols for risk assessment and management in stem cell trials, which are critical for safeguarding participants and ensuring the integrity of research outcomes.

Advocacy groups play a crucial role in shaping the future of stem cell research. These organisations not only promote awareness and education but also influence policy and regulatory frameworks. By collaborating with researchers and regulatory bodies, advocacy groups can help bridge the gap between scientific innovation and public perception, ensuring that research is conducted ethically and transparently. Their involvement is vital in fostering an environment where emerging trends can thrive while adhering to ethical standards.

Finally, education and training programmes for stem cell researchers are integral to the advancement of the field. As technologies evolve, so too must the skill sets of those working in stem cell laboratories. Comprehensive training initiatives can equip researchers with the knowledge necessary to navigate the complexities of new methodologies and regulatory requirements. By prioritising education, the stem cell research community can ensure that future advancements are approached with the utmost care and ethical consideration, ultimately benefiting both science and society.

Anticipating Regulatory Changes

Anticipating regulatory changes in stem cell research is crucial for healthcare personnel and biomedical scientists alike. As the landscape of scientific innovation evolves, so too do the ethical frameworks and compliance guidelines that govern this field. Staying ahead of these changes allows researchers to adapt their practices, ensuring that they not only meet current standards but also anticipate future requirements. This proactive approach can mitigate risks associated with non-compliance and maintain the integrity of research initiatives.

The role of oversight bodies is vital in shaping the regulatory environment surrounding stem cell laboratories. These organisations provide the necessary guard rails that help navigate the complexities of ethical research. By engaging with these bodies, researchers can gain insights into upcoming regulatory shifts and participate in discussions that influence policy development. This collaboration fosters a culture of compliance and encourages best practices across the industry.

Advocacy groups also play a significant role in anticipating regulatory changes. These organisations often act as a bridge between researchers and policymakers, helping to articulate the importance of stem cell research and the need for supportive regulations. By raising awareness of the potential benefits and addressing public concerns, advocacy groups can help shape a regulatory framework that is both ethical and conducive to scientific progress.

In addition to understanding the regulatory landscape, effective education and training programmes for stem cell researchers are essential. Such programmes should incorporate risk assessment and management strategies that align with anticipated regulatory changes. By equipping researchers with the tools to navigate potential challenges, these educational initiatives can enhance compliance and promote ethical research practices within laboratories.

Finally, as the field of stem cell research continues to advance, the ability to anticipate regulatory changes will become increasingly important. Researchers who remain vigilant and adaptable will not only safeguard their work but also contribute to the broader goal of advancing medical science responsibly. This forward-thinking mindset is essential in ensuring that the promise of stem cell research is realised in a manner that prioritises ethical standards and regulatory compliance.

Building a Culture of Compliance and Care

Creating a culture of compliance and care within stem cell laboratories is paramount for ensuring ethical research practices and safeguarding patient welfare. This culture begins with a clear understanding of the regulatory standards that govern stem cell research. Health care personnel and biomedical scientists must be well-versed in these standards, as they form the foundation of ethical frameworks that guide their work. By fostering an environment where compliance is seen as a shared responsibility, laboratories can ensure that all team members are aligned in their commitment to ethical research practices.

Education and training programmes are essential for instilling a culture of compliance and care. These programmes should not only cover the technical aspects of stem cell research but also emphasise the ethical considerations that underpin this work. Regular training sessions can help reinforce the importance of regulatory compliance, informed consent, and risk assessment. Furthermore, engaging advocacy groups in these training initiatives can provide additional insights and support, promoting a more holistic understanding of the implications of stem cell research.

The role of oversight bodies is critical in maintaining a culture of compliance. These organisations provide the necessary guard rails for stem cell research, ensuring that laboratories adhere to established ethical frameworks and regulatory requirements. By implementing regular audits and inspections, oversight bodies can identify areas for improvement and offer guidance to laboratories. This collaboration between oversight bodies and research institutions fosters a proactive approach to compliance and care, ultimately enhancing the integrity of stem cell research.

Best practices for obtaining informed consent are also a vital component of building a culture of compliance and care. Researchers must prioritise transparent communication with participants, ensuring they fully understand the implications of their involvement in stem cell trials. By developing clear consent processes and materials, laboratories can empower participants to make informed decisions about their participation. This not only enhances compliance but also shows respect for the autonomy of individuals involved in research.

Finally, risk assessment and management in stem cell trials should be an ongoing process within laboratories. By regularly evaluating potential risks and implementing strategies to mitigate them, laboratories can uphold a high standard of care. This proactive approach not only protects participants but also reinforces the laboratory's commitment to ethical research practices. Ultimately, fostering a culture of compliance and care is essential for the advancement of stem cell research, ensuring that scientific progress aligns with ethical imperatives.

Conclusion

Summary of Key Points

The key points related to compliance and care within stem cell laboratories, highlighting the importance of regulatory standards and ethical frameworks. In an ever-evolving field like stem cell research, adherence to established guidelines is essential for ensuring the safety and efficacy of research practices. Regulatory compliance not only protects the integrity of the research but also safeguards the rights and welfare of participants involved in stem cell trials.

The role of advocacy groups in stem cell research cannot be overstated. These organisations play a crucial part in promoting ethical practices and supporting researchers in navigating the complex regulatory landscape. By providing resources and education, advocacy groups help to ensure that all parties involved in stem cell research understand their responsibilities and the significance of obtaining informed consent from participants.

Risk assessment and management are also vital components of stem cell trials. Researchers must identify potential risks associated with their studies and implement strategies to mitigate these risks effectively. This proactive approach not only enhances the safety of participants but also contributes to the overall credibility of stem cell research as a legitimate scientific endeavour.

Education and training programmes for stem cell researchers are key to fostering a culture of compliance and ethical responsibility. By equipping researchers with the necessary knowledge and skills, these programmes ensure that they are well-prepared to conduct their work in accordance with regulatory standards. Continuous professional development is essential for keeping pace with the latest advancements and regulatory changes in the field.

In conclusion, the interplay between compliance, ethical frameworks, and best practices is fundamental to the advancement of stem cell research. By adhering to established guidelines and fostering a collaborative environment among all stakeholders, we can ensure that stem cell research continues to progress in a responsible and ethical manner, ultimately benefiting health care and society at large.

The Path Forward for Stem Cell Research

The future of stem cell research is poised at a critical juncture, where advancing scientific inquiry must harmoniously align with robust ethical frameworks and regulatory compliance. As healthcare personnel and biomedical scientists embark on this journey, it is essential to establish clear guard rails that not only protect participants but also foster innovation. Regulatory bodies play a pivotal role in shaping these parameters, ensuring that research adheres to established standards while remaining flexible enough to accommodate new discoveries and methodologies.

Ethics will remain at the forefront of stem cell research, guiding the development of best practices for informed consent. Researchers must prioritise transparency and ensure that participants fully understand the implications of their involvement. This commitment to ethical standards is crucial in maintaining public trust and support, particularly in a field often clouded by controversy. Advocacy groups can serve as invaluable partners in this respect, helping to bridge gaps between researchers and the communities they serve, while promoting an informed dialogue around stem cell therapies.

The landscape of regulatory compliance in stem cell laboratories is continually evolving, necessitating ongoing education and training programmes for researchers. These initiatives should focus not only on the technical aspects of stem cell research but also on the legal and ethical considerations that underpin their work. By fostering a culture of compliance, laboratories can mitigate risks associated with stem cell trials, ensuring that safety and efficacy remain paramount.

Risk assessment and management will be vital as stem cell trials progress from the laboratory to clinical application. Researchers must adopt comprehensive strategies to identify potential risks early in the process, allowing for proactive measures to be implemented. Collaboration with oversight bodies will be essential in navigating these challenges, as they provide the necessary expertise and regulatory insight to guide researchers through the complexities of trial design and execution.

In conclusion, the path forward for stem cell research is one that balances innovation with responsibility. By emphasising ethical frameworks, regulatory compliance, and the importance of informed consent, stakeholders can work together to create a landscape that not only advances scientific knowledge but also prioritises the well-being of participants. Engaging advocacy groups and investing in education will further strengthen this foundation, ensuring that stem cell research continues to thrive in a responsible and ethically sound manner.

Pause for thought

- Stem cell biology is a branch of biomedical science that focuses on the properties and applications of stem cells, which have the unique ability to develop into different cell types.

- The ethical frameworks surrounding stem cell research are essential to guide the responsible use of these powerful cells. Though regulation varies across countries, common thesis includes the necessity for informed consent, respect for human dignity, and the avoidance of commodification of human life.

- Oversight bodies play a pivotal role in ensuring compliance with these ethical standards, which helps to maintain public trust in scientific research and its applications. This ethical landscape is particularly important as it provides guard rails for researchers navigating complex moral dilemmas in stem cell studies.

- Regulatory compliance in stem cell laboratories is vital for ensuring that research is conducted safely and ethically. Laboratories must adhere to stringent guidelines that extend from laboratory practices to management of biological materials. Best practices in consent processes are also paramount, as researchers must ensure that participants are fully informed about the implications of their contributions to stem cell research.

- Clear communication about potential risks and benefits, are essential for fostering transparency and accountability.

- Advocacy groups play an influential role in stem cell research by promoting awareness and supporting policy changes that facilitate scientific progress. These groups bridge the gap between researchers, patients and regulatory bodies and thus ensures that the values of those affected by diseases are heard. They also contribute to education and training programs for stem cell researchers providing crucial resources that enhance knowledge and skills in the field, thereby elevating the overall quality of research and its outcome.

- Risk assessment and management in stem cell trials are critical components of the research process. Researchers must evaluate potential risk to participate to participate and establish protocols to mitigate them.

- Regulatory standards act as guard rails that help researchers navigate the complex ethical landscape inherent in this field. Compliance with regulatory frameworks not only protect the rights of participants but also enhances the credibility of research outcomes, ultimately fostering public trust in scientific advancements.

- Ethical frameworks underpinning regulatory standards are vital for guiding researchers in making informed decisions. They provide a foundation for assessing the moral implications of stem cell research, helping to balance scientific enquiry with respect for human dignity.

- Defining guard rails in stem cell research is essential to ensure that scientific enquiry proceeds ethically and responsibly. These guard rails serve as frameworks within which researchers operate, establishing clear boundaries that protect both participants and the integrity of the research. Through the delineation of acceptable practices, these guidelines assist in navigating the complex ethical landscape inherent in stem cell studies, where the potential for significant medical advancements must be balanced against the risks involved.

Take Home Nuggets

- One of the primary aspects of guard rails is the establishment of frameworks that govern consent procedures. Informed consent is not merely a formality. It is a fundamental component of respect for autonomy and the rights of the participants.

- Best practices in this area necessitate that researchers communicate risks, benefits and the nature of the research in a manner that is comprehensive to participants. This ensures that individuals are truly informed and can make decisions aligned with their values and preferences.

- The introduction of ethical frameworks was a significant milestone in the evolution of regulation. The framework sought to balance the pursuit of scientific knowledge with the moral responsibilities owed to individuals. The key principles which emerged included the necessity for informed consent, respect for autonomy and the minimisation of harm. These ethical considerations helped to shape best practices within laboratories, ensuring that research protocols align with societal values and expectations.

- Advocacy groups have raised public awareness and influenced policymakers by voicing the concerns of various stakeholders, including patients, researchers and ethicist. By engaging in dialogue with regulatory bodies, these groups have contributed to a more informed and responsive regulatory environment, essential for the advancement of stem cell source.

- Key international bodies such as the World Health Organisation and international society for stem cell research have established comprehensive guidelines that address both the scientific and ethical consideration inherent in stem cell research. These guidelines serve as guard rails, providing direction and clarity in an evolving field that holds immense potential for medical advancements.

- Education and training programs for stem cell researchers must incorporate ethical principles prominently. These programs should equip researchers with the knowledge and skills necessary to navigate the complex ethical landscape of their work. Continuous education on ethical issues, informed consent and risk management is vital for fostering a culture of compliance and care within stem cell laboratories. By investing in training, institutions can ensure that their personnel uphold the highest ethical standards, ultimately benefitting both research integrity and patient welfare.

- The ethical framework guiding stem cell research emphasize the importance of informed consent as a safeguard against coercion and exploitation. These frameworks provide guidelines for researchers to follow ensuring that consent is obtained in a manner that is transparent and respectful.

- The rapidly evolving field of stem cell research poses challenges between innovations and ethics, which is a pressing concern for health care personnel, biomedical scientist and regulatory bodies alike. As advancements in technology open new avenues for treatment and research it becomes imperative to establish guard rails that ensure these innovations do not compromise ethical standards. It is therefore a challenge to foster an environment in which scientific progress is balanced with a commitment to ethical practices, safeguarding the rights and welfare of participants involved in stem cell studies.

- In the United Kingdom, the Human Fertility and Embryology (HFEA) is one of the primary regulatory bodies responsible for overseeing activities involving human embryos and stem cells. This agency sets strict guidelines for research protocols, focusing on ethical considerations and safety requirements. By enforcing compliance with these standards, the HFEA ensures that stem cell laboratories operate within a framework that prioritises both scientific advancement and public trust.

- Regulatory compliance in stem cell laboratories encompass various aspects including adherence to local, national, and international regulations. Laboratories must implement best practices for quality assurance and risk management to mitigate potential ethical branches.

Chapter 8
Key Developments in Stem Cell Technology

The field of stem cell technology has witnessed significant advancements over the past few decades, sparking both excitement and ethical dilemmas. One of the most notable developments has been the emergence of induced pluripotent stem cells (iPSCs), which allow adult cells to be reprogrammed into a pluripotent state. This breakthrough has opened new avenues for regenerative medicine, presenting an alternative to the contentious use of embryonic stem cells. However, the ethical implications of iPSCs, including concerns over consent and the potential for commercial exploitation, remain hotly debated among health care professionals and researchers.

In addition to iPSCs, advancements in gene editing technologies, such as CRISPR, have further complicated the ethical landscape of stem cell research. These tools allow for precise modifications of the genome, raising questions about the moral status of genetically altered cells and the long-term effects on human health. Health care professionals must navigate these complex issues, balancing the potential benefits of such technologies against the ethical concerns they evoke. The intersection of scientific innovation and ethical practice is thus a critical area of focus for biomedical scientists and oversight bodies alike.

The commercialisation of stem cell therapies has also emerged as a significant issue, especially in the context of cross-border treatments. Many countries have varying regulations regarding stem cell research and therapies, leading to a patchwork of ethical standards. This situation presents dilemmas for healthcare professionals who may encounter patients seeking treatments that are unavailable or unregulated in their home countries. The ethical challenges posed by these disparities underscore the need for cohesive international guidelines to protect patient rights and ensure ethical practices in stem cell research.

Moreover, the ethical considerations surrounding the use of stem cells from human tissues, especially in relation to minors, demand scrutiny. Consent processes must be robust, ensuring that all participants, particularly vulnerable populations, are adequately informed and protected. This aspect of stem cell research not only highlights the necessity for stringent ethical oversight but also reflects the growing awareness of the rights of individuals involved in research. Health care professionals must remain vigilant in advocating for ethical practices that respect patient autonomy while advancing scientific knowledge.

Finally, religious perspectives on stem cell research add another layer of complexity to the ethical discourse. Various faiths hold differing views on the moral implications of using embryonic stem cells, which can impact public opinion and policymaking. Engaging with these perspectives is crucial for health care professionals, as it fosters a more inclusive dialogue and helps to address the concerns of diverse communities. Ultimately, navigating the ethical waters of stem cell research requires a multifaceted approach that respects both scientific progress and the moral values of society.

Ethical Controversies in Stem Cell Use

Defining Ethical Controversies

The ethical controversies surrounding stem cell research have become a focal point for health care professionals, biomedical scientists, and oversight bodies alike. These controversies often stem from the various sources of stem cells, particularly embryonic stem cells, which pose significant moral and ethical dilemmas. The debate is not just confined to scientific and medical implications but extends into the realms of personal beliefs and societal values, making it a complex issue that requires careful navigation.

Consent is another critical aspect of ethical considerations in stem cell research. The use of stem cells derived from human tissues necessitates informed consent from donors, which raises questions about autonomy and the understanding of potential risks and benefits. Health care professionals must ensure that individuals are fully aware of how their tissue will be used and the implications it may have, especially in cases involving vulnerable populations such as minors.

Religious perspectives significantly influence opinions on stem cell research, particularly regarding the moral status of embryos. Different faiths offer varying viewpoints on when life begins and the sanctity of human life, which directly affects attitudes towards both embryonic stem cell research and the use of induced pluripotent stem cells. This diversity of beliefs complicates the ethical landscape, requiring sensitivity and respect for differing views within clinical and research settings.

The commercialisation of stem cell research also poses ethical challenges, particularly concerning the potential for exploitation and profit-driven motives overshadowing patient welfare. As funding becomes increasingly tied to commercial interests, the risk of compromising ethical standards rises. Oversight bodies must strike a balance between promoting innovation and ensuring that ethical practices remain a priority, especially when vulnerable populations are involved.

Finally, cross-border ethical dilemmas arise as patients seek stem cell treatments that may not be available or legal in their home countries. This situation creates a grey area in terms of patient rights and ethical research practices. Health care professionals must navigate these complexities while advocating for patient safety and adherence to ethical guidelines, ensuring that all stem cell research and treatment protocols are conducted in an ethically sound manner.

Public Perception and Misconceptions

Public perception of stem cell research often diverges sharply from the scientific community's understanding. Misconceptions regarding the nature of stem cells, particularly embryonic stem cells, contribute to a widespread apprehension. Many individuals equate stem cell research with the termination of human life, leading to ethical debates that overshadow the potential benefits of such research. This fear complicates discussions among health care professionals and biomedical scientists, who must navigate these perceptions while advocating for scientific advancements.

The ethical implications surrounding consent in the use of stem cells from human tissues are frequently misunderstood. Many assume that all forms of stem cell research require the destruction of embryos, which is not always the case. Induced pluripotent stem cells (iPSCs), for instance, are derived from adult cells and do not involve embryonic tissues. This misunderstanding can hinder informed consent processes, as potential donors may not fully grasp the implications of their participation in research, leading to ethical dilemmas that health care professionals must address.

Religious perspectives on stem cell research further complicate public perception. Various faith groups have differing views on the sanctity of life, impacting their stance on embryonic versus adult stem cell research. This divergence can create a climate of controversy, making it challenging for biomedical scientists and oversight bodies to establish a consensus. It is essential to engage religious and community leaders in discussions about the potential benefits of stem cell research to mitigate fears and foster a more informed public dialogue.

Commercialisation of stem cell research presents another layer of ethical concern. The potential for profit can sometimes overshadow the ethical considerations that should guide research and treatment protocols. Health care professionals must be vigilant about ensuring that commercial interests do not compromise the integrity of research or the welfare of patients. This is especially critical in the context of cross-border treatments where regulatory frameworks may differ, potentially leading to exploitation of vulnerable populations.

Finally, the ethical challenges surrounding stem cell research involving minors and animal testing are paramount. Minors are particularly vulnerable, raising questions about consent and the potential long-term effects of participation in research. Similarly, animal testing poses ethical dilemmas regarding the treatment of test subjects. It is crucial for health care professionals and researchers to remain cognisant of these issues, ensuring that ethical standards are upheld across all facets of stem cell research and its applications.

The Role of Ethics Committees

Ethics committees play a pivotal role in the realm of stem cell research, providing oversight and guidance to ensure that ethical standards are upheld. These committees, often composed of a diverse group of experts including healthcare professionals, bioethicists, and legal advisors, are tasked with evaluating the moral implications of research projects. Their primary function is to assess proposals for ethical compliance, particularly in areas fraught with controversy, such as the use of embryonic stem cells and the consent processes involving human tissues.

One of the critical functions of ethics committees is to facilitate informed consent, ensuring that participants are fully aware of the implications of their involvement in research. This process is particularly complex in the context of stem cell research, where the potential benefits must be weighed against the ethical concerns surrounding the use of human embryos. Committees are responsible for developing guidelines that protect participants, especially vulnerable groups such as minors, and ensuring that their rights are respected throughout the research process.

The intersection of ethics and commercialisation in stem cell research presents additional challenges for ethics committees. As the field becomes increasingly lucrative, there is a risk that ethical considerations may be overshadowed by profit motives. Committees must remain vigilant in their oversight, ensuring that commercial interests do not compromise the integrity of research practices or the welfare of research subjects.

Moreover, ethics committees are crucial in navigating the diverse religious perspectives on stem cell research. Different faiths hold varying views on the moral status of embryos, which can lead to significant ethical dilemmas. Committees must engage with these perspectives, fostering dialogue between researchers and religious communities to find common ground while respecting individual beliefs and values.

Finally, as stem cell treatments cross borders, ethics committees face the challenge of addressing cross-border ethical dilemmas. Variations in regulatory frameworks and ethical standards can complicate international collaborations and the treatment of patients. Ethics committees must establish protocols that not only comply with local laws but also uphold global ethical standards, ensuring that patient rights are protected regardless of geographical boundaries.

Legislative Responses to Embryonic Stem Cell Research

The legislative responses to embryonic stem cell research have evolved significantly over the past few decades, shaped by ethical concerns and public opinion. Governments worldwide grappled with the implications of using human embryos for scientific advancement, leading to a patchwork of regulations. In the United States, for example, federal funding for embryonic stem cell research faced restrictions under various administrations, reflecting the contentious nature of the debate. These policies not only influence research funding but also impact the scope of scientific inquiry and the potential for breakthroughs in regenerative medicine.

In many countries, ethical considerations surrounding consent play a pivotal role in legislative frameworks. The necessity for informed consent from donors of embryonic tissues highlights the need for transparency and respect for individual autonomy. Legislative bodies often mandate rigorous consent processes to ensure that donors are fully aware of the implications of their contributions. This aspect of legislation is crucial for maintaining public trust and upholding ethical standards in the research community.

Religious perspectives also significantly influence legislative actions concerning embryonic stem cell research. In regions where religious beliefs strongly oppose the destruction of embryos, lawmakers face pressure to enact strict regulations or outright bans on such research. This intersection of faith and policy complicates the legislative landscape, as it requires a balance between scientific advancement and moral considerations. As a result, health care professionals and biomedical scientists must navigate these complex ethical waters while adhering to the laws governing their practice.

The impact of commercialisation on ethical practices in stem cell research cannot be overlooked. As private companies enter the field, the potential for profit can clash with ethical imperatives. Legislative responses often attempt to regulate the commercialisation of stem cell therapies to prevent exploitation, especially in vulnerable populations. Oversight bodies are tasked with ensuring that ethical standards are maintained, which is particularly critical in the context of emerging technologies such as induced pluripotent stem cells.

Lastly, cross-border ethical dilemmas arise as researchers and patients seek stem cell treatments outside their home countries. Different legislative environments can lead to disparities in ethical standards, creating challenges for health care professionals. The intersection of patient rights and research ethics becomes increasingly complex in this global context. Legislators must consider not only the implications for domestic policy but also the international ramifications of their decisions regarding stem cell research, highlighting the need for a cohesive and ethically sound approach.

Consent and the Use of Stem Cells from Human Tissues

Informed Consent in Stem Cell Research

Informed consent serves as a cornerstone of ethical practice in stem cell research, ensuring that participants are fully aware of the implications of their involvement. This process is particularly complex in the context of embryonic stem cell research, where the moral status of the embryo raises significant ethical questions. Health care professionals and biomedical scientists must navigate these dilemmas carefully, balancing the potential benefits of research with the rights and beliefs of individuals involved. Clear communication and education about the nature of the research and its potential outcomes are essential in fostering trust and respect.

The ethical implications of using stem cells derived from human tissues further complicate the informed consent process. Participants must understand not only what their consent entails but also the possible risks associated with the use of their biological materials. Oversight bodies play a crucial role in ensuring that consent forms are comprehensive and transparent, providing individuals with the information necessary to make informed decisions. Consequently, it is vital for researchers to engage with participants sincerely, addressing their concerns and allowing for an open dialogue about the research's ethical dimensions.

Religious perspectives on stem cell research significantly influence public opinion and individual choices regarding consent. Many faith communities have articulated their stances on the moral implications of using embryonic stem cells, often opposing such research on ethical grounds. This presents a challenge for researchers who must respect these beliefs while also advocating for the scientific merits of their work. It is essential for health care professionals to approach these discussions with sensitivity and understanding, recognising that ethical considerations often intersect with deeply held convictions.

Commercialisation of stem cell research introduces additional ethical challenges related to informed consent. As private entities become increasingly involved in this field, the potential for profit may overshadow the ethical responsibilities researchers have towards participants. Ensuring that consent is obtained without coercion and that participants are not exploited for financial gain is paramount. This requires a robust regulatory framework that upholds ethical standards while fostering innovation in stem cell therapies.

Finally, the ethical considerations surrounding stem cell research involving minors necessitate a heightened level of scrutiny when it comes to informed consent. Given the vulnerability of this population, obtaining consent must involve not only the minors themselves but also their guardians. Researchers must be diligent in explaining the research in an age-appropriate manner and ensuring that minors' rights and welfare are prioritised. Navigating these ethical waters requires a commitment to transparency, respect, and a dedication to the well-being of all participants involved in stem cell research.

Challenges in Obtaining Consent

Obtaining consent in stem cell research presents significant challenges that are often compounded by ethical, legal, and social implications. For healthcare professionals and biomedical scientists, the need for transparent and informed consent is paramount, yet the complexities surrounding stem cell sources, particularly embryonic stem cells, can create confusion among potential donors. The process must ensure that individuals fully understand the implications of their consent, including the potential for their donated tissues to contribute to research that might lead to controversial therapeutic applications.

The ethical implications of using human tissues for stem cell research are particularly pronounced when considering the perspectives of various stakeholders, including patients, families, and oversight bodies. Informed consent must go beyond mere documentation; it requires a thorough dialogue about the implications of stem cell use and the potential outcomes of research. This dialogue is further complicated by differing interpretations of what constitutes adequate understanding, as cultural and individual beliefs about stem cell research can significantly influence perceptions of consent.

Religious perspectives also play a critical role in the discourse surrounding consent for stem cell research. Many religious groups hold firm beliefs regarding the sanctity of human life from conception, raising ethical dilemmas about the use of embryonic stem cells. This can lead to situations where potential donors may feel conflicted about providing consent, necessitating healthcare professionals to navigate these sensitive discussions with care and respect for diverse beliefs.

Moreover, the commercialisation of stem cell research introduces an additional layer of complexity to the consent process. As private entities increasingly enter the field, concerns arise about the potential for exploitation and the prioritisation of profit over ethical standards. This commercial landscape may push for expedited consent processes, risking the thoroughness required to ensure that participants are genuinely informed and their rights protected.

Lastly, ethical challenges in obtaining consent are magnified when involving vulnerable populations, such as minors. Special considerations must be taken to ensure that consent is not only obtained from guardians but that the minors themselves comprehend the implications of their participation. Cross-border ethical dilemmas also emerge, where differing regulations and standards of consent can lead to exploitation or misunderstanding in international research contexts. Thus, navigating these challenges requires a robust ethical framework and ongoing dialogue amongst all stakeholders in the stem cell research arena.

The Role of Donor Autonomy

The concept of donor autonomy is pivotal in the realm of stem cell research, particularly when addressing the ethical implications surrounding consent and the use of human tissues. Donors must have the right to make informed decisions about their own biological materials, free from coercion or undue influence. This principle upholds the dignity of the individual and ensures that participants are fully aware of the potential uses of their donated cells, including the risks involved. Health care professionals and biomedical scientists must prioritise clear communication about these aspects to foster a trusting relationship with donors.

In the context of embryonic stem cell research, the issue of donor autonomy becomes even more complex. Donors, often parents facing challenging circumstances, may not fully grasp the long-term implications of their decisions. This raises ethical questions about the extent to which consent is genuinely informed. Oversight bodies play a crucial role in establishing guidelines that promote transparency and protect the interests of donors, ensuring that their autonomy is respected and upheld throughout the research process.

Religious perspectives significantly influence views on donor autonomy and the legitimacy of stem cell research. Many faith traditions advocate for the sanctity of life, which can lead to conflicting opinions on the use of stem cells from embryos. Understanding these diverse viewpoints is essential for health care professionals and researchers as they navigate the ethical landscape. Engaging with religious communities can also provide insights into the moral considerations surrounding donor autonomy, facilitating a more inclusive dialogue on the topic.

The commercialisation of stem cell research poses additional challenges to donor autonomy. As the market for stem cell therapies expands, there is a risk that financial incentives may overshadow ethical considerations. Donors may feel pressured to contribute to research for monetary gain rather than altruistic reasons, potentially compromising their autonomy. It is imperative for oversight bodies to implement regulations that safeguard against exploitation and ensure that donor decisions are made in a context that prioritises ethical practices over profit.

Lastly, the ethical considerations surrounding donor autonomy extend to vulnerable populations, including minors. When involving children in stem cell research, obtaining genuine informed consent becomes paramount. Parents or guardians may advocate for their children's participation, but it is crucial to assess the child's ability to understand the implications of their involvement. This underscores the need for robust ethical frameworks that protect the rights of all donors, ensuring that autonomy remains a cornerstone of ethical stem cell research practices.

Religious Perspectives on Stem Cell Research and Usage

Overview of Major Religious Views

In the discourse surrounding stem cell research, various religious views play a pivotal role in shaping ethical perspectives and policy decisions. Major religious traditions, including Christianity, Judaism, and Islam, have distinct beliefs about the sanctity of life and the moral status of embryos. These beliefs influence not only personal attitudes towards stem cell research but also institutional policies that govern biomedical practices. Understanding these religious frameworks is essential for healthcare professionals and biomedical scientists who navigate the complexities of ethical decision-making in this field.

Christianity, particularly in its Catholic and Protestant branches, often holds the view that human life begins at conception. This belief leads many Christians to oppose embryonic stem cell research, as it involves the destruction of embryos. The Catholic Church has been particularly vocal in its condemnation of practices that it deems to infringe upon the dignity of human life. Conversely, some Protestant denominations may adopt a more permissive stance, suggesting that the potential benefits of stem cell research can justify its ethical implications, especially when considering therapies for debilitating conditions.

Judaism presents a nuanced perspective on stem cell research, rooted in the value placed on saving lives. Many Jewish authorities argue that the potential to alleviate suffering and save lives can override concerns about the destruction of embryos. This view is often supported by the principle of "pikuach nefesh," which prioritises the preservation of human life. Consequently, Jewish bioethics may support the use of embryonic stem cells under specific conditions, highlighting the tension between religious beliefs and scientific advancements.

Islamic perspectives on stem cell research are varied and depend significantly on the interpretation of religious texts and the context of medical ethics. Many Islamic scholars emphasise the importance of intention and the moral implications of using stem cells. While some may prohibit the use of embryonic stem cells due to concerns over the sanctity of life, others may permit their use if they can lead to significant medical benefits. This diversity within the Muslim community reflects the broader ethical dilemmas faced by healthcare professionals when considering the implications of stem cell research across different religious contexts.

Lastly, the commercialisation of stem cell research introduces additional ethical challenges, particularly regarding consent and patient rights. The potential for profit can complicate the ethical landscape, leading to concerns about exploitation and the commodification of human tissues. Moreover, as stem cell treatments increasingly cross borders, healthcare professionals must navigate a complex web of ethical standards influenced by varying religious and cultural views. This intersection of commerce, ethics, and religion underscores the importance of fostering dialogue among stakeholders to ensure that ethical standards are upheld in the pursuit of scientific innovation.

Ethical Conflicts Between Science and Religion

The intersection of science and religion often presents ethical conflicts, particularly in the realm of stem cell research. In healthcare and biomedical fields, professionals grapple with the implications of using embryonic stem cells, which raises questions about the moral status of embryos. Many religious perspectives view the embryo as a life that must be protected, leading to significant ethical dilemmas for researchers who seek to advance medical knowledge and therapies. This ongoing tension highlights the need for dialogue between scientific inquiry and religious beliefs to navigate ethical waters effectively.

Consent is another critical area where ethical conflicts arise in stem cell research. Obtaining informed consent from donors, particularly when using tissues from human embryos or minors, is a complex process that requires careful consideration of ethical standards. Healthcare professionals must ensure that consent is voluntary and informed, while also addressing the concerns of religious groups who may oppose the use of such materials. The challenge lies in balancing the rights of individuals to make choices about their bodies with the ethical implications of those choices in the context of scientific advancement.

The commercialisation of stem cell research adds another layer of ethical complexity. As private companies invest in stem cell therapies, the potential for profit can sometimes overshadow ethical considerations. This commodification can lead to exploitation of vulnerable populations, particularly in cross-border scenarios where regulations may be less stringent. It is essential for oversight bodies to establish robust guidelines that safeguard ethical practices while allowing for scientific innovation. The debate surrounding the commodification of stem cells underscores the need for a cohesive ethical framework that prioritises patient rights and safety.

Furthermore, the emergence of induced pluripotent stem cells (iPSCs) presents new ethical questions regarding their status compared to traditional embryonic stem cells. While iPSCs offer promising avenues for research without the ethical concerns tied to embryos, the long-term implications of their use require thorough examination. Bioethicists and researchers must engage in ongoing discussions to establish consensus on the ethical treatment of these cells, considering both scientific advancements and the moral views held by various religious communities.

Lastly, ethical challenges in animal testing for stem cell therapies must not be overlooked. As researchers explore the efficacy of stem cell treatments, the use of animals in experimentation raises significant moral questions regarding their welfare. Health care professionals and scientists must consider alternative methods to reduce animal suffering while adhering to ethical standards. The dialogue between scientific progress and ethical responsibility remains critical, particularly as society navigates the complex landscape of stem cell research and its implications for both human and animal rights.

Interfaith Dialogues on Stem Cell Research

The topic of stem cell research has ignited passionate debates across various sectors, notably within the realms of healthcare, ethics, and religion. Interfaith dialogues have emerged as a vital platform for discussing the ethical implications of embryonic stem cell research. These discussions often highlight the diverse perspectives held by different faith traditions regarding the sanctity of life, the moral status of embryos, and the potential benefits of stem cell treatments. By fostering understanding and respect among differing beliefs, interfaith dialogues aim to create a more cohesive approach to stem cell research that acknowledges and incorporates these varied viewpoints.

Religious perspectives play a significant role in shaping public opinion on stem cell research. Many religious groups express concerns about the moral implications of using human embryos for research purposes, viewing it as a violation of the sanctity of life. However, some faith communities are more open to the possibilities of stem cell therapies, particularly when they can alleviate suffering and improve quality of life. Interfaith dialogues provide an opportunity for these groups to express their views, challenge misconceptions, and explore common ground, ultimately contributing to a more nuanced understanding of the ethical complexities involved in stem cell research.

Consent and the use of stem cells from human tissues is another critical area explored in interfaith dialogues. The ethical considerations surrounding informed consent are paramount, particularly when it involves vulnerable populations such as minors. Religious leaders can play an essential role in educating their communities about the importance of consent and the ethical implications of using human tissues in research. By addressing these concerns collaboratively, interfaith dialogues can help establish guidelines that respect individual rights while promoting scientific advancement.

The impact of commercialisation on ethical practices in stem cell research is also a focal point in these discussions. As the market for stem cell therapies expands, ethical considerations must be carefully examined to prevent exploitation and ensure equitable access. Interfaith dialogues can address the potential dangers of commodifying human life and encourage a collective commitment to ethical standards that prioritise human dignity over profit. By engaging diverse perspectives, these discussions can help shape policies that balance innovation with ethical integrity.

Lastly, interfaith dialogues on stem cell research can provide a forum for discussing cross-border ethical dilemmas in stem cell treatments. As patients seek care globally, differing ethical standards can lead to complications in treatment and patient rights. Engaging in these conversations allows stakeholders to reflect on the implications of their practices and consider how international cooperation can foster ethical consistency in stem cell research. Through collaboration and mutual respect, interfaith dialogues can enhance the ethical landscape of stem cell research and advocate for the welfare of all individuals involved.

The Impact of Commercialisation on Ethical Practices in Stem Cell Research

The Commercial Landscape of Stem Cell Research

The commercial landscape of stem cell research has evolved significantly over the past few decades, driven largely by advancements in technology and an increasing demand for innovative therapies. This burgeoning market has attracted the attention of various stakeholders, including private investors, pharmaceutical companies, and academic institutions. As these players vie for a share of the market, ethical concerns associated with the commercialization of stem cell research have become more pronounced, particularly regarding the implications of profit-driven motives on research integrity and patient care.

One of the most contentious issues within this landscape is the ethical implications of embryonic stem cell research. The use of human embryos raises profound moral questions, particularly about the status of the embryo and the rights of potential human life. This has led to heated debates not only within the scientific community but also across various religious and cultural groups. As commercial interests push for the advancement of embryonic stem cell therapies, the need for clear ethical guidelines becomes increasingly critical.

Consent plays a pivotal role in stem cell research, especially in light of the complexities surrounding human tissues. The process of obtaining informed consent from donors must be transparent and respectful, ensuring that individuals understand the implications of their contributions. This is particularly vital in cases involving vulnerable populations, such as minors, where additional ethical considerations must be taken into account. The intersection of patient rights and stem cell research ethics poses ongoing challenges for healthcare professionals and oversight bodies alike.

The emergence of induced pluripotent stem cells (iPSCs) has added another layer to the ethical debate. While iPSCs offer a promising alternative to embryonic stem cells, questions regarding their ethical status and the implications of their use continue to surface. The potential for commercial exploitation of iPSCs also raises concerns about the motivations behind their development and the possible prioritisation of profit over patient welfare.

Lastly, cross-border ethical dilemmas in stem cell treatments present significant challenges. Different countries maintain varying regulations and ethical standards, which can lead to discrepancies in treatment availability and quality. This situation complicates the landscape for healthcare professionals and researchers who must navigate these differences while upholding ethical practices in stem cell research. The commercialisation of stem cell therapies must therefore be approached with caution, ensuring that ethical standards are maintained across all levels of research and application.

Ethical Implications of Profit Motives

The ethical implications of profit motives in stem cell research are complex and multifaceted, especially as advancements in biomedical sciences continue to evolve. Health care professionals and biomedical scientists must navigate a landscape where profit can sometimes overshadow ethical considerations. The drive for profit can lead to prioritising commercial interests over patient welfare, raising questions about the integrity of research and the potential exploitation of vulnerable populations, particularly in terms of consent and the use of human tissues in research.

One significant ethical concern arises when profit motives intersect with the use of embryonic stem cells. The commodification of these cells can lead to contentious debates about the moral status of embryos and the implications of treating them as mere biological resources. This raises profound ethical questions, particularly within religious communities that hold specific beliefs about the sanctity of life. The challenge lies in balancing scientific advancement with respect for diverse moral perspectives while ensuring that research is conducted in a manner that aligns with ethical standards.

The impact of commercialisation on ethical practices in stem cell research cannot be understated. As companies seek to profit from breakthroughs in stem cell therapies, there is a risk that ethical guidelines may be bent or overlooked. This commercial pressure can lead to unethical practices, such as inadequate informed consent processes or the exploitation of patients, especially minors, who may not fully understand the implications of participation in research. It is crucial for oversight bodies to enforce strict regulations that uphold ethical standards while fostering innovation in the field.

Cross-border ethical dilemmas further complicate the landscape of stem cell research. Different countries have varying regulations regarding the use of stem cells, leading to situations where researchers may seek less stringent environments to conduct controversial studies. This creates ethical challenges, as patients may travel abroad for treatments that are deemed unethical or unproven in their home countries. Health care professionals must be aware of these disparities and advocate for ethical practices that protect patient rights and ensure safe, responsible research.

Finally, the debate over induced pluripotent stem cells (iPSCs) presents an additional layer of ethical complexity. While iPSCs offer significant potential for therapeutic applications without the ethical concerns associated with embryonic stem cells, their status and the implications of their use remain contentious. The intersection of patient rights and stem cell research ethics demands ongoing dialogue among stakeholders, ensuring that as science progresses, ethical considerations remain at the forefront of research and application in this rapidly evolving field.

Regulation of Commercial Stem Cell Practices

The regulation of commercial stem cell practices is a critical area of consideration for health care professionals and biomedical scientists. As the field of stem cell research has expanded, so too have the ethical controversies surrounding its application. Regulatory frameworks must address the complexities of consent, especially concerning the use of human tissues and the implications of embryonic stem cell research. Furthermore, the intersection of commercialisation and ethical practices raises significant concerns regarding the motives behind stem cell therapies and their availability to patients.

One of the primary ethical issues involves obtaining informed consent from donors of human tissues used in research. Health care professionals must ensure that donors fully understand the implications of their contributions, particularly when it comes to embryonic stem cells. Additionally, the ethical implications of using stem cells from minors require careful consideration, as the capacity for informed consent is limited. This necessitates a clear regulatory framework that safeguards the rights of vulnerable populations while allowing for scientific advancement.

Religious perspectives also play a significant role in shaping the ethical landscape of stem cell research. Different faiths hold varying views on the sanctity of life and the moral status of embryos, which can influence public policy and regulatory decisions. It is essential for oversight bodies to engage with these diverse perspectives to create regulations that are respectful of religious beliefs while promoting scientific progress.

The commercialisation of stem cell therapies presents a unique set of ethical challenges, particularly in terms of the potential for exploitation and inequity in access to treatments. The debate over induced pluripotent stem cells further complicates the regulatory environment, as these cells present a promising alternative to embryonic stem cells without the associated ethical concerns. However, the ethical status of these cells remains contentious, necessitating ongoing dialogue among stakeholders in the field.

Cross-border ethical dilemmas also arise as patients seek stem cell treatments in countries with less stringent regulations. This raises questions about the intersection of patient rights and the ethical responsibilities of health care providers. It is crucial for professionals in the field to navigate these complex issues thoughtfully, ensuring that ethical considerations remain at the forefront of commercial stem cell practices, ultimately fostering trust and integrity in the research community.

Ethical Considerations in Stem Cell Research Involving Minors

Vulnerability of Minors in Research

The vulnerability of minors in research, particularly in the context of stem cell studies, raises significant ethical concerns that must be carefully navigated. Minors are not fully capable of providing informed consent, which is a cornerstone of ethical research practices. This inability to consent independently makes them particularly susceptible to exploitation and raises questions about the validity of any consent obtained from parents or guardians. Therefore, it is essential for healthcare professionals and oversight bodies to ensure that the rights and welfare of these young participants are rigorously protected throughout the research process.

One of the primary ethical dilemmas in involving minors in stem cell research is the balance between potential benefits and risks. Researchers may argue that the advancements in stem cell therapies could lead to significant medical breakthroughs that benefit society as a whole. However, the risks to minors, including physical harm or psychological distress, must be weighed heavily against these potential benefits. The ethical principle of minimising harm is particularly pertinent, as minors may not fully understand the implications of their participation, thus necessitating a cautious approach in their inclusion in such studies.

Moreover, the involvement of minors in stem cell research often intersects with complex family dynamics and societal values. Parents or guardians may feel pressured to consent to their child's participation due to the promise of innovative treatments, especially in cases where traditional therapies have failed. This pressure can create ethical conflicts, as the child's best interests may not align with the desires of the parents. Thus, it is crucial for researchers and ethical review boards to engage in thorough discussions about the motivations behind parental consent and to consider the minor's perspective in these decisions.

The issue of commercialisation also plays a significant role in the ethical landscape surrounding minors in stem cell research. As the field progresses, the potential for profit can overshadow ethical considerations, leading to situations where the welfare of young participants is compromised for financial gain. This commercial pressure can further complicate the already delicate balance between innovation and ethical responsibility, necessitating stringent regulations that prioritise the rights of minors above commercial interests.

Ultimately, the ethical considerations surrounding minors in stem cell research are multifaceted and require a collaborative approach from healthcare professionals, researchers, and oversight bodies. Establishing robust ethical guidelines that address informed consent, risk assessment, and the potential for exploitation is essential. Only through careful attention to these issues can the field of stem cell research navigate the complex waters of ethics while still striving for scientific advancement that respects and protects its most vulnerable participants.

Consent and Assent in Paediatric Research

The intricacies of consent and assent in paediatric research present unique ethical challenges, particularly in the realm of stem cell research. Given that minors are not legally able to provide informed consent, it falls upon parents or guardians to make decisions on their behalf. However, it is essential to recognise the importance of involving young participants in the decision-making process to the extent that their maturity allows. This dual-layer of consent not only respects the rights of the child but also promotes a sense of agency that is crucial for their emotional and psychological development.

In the context of stem cell research, the ethical implications of obtaining consent become even more pronounced. Researchers must navigate the sensitive terrain of parental authority versus the child's developing autonomy. Furthermore, the nature of the research—often involving potentially life-altering treatments—adds a layer of urgency to these decisions. Ensuring that parents fully understand the implications of their choices, as well as the potential risks and benefits to their child, is paramount in adhering to ethical research practices.

Assent, as a complement to consent, is a vital component in engaging minors in research. It acknowledges their capacity to comprehend the basic elements of the study and to express their willingness to participate, even when they are not legally able to provide consent. Researchers must develop age-appropriate methods to explain the study, ensuring that the language used is accessible and that the child's questions are adequately addressed. This approach not only enhances the ethical integrity of the research but also fosters trust between the researcher and the young participant.

The ethical considerations surrounding consent and assent are further complicated by the commercialisation of stem cell research. As the field evolves, the involvement of for-profit entities may lead to conflicts of interest that could undermine the ethical treatment of child participants. It is crucial for oversight bodies to implement stringent guidelines that ensure the protection of minors, particularly in studies funded or conducted by commercial enterprises. Maintaining a focus on ethical practices amidst financial incentives is an ongoing challenge that requires vigilance from all stakeholders involved.

Ultimately, the discourse on consent and assent in paediatric research highlights the intersection of ethical principles, child rights, and the evolving landscape of stem cell research. Health care professionals, biomedical scientists, and oversight bodies must collaborate to create frameworks that prioritise the well-being of young participants while advancing scientific knowledge. The commitment to ethical standards in research involving minors not only safeguards their rights but also strengthens the integrity of the scientific community as a whole.

Ethical Guidelines for Research Involving Minors

The ethical guidelines for research involving minors are crucial in maintaining the integrity and welfare of young participants in stem cell research. Given the vulnerabilities of this population, it is imperative that researchers adhere to stringent ethical standards that protect minors from potential harm. This includes ensuring that the research is scientifically valid, necessary, and conducted in a manner that prioritises the well-being and rights of the child. Researchers must recognise the unique challenges presented when working with minors and the importance of safeguarding their interests throughout the research process.

Informed consent is a cornerstone of ethical research, yet obtaining consent from minors requires special considerations. While parents or guardians typically provide consent for the involvement of minors in research, it is essential to also seek the assent of the minors themselves. This process involves communicating the research purpose, procedures, risks, and benefits in an age-appropriate manner, allowing minors to express their willingness to participate. This dual layer of consent not only respects the autonomy of the child but also reinforces the ethical commitment of researchers to uphold the rights of their participants.

The potential for coercion or undue influence must be carefully managed when involving minors in stem cell research. Researchers should be vigilant in ensuring that participation is entirely voluntary and that minors do not feel pressured to take part due to parental expectations or possible rewards. Ethical guidelines dictate that researchers must create an environment where minors can freely voice their concerns or decline participation without fear of negative repercussions. This encourages a culture of respect and care, which is fundamental in research settings involving vulnerable populations.

Moreover, researchers must navigate the complexities of balancing scientific advancement with ethical responsibilities. The benefits of stem cell research involving minors can be significant, particularly in addressing rare diseases or conditions that affect children. However, the potential for exploitation or harm raises ethical concerns that must be addressed proactively. Oversight bodies play a vital role in ensuring that research protocols are rigorously evaluated for compliance with ethical standards, thereby safeguarding the interests of young participants while facilitating advancements in medical science.

Finally, as the field of stem cell research continues to evolve, ongoing dialogue among health care professionals, biomedical scientists, and oversight bodies is essential. Ethical guidelines must be regularly revisited and updated to reflect new findings, societal values, and technological advancements. This collaborative approach ensures that the ethical implications of research involving minors are continually assessed, fostering an environment of trust and integrity in the scientific community while promoting the welfare of the youngest and most vulnerable participants.

The Debate Over Induced Pluripotent Stem Cells and Their Ethical Status

Understanding Induced Pluripotent Stem Cells

Induced pluripotent stem cells (iPSCs) represent a significant advancement in regenerative medicine, providing a unique alternative to embryonic stem cells. By reprogramming somatic cells to an embryonic-like state, scientists can generate cells capable of differentiating into any cell type. This breakthrough not only opens new avenues for disease modelling and drug screening but also raises a host of ethical questions regarding their use and implications. As healthcare professionals and biomedical scientists explore the potential of iPSCs, they must navigate these complex ethical waters carefully.

The ethical controversy surrounding stem cell research primarily stems from the use of embryonic stem cells, which involves the destruction of human embryos. iPSCs circumvent this issue, as they can be derived from adult tissues, thus avoiding the moral dilemmas associated with embryo use. Nevertheless, the generation of iPSCs still necessitates a thorough understanding of consent, particularly when human tissues are involved. Ethical guidelines must be established to ensure that individuals donating tissue for iPSC research provide informed consent, recognising the potential future uses of their biological materials.

Religious perspectives on stem cell research further complicate the ethical landscape. Many religious groups oppose the use of embryonic stem cells based on beliefs about the sanctity of life. While iPSCs offer a solution to some of these concerns, they do not fully resolve the underlying ethical debates. Healthcare professionals must engage with these perspectives to foster a comprehensive dialogue around iPSC research, ensuring that ethical considerations are respected across different belief systems.

The commercialisation of iPSC technology presents additional ethical challenges, particularly concerning the accessibility and fairness of treatments derived from this research. As companies invest in iPSC therapies, there is a risk of prioritising profit over ethical practices, potentially leading to inequities in healthcare access. Oversight bodies play a crucial role in regulating these developments, ensuring that patient rights are upheld and ethical guidelines are adhered to in the pursuit of innovation.

Finally, the intersection of iPSC research ethics with vulnerable populations, such as minors, necessitates careful consideration. The ethical implications of using stem cells from minors, alongside cross-border dilemmas related to stem cell treatments, highlight the need for robust ethical frameworks. As the field progresses, ongoing dialogue among healthcare professionals, scientists, and oversight bodies will be essential to address these challenges, ensuring that iPSC research advances responsibly and ethically.

Ethical Comparisons with Embryonic Stem Cells

The ethical comparisons surrounding embryonic stem cells (ESCs) remain a contentious topic within the biomedical community. Health care professionals and biomedical scientists frequently grapple with the moral implications of using human embryos for research purposes. Proponents argue that the potential benefits of ESCs in treating debilitating diseases justify their use, while opponents raise concerns about the sanctity of human life and the moral status of embryos. This dichotomy creates a complex landscape for oversight bodies tasked with regulating stem cell research and ensuring ethical standards are upheld.

Consent is a pivotal issue in the discourse on stem cell research, particularly concerning the sourcing of embryonic stem cells. Ethical considerations necessitate that donors are fully informed about the implications of their contributions. The process of obtaining consent must be transparent and respect the autonomy of individuals, particularly when it involves sensitive issues surrounding reproduction and potential exploitation. The challenge lies in balancing the need for scientific advancement with the ethical obligation to protect donor rights and ensure informed decision-making.

Religious perspectives significantly influence the ethical landscape of embryonic stem cell research. Various faith traditions have distinct views on the moral status of embryos, which can shape public opinion and policy decisions. For instance, some religious groups advocate for the use of stem cells derived from excess embryos created during in vitro fertilisation, while others categorically oppose any research involving embryos. This intersection of ethical considerations and religious beliefs underscores the need for inclusive dialogue that respects diverse viewpoints while striving for the common good in health care.

The commercialisation of stem cell research presents additional ethical challenges, particularly regarding the potential for profit-driven motives to overshadow patient welfare. As new therapies emerge, there is a risk that financial gains could compromise ethical practices, leading to exploitation of vulnerable populations. Oversight bodies must remain vigilant to ensure that the pursuit of innovation does not come at the expense of ethical standards and patient rights, particularly in cases where treatments are marketed without sufficient evidence of safety and efficacy.

Lastly, the debate surrounding induced pluripotent stem cells (iPSCs) adds another layer of complexity to ethical discussions in stem cell research. While iPSCs offer a promising alternative that circumvents the ethical dilemmas associated with embryonic cells, their status and implications are still being explored. Ethical considerations involving minors and cross-border treatments further complicate the narrative, necessitating ongoing dialogue among health care professionals, scientists, and ethicists to navigate these multifaceted issues responsibly. The intersection of patient rights and the ethical implications of stem cell research continue to evolve, highlighting the importance of ethical vigilance in advancing medical science.

Regulatory Framework for Induced Pluripotent Stem Cells

The regulatory framework for induced pluripotent stem cells (iPSCs) is a complex interplay of laws, guidelines, and ethical considerations that govern their research and application. Health care professionals and biomedical scientists must navigate this landscape carefully, as the use of iPSCs raises significant ethical questions. The framework varies significantly across countries, with some jurisdictions establishing rigorous oversight bodies that monitor stem cell research while others adopt a more permissive approach. Understanding these regulatory mechanisms is crucial for researchers and practitioners involved in stem cell therapies, as they directly impact ongoing research initiatives and clinical applications.

Central to the ethical discourse surrounding iPSCs is the question of consent and the use of human tissues. Unlike embryonic stem cells, which often involve contentious debates about the moral status of embryos, iPSCs are derived from adult somatic cells, raising different ethical considerations. Health care professionals must ensure that consent is obtained transparently from donors, particularly when dealing with sensitive tissues. This aspect of the regulatory framework is vital in upholding patient rights and fostering trust between researchers and the communities they serve.

The commercialisation of stem cell research introduces another layer of ethical complexity. As iPSCs have significant potential for therapeutic applications, the interests of commercial entities can sometimes conflict with ethical practices in research. Oversight bodies play a crucial role in ensuring that commercial interests do not compromise ethical standards, particularly in the context of patient safety and informed consent. This tension necessitates ongoing dialogue among stakeholders, including scientists, ethicists, and commercial entities, to establish a balanced approach that prioritises ethical integrity.

Religious perspectives also play a pivotal role in shaping the regulatory landscape for iPSCs. Different faith traditions offer diverse interpretations of the moral implications of stem cell research, influencing public opinion and policy decisions. It is essential for health care professionals and oversight bodies to engage with these perspectives to foster an inclusive dialogue about the ethical status of iPSCs. This engagement can help mitigate cross-border ethical dilemmas, particularly in regions where religious beliefs significantly influence health care practices.

Finally, the ethical challenges associated with animal testing in stem cell research cannot be overlooked. As researchers explore the potential of iPSCs for therapeutic applications, they must consider the implications of animal models in their studies. This aspect of the regulatory framework demands rigorous ethical scrutiny to ensure that animal welfare is upheld while advancing scientific knowledge. Biomedical scientists must remain vigilant in their commitment to ethical research practices, particularly as the field of stem cell research continues to evolve.

Cross-Border Ethical Dilemmas in Stem Cell Treatments

Global Variations in Stem Cell Regulations

The regulation of stem cell research varies significantly across the globe, influenced by cultural, ethical, and legal frameworks unique to each region. In the United States, for example, federal funding for embryonic stem cell research is restricted, while private funding can pursue more liberal avenues. This dichotomy creates a complex landscape where the ethical implications and public perception of stem cell use clash with scientific advancement. As healthcare professionals and biomedical scientists navigate this terrain, understanding these regulations is vital for compliance and ethical practice.

In Europe, the regulations on stem cell research are often stricter, particularly in countries like Germany and France, where the use of embryonic stem cells is tightly controlled. These regulations stem from deep-rooted ethical concerns and religious perspectives that influence public policy. In contrast, nations like the United Kingdom have adopted a more permissive stance, allowing embryonic stem cell research under stringent oversight by bodies such as the Human Fertilisation and Embryology Authority (HFEA). This variation showcases the need for international dialogue and harmonisation of guidelines to ensure ethical standards in stem cell research.

Moreover, the commercialisation of stem cell therapies poses additional ethical challenges, particularly regarding consent and the use of human tissues. As private companies seek to profit from stem cell interventions, the potential for exploitation and misinformed consent becomes a pressing concern. This commercial aspect can lead to ethical dilemmas, especially when considering vulnerable populations, such as minors, and their ability to consent to experimental treatments. The intersection of patient rights and research ethics is crucial in navigating these murky waters.

The debate around induced pluripotent stem cells (iPSCs) further complicates the regulatory environment. While iPSCs offer promising alternatives to embryonic stem cells, their ethical status remains contested. The potential for these cells to replicate the capabilities of embryonic cells raises questions about the moral considerations of their use. As researchers and oversight bodies grapple with these issues, they must remain attuned to the evolving scientific landscape and its ethical implications.

Finally, cross-border ethical dilemmas in stem cell treatments warrant attention as patients often seek therapies unavailable in their home countries. This trend can lead to a patchwork of regulations, where patients become embroiled in ethical grey areas. Healthcare professionals must understand these global variations to provide informed guidance and ensure ethical practices are maintained, regardless of the regulatory environment in which they operate.

Ethical Issues in Medical Tourism

Medical tourism presents a complex landscape of ethical issues, particularly in the realm of stem cell research and treatment. As patients travel across borders seeking advanced therapies, the question of informed consent becomes paramount. Many individuals may not fully understand the risks associated with procedures that are often unregulated in the host countries. This lack of transparency can lead to exploitation and ethical dilemmas, especially when vulnerable populations are involved.

Another critical ethical issue in medical tourism is the disparity in healthcare quality and standards. Patients may be lured by the promise of innovative treatments at a lower cost, but they often overlook the fact that these treatments may not adhere to the rigorous ethical guidelines established in their home countries. The commercialisation of stem cell therapies can exacerbate this issue, as profit motives may overshadow patient welfare, leading to the prioritisation of financial gain over ethical responsibility.

The intersection of patient rights and stem cell research ethics is particularly pronounced in medical tourism. Patients travelling for treatments often relinquish certain rights, such as access to their medical history and follow-up care, which can compromise their overall health outcomes. This raises questions about the ethical obligations of healthcare providers to ensure that patients are not only informed but also protected throughout their medical journeys.

Moreover, the ethical implications of embryonic stem cell research can become entangled with the practices of medical tourism. In some regions, the sourcing of stem cells may not meet the ethical standards expected in more regulated environments. This can lead to contentious debates surrounding the use of human tissues and the moral status attributed to embryos, further complicating the ethical landscape for healthcare professionals involved in this field.

Lastly, the challenges of addressing ethical issues in the context of medical tourism are compounded when considering the involvement of minors. The ethical considerations surrounding consent become particularly sensitive when dealing with young patients. Healthcare professionals must navigate a landscape where the rights of minors, parental consent, and the potential for exploitation intersect, making it crucial to establish robust ethical frameworks that protect these vulnerable individuals in the realm of stem cell treatments.

International Collaboration and Ethical Standards

International collaboration in stem cell research is essential for advancing scientific knowledge and improving therapeutic outcomes. Researchers across the globe are increasingly recognising that sharing expertise, resources, and findings can lead to significant breakthroughs in understanding stem cells and their applications. However, this collaboration also raises complex ethical questions that must be addressed to ensure responsible practices.

The ethical implications of embryonic stem cell research vary greatly across different cultures and legal frameworks. Some countries have strict regulations guiding the use of embryonic stem cells, while others have more lenient approaches. This disparity can lead to ethical dilemmas when researchers from countries with stringent guidelines engage in partnerships with those from more permissive environments. It is crucial for international collaborators to navigate these differences sensitively and ethically to maintain integrity in their research.

Consent remains a fundamental aspect of ethical practices in stem cell research. The collection of human tissues for stem cell use necessitates informed consent from donors, which must be obtained transparently. However, the complexities of consent become even more pronounced when involving vulnerable populations, such as minors. Researchers must ensure that ethical considerations surrounding consent are prioritised, thereby safeguarding the rights and autonomy of all individuals involved in the research process.

Religious perspectives also play a significant role in shaping attitudes towards stem cell research. Different faiths have varying beliefs regarding the moral status of embryos and the acceptability of using stem cells derived from them. As international collaborations often bring together researchers from diverse religious backgrounds, it is vital to engage in open discussions about these perspectives. This dialogue can foster mutual understanding and respect, ultimately enhancing the ethical framework guiding stem cell research.

The commercialisation of stem cell therapies presents additional ethical challenges that researchers must confront. As the demand for stem cell treatments grows, the potential for profit-driven motives may conflict with ethical standards. It is essential for oversight bodies to establish clear guidelines that prioritise patient safety and ethical integrity over financial gain. By promoting transparency and accountability in commercial ventures, the international community can help uphold ethical standards in stem cell research.

The Intersection of Patient Rights and Stem Cell Research Ethics

Patient Rights in the Context of Stem Cell Research

In the realm of stem cell research, patient rights stand as a fundamental pillar that must be respected and upheld. Health care professionals and biomedical scientists are tasked with ensuring that patients are not only informed about the procedures involving stem cells but also actively involved in the decision-making process. This is particularly crucial when it comes to the use of embryonic stem cells, where ethical controversies often arise surrounding the origin and status of these cells. Patients must be made aware of their rights to consent, refuse treatment, and seek clarification on the implications of their participation in research.

The ethical implications of consent are magnified in the context of stem cell research. Obtaining informed consent is not merely a procedural formality; it is an ethical obligation that ensures patients comprehend the potential risks and benefits associated with their involvement. This is especially pertinent when considering the collection of stem cells from human tissues, where patients must understand the long-term consequences of their contributions. Health care professionals must navigate these conversations delicately, ensuring that patients feel empowered rather than coerced into participation.

Religious perspectives on stem cell research further complicate the landscape of patient rights. Different faiths hold varied beliefs regarding the sanctity of life and the moral status of embryos, which can significantly influence a patient's willingness to engage in such research. Health care professionals must be sensitive to these perspectives, accommodating patients' beliefs while also providing comprehensive information about the scientific aspects of stem cell research. This balance is essential in fostering an environment of trust and respect between patients and medical providers.

The commercialisation of stem cell therapies also raises ethical concerns regarding patient rights. As the market for stem cell treatments expands, the potential for exploitation of vulnerable patients increases. Oversight bodies must remain vigilant in ensuring that ethical practices are upheld, preventing scenarios where patients are prioritised as mere commodities. This is particularly critical in cross-border treatments, where regulatory frameworks may differ significantly, placing patients at risk of unethical practices.

Finally, ethical considerations in stem cell research involving minors highlight the need for robust protections and advocacy for younger patients. Minors may lack the capacity to fully understand the implications of their involvement in research, necessitating the involvement of guardians or advocates to safeguard their rights. Health care professionals must be well-versed in these dynamics, ensuring that the best interests of minors are always at the forefront of any stem cell research protocol. This commitment to patient rights not only enhances ethical standards but also fosters public trust in the ongoing developments in stem cell science.

Balancing Patient Rights with Research Objectives

The intersection of patient rights and research objectives is a critical aspect of stem cell research that requires careful consideration. As healthcare professionals and biomedical scientists pursue innovative therapies, they must ensure that patient autonomy is respected and upheld. This balance becomes particularly complex when dealing with controversial areas such as the use of embryonic stem cells, where ethical implications are often at the forefront of public debate.

Consent plays a pivotal role in maintaining this balance. It is essential for researchers to obtain informed consent from patients or donors, particularly when human tissues are involved. The process of obtaining consent must be transparent, ensuring that individuals fully understand the potential risks and benefits of participating in research. This is especially crucial when considering vulnerable populations, such as minors, who may not be able to provide informed consent independently.

Religious perspectives further complicate the ethical landscape of stem cell research. Different belief systems have varying opinions on the moral status of embryos and the appropriateness of using human tissues for research purposes. Researchers must navigate these perspectives sensitively, acknowledging the diverse viewpoints that can influence patient decisions and societal acceptance of stem cell therapies.

The impact of commercialisation on ethical practices cannot be overlooked. As stem cell research becomes increasingly intertwined with commercial interests, there is a danger that the pursuit of profit may overshadow ethical considerations. Oversight bodies must actively monitor this dynamic to ensure that patient rights are not compromised in the quest for financial gain, thereby safeguarding the integrity of the research process.

In conclusion, the balance between patient rights and research objectives is a delicate one that requires ongoing dialogue among healthcare professionals, scientists, and ethical oversight bodies. As advancements in stem cell research continue to evolve, it is imperative that all stakeholders prioritise ethical considerations, ensuring that patient welfare remains at the heart of research endeavours. Only through such commitment can we hope to navigate the complex ethical waters surrounding stem cell research effectively.

Ethical Advocacy for Patients

Ethical advocacy for patients in the context of stem cell research is paramount, particularly as advancements continue to raise complex moral questions. Health care professionals and biomedical scientists must navigate these ethical waters with a commitment to patient welfare at the forefront of their practices. This involves not only recognising the potential benefits of stem cell therapies but also understanding the ethical implications surrounding their use, especially concerning embryonic stem cells. The balance between innovation and ethical responsibility is delicate and requires ongoing dialogue and education among stakeholders.

Informed consent lies at the heart of ethical patient advocacy. Patients should be fully educated about the types of stem cells being used, including those derived from human tissues and the potential risks involved. This is particularly crucial when considering vulnerable populations, such as minors, who may not fully grasp the implications of their participation in research. Ensuring that consent processes are transparent and respectful is essential to uphold the dignity and autonomy of patients while also maintaining ethical standards in research.

Religious perspectives on stem cell research add another layer of complexity to the ethical landscape. Different faiths interpret the sanctity of life and the moral status of embryos in varied ways, which can influence public opinion and policy decisions. Health care professionals must be aware of these diverse viewpoints and engage with them sensitively, facilitating discussions that respect individual beliefs while advocating for ethical practices in scientific research.

The commercialisation of stem cell therapies poses significant ethical challenges as well. The potential for profit can sometimes overshadow patient welfare, leading to practices that may exploit vulnerable individuals seeking cures. As oversight bodies work to regulate the field, it is crucial that they prioritise ethical considerations and ensure that commercial interests do not compromise the integrity of stem cell research. This requires a collaborative effort among scientists, ethicists, and policymakers to establish guidelines that protect patients.

Lastly, the debate over induced pluripotent stem cells (iPSCs) and their ethical standing highlights the evolving nature of this field. iPSCs offer promising alternatives that may bypass some of the ethical concerns associated with embryonic stem cells. However, ongoing discussions surrounding their use underscore the necessity for continuous ethical reflection and advocacy. Health care professionals must remain engaged in these debates, promoting a culture of ethical consideration that prioritises patient rights and welfare in all aspects of stem cell research.

Ethical Challenges in Animal Testing for Stem Cell Therapies

The Role of Animal Testing in Stem Cell Research

The role of animal testing in stem cell research is a contentious issue, particularly among health care professionals and biomedical scientists. Animal models have historically been utilised to study the safety and efficacy of new treatments derived from stem cells. This practice raises significant ethical questions, especially regarding the welfare of the animals involved and the justification for their use in research that could potentially lead to human therapies.

In the context of embryonic stem cell research, the necessity of animal testing often comes under scrutiny. Critics argue that the moral implications of using animals, especially those derived from embryos, parallel the ethical debates surrounding human embryonic stem cells. This duality invites a complex dialogue about the rights of all sentient beings, pushing researchers to consider alternative methods that could reduce or eliminate the need for animal testing.

Consent is another critical aspect when discussing animal testing in stem cell research. Just as obtaining informed consent from human donors is paramount, the ethical treatment of animals requires stringent guidelines. Regulatory bodies must ensure that any research involving animals adheres to ethical standards that respect their well-being and promote humane treatment throughout the research process.

Moreover, the commercialisation of stem cell research introduces additional ethical dilemmas regarding animal testing. As the demand for effective therapies grows, the pressure to expedite research can lead to compromises in ethical practices. It is essential for oversight bodies to continuously evaluate the practices surrounding animal testing, ensuring that they align with ethical considerations while still advancing scientific knowledge.

Finally, the intersection of patient rights and the ethics of animal testing in stem cell therapies is an area ripe for exploration. Patients often seek innovative treatments with the hope of improved health outcomes, yet how these therapies are developed must be ethically sound. As the field evolves, ongoing dialogue among health care professionals, scientists, and ethicists will be crucial in navigating these complex issues, ensuring that the rights of both patients and animals are upheld in the pursuit of scientific advancement.

Ethical Justifications for Animal Use

The ethical justifications for animal use in research, particularly in the context of stem cell studies, are often framed within the broader discourse of scientific advancement and public health benefits. Many healthcare professionals and biomedical scientists argue that the use of animals in research is essential for gaining insights into complex biological processes that cannot be replicated in vitro. This justification hinges on the belief that the potential benefits to human health and the advancement of medical science outweigh the moral considerations regarding animal welfare. The necessity of using animals is particularly pronounced in the early stages of stem cell research, where understanding the biological implications of stem cells requires living models.

Moreover, ethical frameworks such as utilitarianism often play a significant role in justifying animal research. Utilitarian principles advocate for actions that maximise overall happiness or benefit, suggesting that if animal research leads to significant medical advancements and improved health outcomes for humans, it may be morally permissible. This perspective is frequently invoked in discussions surrounding embryonic stem cell research, where the potential to alleviate human suffering is weighed against the ethical concerns associated with the destruction of embryos. Such utilitarian arguments are contentious but prevalent in debates among healthcare professionals and bioethicists.

In addition to utilitarianism, the concept of the social contract also offers an ethical justification for the use of animals in research. This perspective posits that society has an implicit agreement to conduct research that may involve animal testing in pursuit of knowledge and health benefits. In this view, as long as researchers adhere to strict ethical standards and regulations designed to minimise animal suffering, the use of animals can be ethically justified. Oversight bodies play a crucial role in enforcing these standards, ensuring that animal welfare is prioritised in the research process while still allowing for scientific exploration.

Religious perspectives often complicate the ethical landscape surrounding animal use in research. Various faith traditions have differing views on the moral status of animals, which can influence opinions on the acceptability of using animals for scientific purposes. For instance, some religious groups may advocate for the protection of all sentient beings, while others may support research if it leads to significant benefits for humanity. This diversity of beliefs can create challenges for researchers and oversight bodies trying to navigate the ethically charged waters of stem cell research, emphasising the need for inclusive dialogue among stakeholders.

Ultimately, the debate over the ethical justifications for animal use in stem cell research highlights the tension between scientific progress and moral responsibility. As healthcare professionals and biomedical scientists grapple with these issues, it becomes increasingly important to engage in interdisciplinary discussions that consider not only the scientific implications but also the ethical ramifications of animal research. Addressing these complexities is essential to fostering a responsible research environment that respects both human and animal welfare, ensuring that advancements in stem cell research are achieved ethically and sustainably.

Alternatives to Animal Testing in Stem Cell Research

The ethical concerns surrounding animal testing in stem cell research have prompted scientists and researchers to seek alternatives that can yield reliable results without compromising animal welfare. One promising approach involves the use of in vitro models, such as organoids and tissue-engineered constructs, which can mimic the complexity of human tissues. These models provide a platform for studying diseases and testing potential therapies while reducing the reliance on animal subjects. By leveraging advancements in biotechnology, researchers can create more relevant and ethical experimental designs that align with the growing demand for humane research practices.

Moreover, the advent of induced pluripotent stem cells (iPSCs) presents another alternative that holds significant promise. iPSCs can be derived from adult tissues, allowing researchers to create patient-specific cell lines without the ethical complications associated with embryonic stem cells. This technology not only circumvents the need for animal testing but also enables the exploration of personalised medicine, where treatments can be tailored to individual genetic backgrounds. The use of iPSCs enhances the ethical landscape of stem cell research, reinforcing the commitment to patient rights and informed consent.

In addition, computer modelling and simulations have emerged as powerful tools in the realm of biomedical research. These digital platforms can predict cellular behaviours and the outcomes of various treatments, thus reducing the need for preliminary animal studies. By integrating data from existing research, scientists can create sophisticated models that inform experimental designs and anticipate the efficacy of new therapies. This shift towards computational methods aligns with a broader movement towards transparency and reproducibility in scientific research, addressing some of the ethical dilemmas associated with animal testing.

Collaborative efforts between researchers and regulatory bodies have also led to the establishment of guidelines and frameworks that promote alternative methods in stem cell research. These initiatives encourage scientists to adopt non-animal testing strategies and provide funding for the development of innovative technologies. By fostering a culture of ethical responsibility and scientific integrity, the scientific community can work towards a future where animal testing is no longer a necessity in stem cell research.

In conclusion, the exploration of alternatives to animal testing in stem cell research not only enhances scientific outcomes but also addresses ethical concerns that have long plagued the field. By embracing in vitro models, iPSCs, and computational technologies, researchers can pave the way for more humane and effective research practices. Ultimately, the ongoing dialogue surrounding these alternatives will shape the future of stem cell research and influence the ethical standards that govern it.

Conclusion and Future Directions in Stem Cell Research Ethics

Summary of Ethical Challenges

The ethical landscape surrounding stem cell research is fraught with challenges that provoke intense debate among health care professionals, biomedical scientists, and oversight bodies. One of the primary concerns revolves around the use of embryonic stem cells, which raises questions about the moral status of human embryos. The potential for life and the rights of the unborn are hotly contested issues that invoke various perspectives, including religious beliefs and philosophical viewpoints. As a result, the ethical implications of this research extend beyond scientific inquiry and touch upon deep-seated moral convictions.

Consent is another critical ethical challenge in the realm of stem cell research. The use of stem cells derived from human tissues necessitates clear and informed consent from donors, especially when it involves vulnerable populations such as minors. Health care professionals must navigate the complexities of obtaining consent while ensuring that donors are fully aware of the potential risks and benefits. This becomes particularly complicated when considering the implications of commercialisation, where the profit motive may overshadow ethical considerations, leading to potential exploitation of donors.

Religious perspectives also play a significant role in shaping the ethical discourse surrounding stem cell research. Many faith-based organisations express strong opposition to the use of embryonic stem cells, advocating for alternative methods that align with their moral teachings. This divergence in beliefs not only influences public opinion but also impacts policy-making and funding for research initiatives. Health care professionals must be cognisant of these perspectives as they engage in discussions about stem cell research and its applications.

The debate over induced pluripotent stem cells (iPSCs) introduces further complexity into the ethical considerations of stem cell research. While iPSCs offer promising avenues for regenerative medicine without the ethical concerns associated with embryonic stem cells, questions regarding their manipulation and long-term effects on human health remain. This ongoing discourse illustrates the need for continued ethical scrutiny as new technologies emerge, ensuring that patient rights are upheld and that research practices remain aligned with ethical standards.

Cross-border ethical dilemmas further complicate the landscape of stem cell treatments. Variations in regulatory frameworks and ethical guidelines across countries can lead to a disparity in treatment options and ethical practices. Health care professionals must be vigilant in addressing these disparities, advocating for consistent ethical standards that prioritise patient safety and rights. As the field of stem cell research continues to evolve, navigating these ethical challenges will be crucial for fostering trust and integrity in biomedical research and healthcare delivery.

Emerging Trends and Future Considerations

The landscape of stem cell research is rapidly evolving, marked by emerging trends that pose both opportunities and ethical dilemmas. One significant trend is the advancement of induced pluripotent stem cells (iPSCs), which allow for the reprogramming of somatic cells into a pluripotent state. This innovation not only expands the potential for patient-specific therapies but also raises critical ethical questions regarding the source of human tissues and the implications of consent. As healthcare professionals and biomedical scientists navigate these waters, they must remain vigilant about the ethical frameworks guiding their research and applications.

Another pressing consideration is the commercialisation of stem cell technologies. The increasing interest from private sectors can accelerate research and development, but it also risks prioritising profit over ethical standards. Oversight bodies need to establish robust regulations to ensure that commercial interests do not undermine the ethical principles of beneficence, non-maleficence, and respect for patient autonomy. The balance between innovation and ethical integrity is crucial as the market for stem cell therapies expands globally.

Moreover, the intersection of religious perspectives with stem cell research cannot be overlooked. Various faith-based organisations hold distinct views on the use of embryonic stem cells, often opposing research that involves the destruction of embryos. This moral landscape complicates policy-making and public acceptance of stem cell technologies. Health care professionals must engage with these perspectives to foster a more inclusive dialogue that respects diverse beliefs while advocating for scientific progress.

Ethical considerations extend to vulnerable populations, including minors, who may be involved in stem cell research. Protecting their rights and ensuring informed consent is paramount. The potential for exploitation or coercion in such scenarios raises alarms about the ethical responsibilities of researchers and practitioners. Guidelines must be established to safeguard these individuals while still allowing for the advancement of crucial medical research.

Lastly, the global nature of stem cell treatments introduces cross-border ethical dilemmas. Patients seeking unapproved therapies may travel to countries with less stringent regulations, complicating the ethical landscape. This phenomenon prompts a reevaluation of patient rights and the responsibilities of healthcare providers in ensuring safe and ethical practices. As the field continues to evolve, it is essential for all stakeholders to remain engaged in ongoing discussions about the ethical implications of their work.

The Role of Stakeholders in Ethical Governance

Stakeholders play a crucial role in ethical governance, particularly in complex fields such as stem cell research. These stakeholders include healthcare professionals, biomedical scientists, oversight bodies, and even the public. Each group brings unique perspectives and expertise that contribute to informed decision-making. Their involvement is essential for navigating the ethical controversies surrounding stem cell usage, which often encompasses issues like consent, commercialization, and the moral implications of embryonic stem cell research.

Healthcare professionals are at the forefront of stem cell research and its applications. Their clinical insights and ethical training equip them to address the nuances of patient rights and welfare. They must grapple with the implications of using stem cells derived from human tissues, ensuring that informed consent processes are robust and transparent. Furthermore, healthcare professionals must also consider the ethical challenges that arise when dealing with vulnerable populations, including minors, who may be involved in such research.

Biomedical scientists, as primary researchers, have a responsibility to maintain ethical standards in their work. They must navigate the delicate balance between scientific advancement and ethical considerations, particularly concerning induced pluripotent stem cells and their status. This requires a thorough understanding of both the scientific and ethical landscapes, as well as engagement with the broader community to foster transparency and trust. Their findings can significantly influence public perception and policy regarding stem cell research.

Oversight bodies play a pivotal role in ensuring that ethical governance frameworks are established and maintained. These organizations are tasked with creating guidelines that govern research practices while promoting ethical standards. They must also address cross-border ethical dilemmas in stem cell treatments, which can arise when different countries have varying regulations and ethical norms. This global perspective is vital in fostering an environment where ethical practices can thrive in an increasingly commercialised landscape.

Lastly, the intersection of various stakeholders creates a dynamic dialogue that is essential for ethical governance in stem cell research. Engaging religious perspectives adds another layer of complexity, as beliefs deeply influence views on the moral status of stem cells. The collaborative efforts of all stakeholders, through open communication and shared values, are crucial for resolving the ethical challenges that arise in this evolving field, ultimately ensuring that stem cell research progresses responsibly and ethically.

Pause for Thought

- Despite the hope for and significant advancement in regenerative medicine offered by stem cell research, the area has been steeped in ethical controversy, since stem cells were isolated from human embryo in 1998.

- The hope of treating previously incurable diseases, as stem cell research developed, the ethical concerns raised is with regards to the source of these cells and the moral status of embryos, necessitated the development of guard rails to maintain research integrity and respect human dignity.

- The debate continues, with those of a cultural norms utilitarian view arguing that the potential benefits of treating debilitating conditions such as Parkinson's disease and spinal cord injuries far outweighs the moral dilemmas posed by research using embryonic cells.

- Others with a religious leaning highlight the sanctity of life, arguing that the destruction of embryo's is ethically indefensible.

- The influence of religion, social edits and cultural norms, coupled with patient rights, the advancement of stem cells research requires ongoing dialogue among health care professionals, scientist and ethicist to effectively navigate these challenging waters.

- With the advent of the induced pluripotent stem cells, much of the ethical dilemma around embryonic stem cell research were by passed, however new and different ethical concerns arose, those dealing with consent and commercialization of stem cells.

- The commercialisation of stem cell therapies is a significant issue, in the context of cross border treatments. Many countries have varying regulations regarding stem cell research and therapies, which leads to a patch work of ethical standards. This may present a dilemma for health care professionals who may encounter patients seeking treatments that are unavailable or unregulated in their home countries. These ethical challenges underscore the need for cohesive international guidelines to protect patient rights and ensure ethical practices in stem cell research.

- Consent processes must be robust ensuring that all participants, particularly vulnerable populations, are adequately informed and protected.

- The ethical controversies surrounding stem cell research have become a focal point for health care professionals, biomedical scientist and oversight bodies. These controversies usually arise from the various sources of stem cells, particularly embryonic stem cells which pose significant moral and ethical dilemmas. This debate extends beyond the scientific and medical implications but extends into the realms of personal beliefs and societal values thus rendering it as a complex issue that requires careful navigation.

- Public perception of stem cells research often diverges sharply from the scientific community's understanding. Misconceptions regarding the nature of stem cells, particularly embryonic stem cells, contribute to widespread apprehension. Many equate stem cell research with the termination of human life which triggers ethical debates that overshadow the potential benefits of such research.

Take Home Nuggets

- Ethical committees play a pivotal role in the realm of stem cell research providing oversight and guidance to ensure that ethical standards are upheld. These committees, often composed of a diverse group of experts including health professional, bioethicist, and legal advisors, are tasked with evaluating the moral implications of research projects. Their primary function is to assess proposals for ethical compliance, particularly in areas fraught with controversy such as the use of embryonic stem cells and consent processes involving human tissues.

- One of the critical functions of the ethics committee is to facilitate informed consent , ensuring that participants are fully aware of the implications of their involvement in research. Here the potential benefits must be weighed against the ethical concerns surrounding the use of human embryos.

- As the field of stem cells use become increasingly lucrative, there is a risk that ethical considerations may be overshadowed by profit motives.

- The moral status of the embryo remains one of the most contentious issues in the realm of stem cell research. It has a central focus, which revolves around the question, when does life begin and the ethical implications of manipulating human embryos for scientific purposes. This debate influences both research practices and patient care.

- The legislative responses to embryonic stem cell research have evolved significantly over the past few decades, shaped by ethical concerns and public opinion. Governments worldwide grappled with the implications of using human embryos for scientific advancement, leading to a patchwork of regulations. In the United States of America for example funding for embryonic stem cell research faced restrictions under various administrations reflecting the contentious nature of the debate.

- What is informed consent? We believe that informed consent serves as a cornerstone of ethical practice, ensuring that participants are fully aware of the implications of their involvement. This process is made difficult in embryonic stem cells where moral status of the embryo raises significant ethical questions

- As private entities become increasingly involved in this field , the potential for profit may overshadow the ethical responsibilities researchers have towards participants. It is thus imperative to ensure that consent is obtained without coercion and that participants are not exploited for financial gain.

- Obtaining consent in stem cell research presents significant challenges that are often compounded by ethical, legal and social implications. For healthcare professionals and biomedical scientist, the need for transparent and informed consent is paramount, yet the complexities surrounding stem cell sources, particularly embryonic stem cells can create confusion among potential donors.

- Ethical challenges in obtaining consent are magnified when involving vulnerable populations such as miners. Special considerations must be taken to ensure that consent is not only obtained from guardians but that the minor themself comprehend the implications of their participation.

- Donors must have the right to make informed decisions about their own biological materials free from coercion or undue influence. This principle upholds the dignity of the individual and ensures that participants are fully aware of the potential uses of their donated cells including any risks involved. Patients must be made aware of their rights to consent, refuse treatment, and seek clarification on the implications of their participation in research.

Chapter 9
Safety Considerations

Preclinical Safety Assessments

Preclinical safety assessments are a critical step in the development of stem cell therapies, ensuring that any potential risks are identified and mitigated before clinical trials commence. These assessments typically involve a series of laboratory studies and animal testing designed to evaluate the biological behaviour of stem cells and their derivatives. Understanding how these cells interact with the host organism is paramount, especially as the therapeutic applications of stem cells expand. By carefully examining the safety profile of these therapies, researchers can provide essential data that supports regulatory approval and patient safety.

One of the key components of preclinical safety assessments is the evaluation of the long-term effects of stem cell transplantation. This includes monitoring for any adverse events, such as tumour formation or immune reactions, which may not become apparent until months or years after the initial treatment. Longitudinal studies are often conducted in animal models to assess the persistence of stem cells and their impact over time. The findings from these studies help inform healthcare providers about the potential risks and benefits associated with stem cell therapies in patients with chronic health conditions.

Additionally, the characterisation of the stem cell product itself is essential. This involves assessing the purity, potency, and identity of the cells used in therapies. Comprehensive testing ensures that the stem cells are free from contaminants and possess the necessary characteristics to achieve the desired therapeutic outcomes. Quality control measures are vital to maintain consistency across batches, and any deviations can significantly influence the safety and efficacy of the treatment. Thus, robust characterisation is a cornerstone of preclinical safety assessments.

Moreover, ethical considerations play a significant role in the preclinical phase. Researchers must navigate complex ethical landscapes, particularly concerning the sourcing of stem cells and the implications of their use in research. Informed consent from donors is crucial, and researchers must ensure that their studies comply with established ethical guidelines. Balancing scientific progress with ethical responsibility is key to fostering trust within the community and ensuring that stem cell therapies can be safely and effectively translated into clinical practice.

In conclusion, preclinical safety assessments are indispensable in the journey toward safe and effective stem cell therapies. They provide critical insights into potential risks, inform ethical practices, and guide the development of effective treatment protocols. As the field continues to evolve, ongoing research and collaboration among healthcare providers, biomedical engineers, and regulatory bodies will be essential to ensure that the promise of stem cell therapies is realised without compromising patient safety.

Clinical Trial Phases and Safety Monitoring

Clinical trials are essential in the development of stem cell therapies, ensuring that treatments are both safe and effective before they reach the market. They typically progress through several phases, each designed to gather specific data on the therapy's performance and safety profile. Phase I trials primarily focus on safety, involving a small number of participants to assess the treatment's tolerability and initial efficacy. These early phases are critical for identifying any immediate adverse effects that could arise from the intervention.

As the trials advance into Phase II, the emphasis shifts from merely assessing safety to evaluating the treatment's efficacy in a larger group of patients. This phase often includes a control group to provide a comparative analysis of the outcomes, allowing researchers to determine the optimal dosage and treatment protocols. Monitoring continues to be rigorous, as this stage can uncover more subtle side effects and provide valuable insights into the therapy's potential benefits and risks.

Phase III trials are the final stage before a treatment is approved for general use and involve thousands of participants across multiple centres. This phase aims to confirm the therapy's effectiveness, monitor side effects in a larger population, and compare the new treatment with standard therapies. The data collected during this phase is critical for regulatory approval and must demonstrate not only that the treatment works but that it is safe for widespread use.

Throughout all phases of clinical trials, safety monitoring is paramount. Independent safety monitoring boards are often established to review data at regular intervals, ensuring that any serious adverse events are addressed promptly. This oversight is crucial, as it allows for adjustments to be made to the trial protocols if necessary, safeguarding the participants and maintaining the integrity of the research.

The importance of long-term safety monitoring cannot be overstated, especially in the context of stem cell therapies. Once a therapy is approved, ongoing studies are essential to track the long-term effects on patients, as some adverse events may not manifest until years after treatment. Regular follow-ups and registries help to gather this vital information, contributing to a deeper understanding of the therapy's long-term efficacy and safety, ultimately guiding future practices in stem cell research and treatment.

Long-term Safety Profiles

Long-term safety profiles of stem cell therapies are becoming increasingly important as these treatments advance and are integrated into clinical practice. Understanding the potential risks and benefits over extended periods is crucial for healthcare providers and patients alike. As stem cell therapies evolve, monitoring their long-term effects will allow for better risk management and informed decision-making in patient care. The data collected from ongoing studies will serve as a foundational element to establish safe protocols for future applications of these therapies.

Research has indicated that while initial outcomes from stem cell therapies can be promising, the long-term implications require scrutiny. A variety of factors, including the source of stem cells, the method of administration, and the underlying condition being treated, can influence the safety profile. It is essential for biomedical engineers and researchers to work collaboratively to gather and analyse longitudinal data that track patients over time. This vigilance will help to identify any delayed adverse effects that may not be immediately apparent following treatment.

Moreover, the ethical considerations surrounding long-term safety cannot be overlooked. Patients with chronic health concerns often have limited options, making the allure of stem cell therapies particularly strong. However, it is the responsibility of healthcare providers to ensure that patients are fully informed about the uncertainties and potential risks associated with long-term outcomes. Transparent communication and patient education play pivotal roles in managing expectations and fostering trust between patients and providers.

As regulatory frameworks evolve, they must incorporate guidelines for the long-term monitoring of patients receiving stem cell therapies. This includes establishing registries and databases that can track patient outcomes and adverse events over time. Such initiatives will not only enhance the understanding of long-term safety profiles but also contribute to the overall body of knowledge regarding the efficacy of these therapies. Stakeholders across healthcare and research sectors must recognise the importance of these efforts in shaping the future landscape of stem cell treatment.

In conclusion, the pursuit of long-term safety profiles for stem cell therapies is an ongoing journey that demands rigorous scientific inquiry and ethical consideration. As the field continues to grow, it is imperative that healthcare providers, researchers, and patients work together to navigate the complexities associated with these innovative treatments. By prioritising long-term safety and efficacy, we can foster an environment where stem cell therapies become a viable and trusted option for patients with chronic health concerns.

Efficacy of Stem Cell Therapies

Evidence from Clinical Trials

Clinical trials play a pivotal role in assessing the safety and efficacy of stem cell therapies, providing the necessary evidence to support their use in various medical conditions. These trials are meticulously designed to evaluate not only the immediate outcomes but also the long-term effects of such treatments. Rigorous protocols ensure that data collected is both reliable and valid, allowing healthcare providers to make informed decisions based on empirical evidence rather than anecdotal reports.

The results from numerous clinical trials have shown promising outcomes for patients suffering from chronic health issues such as neurodegenerative diseases and severe injuries. For instance, studies involving stem cell transplants for conditions like multiple sclerosis and spinal cord injuries have demonstrated significant improvements in patients' quality of life. However, these findings must be interpreted with caution, as the long-term implications of stem cell therapies are still being explored.

Moreover, ongoing clinical trials continue to refine our understanding of the optimal conditions under which stem cell therapies are most effective. Variations in the source of stem cells, the delivery methods, and the specific patient populations involved can all influence treatment outcomes. As research evolves, it is crucial for healthcare providers to stay abreast of the latest findings and adapt their practices accordingly to ensure the best possible patient care.

The ethical considerations surrounding stem cell therapies also emerge as a critical component of clinical trials. Transparency in reporting results, informed consent, and the equitable selection of trial participants must be upheld to maintain public trust and ensure that these therapies are accessible to all who may benefit. This ethical lens is vital, especially as the field of stem cell research continues to advance rapidly.

In conclusion, evidence from clinical trials is essential for validating the safety and efficacy of stem cell therapies. As more data becomes available, healthcare providers and biomedical engineers must work collaboratively to interpret these findings and address any potential risks involved. By doing so, they can contribute to the responsible development and implementation of stem cell therapies, ultimately improving outcomes for patients with chronic health concerns.

Success Rates for Various Conditions

The success rates of stem cell therapies vary significantly depending on the condition being treated. For instance, in the case of acute leukaemia, clinical trials have shown that stem cell transplants can result in remission rates exceeding 60%. This high success rate highlights the potential of stem cell therapies in haematological disorders, where traditional treatments may fall short. As research continues, the refinement of these therapies promises even better outcomes for patients suffering from such malignancies.

Conversely, conditions like spinal cord injuries present a more complex scenario. Current studies indicate that while there is some promise, the success rates for restoring significant motor function remain relatively low, often below 20%. This disparity underscores the challenges faced in repairing nerve tissue and the need for further advancements in the field. The ongoing exploration of different stem cell types and delivery methods may eventually lead to improved therapeutic strategies.

In treating degenerative diseases such as Parkinson's disease, the reported success rates have been more optimistic, with some studies showing benefits in symptom management for up to 50% of patients. These findings suggest that stem cell therapies could play a crucial role in altering disease progression rather than merely alleviating symptoms. However, long-term efficacy and safety remain subjects of rigorous investigation, as the potential for adverse effects must be fully understood before widespread clinical application.

Moreover, the treatment of heart diseases using stem cells has yielded varying results, with success rates reported between 20% to 40%. These therapies have shown promise in improving heart function and reducing the risk of further cardiac events. Nevertheless, the heterogeneity of patient responses necessitates a more personalised approach, considering individual health profiles and specific cardiac conditions.

Finally, the ethical considerations surrounding the use of stem cells also influence their success rates. As healthcare providers and researchers navigate these complex ethical landscapes, transparent communication with patients regarding potential risks and benefits is essential. By fostering an informed patient base, the acceptance and utilisation of stem cell therapies can be enhanced, ultimately leading to better patient outcomes in various health conditions.

Factors Influencing Efficacy

The efficacy of stem cell therapies is influenced by a multitude of factors that must be carefully considered by health care providers and researchers alike. One of the primary factors is the source of the stem cells used in treatment. Adult, embryonic, and induced pluripotent stem cells each have unique properties that can affect their ability to differentiate into the desired cell types and integrate into the host tissue. Understanding these differences is crucial for optimising therapeutic outcomes and ensuring patient safety.

Another significant factor is the method of administration. The route by which stem cells are delivered, whether intravenously, locally injected, or via other techniques, can significantly impact their efficacy. Each method has its own advantages and challenges, influencing the cells' survival, migration, and engraftment rates. Health care providers must evaluate the most appropriate delivery method for each patient based on their specific condition and overall health status.

The microenvironment into which stem cells are introduced also plays a vital role in their efficacy. Factors such as inflammation, the presence of growth factors, and the overall health of the surrounding tissue can either facilitate or hinder stem cell function. Biomedical engineers must consider these environmental factors when designing therapies and creating biomaterials that support stem cell survival and integration.

Patient-specific factors, including age, genetic background, and pre-existing health conditions, can further complicate the effectiveness of stem cell therapies. Individual variations can influence the body's immune response to the transplanted cells and their ability to regenerate damaged tissues. Tailoring treatments to account for these variations are essential for improving long-term outcomes and ensuring the safety of patients undergoing stem cell therapies.

Finally, ongoing research and clinical trials are essential to better understand these influencing factors and refine treatment strategies. Continuous evaluation of safety and efficacy through rigorous scientific inquiry will not only enhance the reliability of stem cell therapies but also foster public trust in these innovative treatments. As the field progresses, collaboration among health care providers, researchers, and patients will be fundamental in navigating the complexities of stem cell therapy efficacy.

Ethical Considerations

Ethical Frameworks in Stem Cell Research

The exploration of ethical frameworks within stem cell research is essential for guiding practices that ensure the safety and efficacy of therapies. As health care providers and biomedical engineers delve into the complexities of stem cell applications, they must navigate a landscape that is often fraught with moral dilemmas. The use of embryonic stem cells, for instance, raises significant ethical concerns regarding the status of the embryo and the implications of its use in research. Understanding these frameworks not only informs decision-making but also aligns practices with societal values and expectations.

Informed consent plays a pivotal role in the ethical conduct of stem cell research. Patients and donors must be adequately informed about the procedures, risks, and potential outcomes associated with stem cell therapies. This transparency fosters trust and empower individuals to make choices that align with their beliefs and health needs. Moreover, ethical frameworks advocate for the continuous oversight of research practices, ensuring that informed consent is not merely a formality but a fundamental principle guiding interactions with participants.

The principle of beneficence, which emphasises the obligation to maximise benefits while minimising harm, is particularly relevant in stem cell therapies. Researchers and practitioners must critically assess the long-term safety and efficacy of treatments, balancing innovation with the potential risks involved. This involves rigorous clinical trials and post-market surveillance to monitor adverse effects and long-term outcomes, thereby reinforcing the ethical commitment to patient welfare.

Equity in access to stem cell therapies also emerges as a vital ethical consideration. Disparities in healthcare provision can lead to unequal opportunities for patients with chronic health concerns. Ethical frameworks advocate for policies that promote fair distribution of resources and access to cutting-edge therapies, ensuring that all patients, regardless of socioeconomic status, can benefit from advancements in stem cell research.

Ultimately, the integration of ethical frameworks into stem cell research not only enhances the credibility of scientific endeavour but also fosters a culture of responsibility and trust. As the field continues to evolve, ongoing dialogue among stakeholders—health care providers, researchers, patients, and ethicists—will be crucial in refining these frameworks. This collaboration is essential for navigating the complexities of stem cell therapies and ensuring that they are safe, effective, and ethically sound.

Informed Consent and Patient Autonomy

Informed consent is a fundamental principle in healthcare, particularly in the realm of stem cell therapies. It is essential that patients fully understand the potential risks and benefits of the treatments they are considering. This understanding empowers patients to make decisions that align with their values and preferences, thereby fostering a sense of autonomy in their healthcare journey. As healthcare providers, it is our responsibility to ensure that this process is not only thorough but also respectful of the patient's right to make informed choices.

Patient autonomy is closely linked to the concept of informed consent. Autonomy is the right of patients to govern themselves and make decisions about their own bodies and healthcare. In the context of stem cell therapies, this means that patients should have access to all relevant information, including the experimental nature of certain treatments and the long-term safety and efficacy data. By promoting patient autonomy, we not only adhere to ethical standards but also improve patient satisfaction and outcomes.

The complexity and evolving nature of stem cell research pose unique challenges in the informed consent process. As new discoveries emerge, the information provided to patients must be updated regularly. This dynamic landscape requires healthcare providers to be well-versed in the latest research findings and to communicate these effectively. Failure to do so can lead to misunderstandings and may undermine the trust that is essential in the patient-provider relationship.

Moreover, special attention must be given to vulnerable populations who may require additional support in the decision-making process. Patients with chronic health concerns may feel pressured to pursue novel therapies without fully understanding the implications. It is crucial for healthcare providers to create a supportive environment where these patients feel comfortable asking questions and expressing their concerns. This approach not only facilitates informed consent but also enhances the overall therapeutic experience.

In conclusion, informed consent and patient autonomy are vital components in the ethical administration of stem cell therapies. By prioritising these principles, healthcare providers can help ensure that patients are well-informed, respected, and empowered in their treatment decisions. As we navigate the future of stem cell therapies, it is imperative that we remain committed to these ethical standards, ultimately leading to better healthcare outcomes and patient trust.

Regulatory Oversight and Guidelines

Regulatory oversight plays a crucial role in the development and application of stem cell therapies. It ensures that these innovative treatments adhere to established safety and efficacy standards designed to protect patients. Regulatory bodies, such as the Food and Drug Administration (FDA) in the United States and the Medicines and Healthcare products Regulatory Agency (MHRA) in the UK, are tasked with evaluating the scientific evidence behind stem cell interventions. By reviewing clinical trial data and manufacturing processes, these organisations help to mitigate risks associated with new therapies before they reach the market.

In addition to evaluating the safety of stem cell therapies, regulatory guidelines also focus on the ethical considerations surrounding their use. This encompasses informed consent, the source of stem cells, and the potential for exploitation or harm to vulnerable populations. Ethical guidelines are intended to ensure that patients are fully aware of the risks and benefits involved in their treatment options. The involvement of ethical review boards is also pivotal in maintaining oversight, as they evaluate proposals to ensure compliance with ethical standards.

Moreover, the landscape of regulatory oversight is constantly evolving, particularly as advancements in stem cell research emerge. This necessitates ongoing dialogue between regulatory agencies, researchers, and healthcare providers. Collaborative efforts can lead to the formulation of adaptive regulations that accommodate innovative therapies while still safeguarding patient safety. As stem cell applications expand, such discussions are essential to ensure that regulations remain relevant and effective.

Long-term safety and efficacy are paramount considerations in the regulation of stem cell therapies. Regulatory agencies require comprehensive data from clinical trials to ascertain not only the immediate effects of treatments but also their long-term impacts on health. This includes monitoring patients over extended periods to identify any delayed adverse effects or unexpected outcomes. Such vigilance is essential for building public trust and ensuring that these therapies are genuinely beneficial in the long run.

Lastly, as stem cell therapies gain popularity, the global regulatory landscape must also consider international collaboration in oversight. Harmonising regulations across borders can facilitate research and access to therapies, while also ensuring that safety standards are upheld universally. By establishing international guidelines, regulatory bodies can work together to address the complexities of stem cell science and maintain a high standard of care for patients worldwide.

Current Applications of Stem Cell Therapies

Treatment of Chronic Diseases

Chronic diseases remain a significant global health challenge, affecting millions of individuals and placing immense strain on healthcare systems. As the demand for innovative treatments grows, stem cell therapies have emerged as a promising avenue for addressing these persistent health issues. These therapies offer the potential to regenerate damaged tissues, restore function, and improve patients' quality of life. However, understanding the long-term safety and efficacy of these interventions is paramount for healthcare providers and biomedical engineers involved in stem cell research.

The treatment of chronic diseases using stem cell therapies involves various approaches, including the use of embryonic stem cells, adult stem cells, and induced pluripotent stem cells. Each type of stem cell has unique properties and potential applications, making it essential for healthcare professionals to stay informed about the latest developments in this rapidly evolving field. This knowledge allows them to make informed decisions about patient care and to communicate effectively with patients regarding the risks and benefits of these therapies.

Long-term follow-up studies are crucial in assessing the safety profile of stem cell therapies. Concerns regarding tumorigenesis, immune rejection, and the potential for unintended consequences highlight the need for rigorous clinical trials and post-marketing surveillance. Healthcare providers must be diligent in monitoring patients who have undergone such treatments to ensure that any adverse effects are promptly addressed and managed. This ongoing assessment is vital for building trust and confidence in stem cell therapies among patients and the broader medical community.

Efficacy is another critical aspect of stem cell treatment for chronic diseases. Research continues to explore which conditions respond best to stem cell therapies, ranging from autoimmune disorders to neurodegenerative diseases. The development of standardised protocols and outcome measures is essential for evaluating the success of these interventions. Healthcare providers must remain engaged with current research to offer evidence-based recommendations and ensure that patients receive the most effective treatments available.

Ultimately, the treatment of chronic diseases through stem cell therapies represents a significant advance in medical science, but it is accompanied by ethical considerations that cannot be overlooked. Informed consent, equitable access to therapies, and the moral implications of stem cell sourcing are critical discussions that healthcare providers and researchers must navigate. By fostering an environment of transparency and collaboration, the medical community can work towards a future where stem cell therapies are safe, effective, and ethically sound, providing hope for those living with chronic health concerns.

Regenerative Medicine

Regenerative medicine represents a revolutionary approach to treating chronic health conditions by leveraging the body's own repair mechanisms. It encompasses a range of therapies, including stem cell treatments, which have shown promise in regenerating damaged tissues and organs. As healthcare providers and biomedical engineers explore these innovative solutions, understanding the long-term safety and efficacy of stem cell therapies becomes paramount. This emerging field not only holds the potential to alleviate symptoms but also aims to address the underlying causes of diseases, transforming patient care.

The use of stem cells in regenerative medicine is particularly noteworthy due to their unique ability to differentiate into various cell types. This characteristic allows for targeted treatments tailored to individual patient needs, offering hope to those with previously untreatable conditions. However, as these therapies are developed and implemented, rigorous clinical trials and post-market surveillance are essential to ensure their safety and effectiveness over time. The challenge remains in balancing rapid innovation with the need for thorough evaluation of long-term outcomes.

Ethical considerations play a crucial role in the advancement of regenerative medicine. The source of stem cells—whether from embryos, adult tissues, or induced pluripotent stem cells—raises significant moral questions that must be addressed by healthcare providers and researchers alike. Transparent communication with patients regarding the origins of stem cells and the potential risks associated with therapies is essential in fostering trust and informed consent. As the field evolves, ongoing dialogue about ethical practices will help shape the future landscape of stem cell research.

Furthermore, the integration of advanced technologies, such as biomaterials and 3D bioprinting, is enhancing the field of regenerative medicine. These innovations enable the creation of more effective delivery systems for stem cell therapies, improving their localisation and impact within the body. By harnessing these technologies, biomedical engineers can develop more precise and personalised treatment plans, ultimately leading to improved patient outcomes. The collaboration between engineers and clinicians is vital in pushing the boundaries of what regenerative medicine can achieve.

In conclusion, the future of regenerative medicine is bright, yet complex. As we navigate the uncharted waters of stem cell therapies, it is imperative to prioritise long-term safety and efficacy while addressing ethical concerns. By fostering collaboration among healthcare providers, researchers, and patients, we can ensure that the benefits of regenerative medicine are realised in a responsible and effective manner. The journey toward fully understanding and harnessing the potential of stem cell therapies is just beginning, but it promises to redefine the treatment of chronic health conditions as we know them.

Innovations in Biomedical Engineering

Innovations in biomedical engineering have significantly transformed the landscape of stem cell therapies, presenting exciting possibilities for treating chronic health conditions. Advances in biomaterials, for instance, have led to the development of scaffolds that support the growth and differentiation of stem cells. These scaffolds not only enhance the survival of transplanted cells but also improve their functionality, paving the way for more effective treatments.

Moreover, the integration of nanotechnology in biomedical engineering has opened new avenues for targeted drug delivery systems that can work in conjunction with stem cell therapies. By utilising nanoparticles, researchers can deliver therapeutic agents directly to the site of injury or disease, minimising side effects and maximising efficacy. This precision in treatment is crucial, particularly for patients with chronic conditions where standard therapies may fall short.

Additionally, advancements in imaging technologies have revolutionised how we monitor stem cell therapies. Techniques such as magnetic resonance imaging (MRI) and positron emission tomography (PET) allow for real-time observation of stem cell behaviour within the body, providing invaluable data on their integration and efficacy over time. Such innovations are essential for ensuring the long-term safety and effectiveness of these therapies, as they enable healthcare providers to make informed decisions based on concrete evidence.

Ethical considerations also play a significant role in the ongoing innovations within biomedical engineering. As new technologies emerge, it is imperative to balance the potential benefits of stem cell therapies with their ethical implications, including issues surrounding consent and the sourcing of stem cells. Continuous dialogue among engineers, healthcare providers, and ethicists is essential to navigate these challenges effectively.

In conclusion, the innovations in biomedical engineering not only enhance the safety and efficacy of stem cell therapies but also foster a more nuanced understanding of their implications. As we move forward, it is crucial for healthcare providers and biomedical engineers to stay abreast of these developments to ensure the best possible outcomes for patients suffering from chronic health concerns. The future of stem cell therapies is bright, with promising advancements that could redefine patient care.

Future Directions

Advances in Stem Cell Research

Recent advances in stem cell research have opened new avenues for treating chronic health conditions, marking significant progress in the field. Researchers have developed innovative methods for deriving stem cells, such as induced pluripotent stem cells (iPSCs), which have demonstrated potential for patient-specific therapies. These advancements not only enhance the understanding of disease mechanisms but also pave the way for personalised medicine, allowing healthcare providers to tailor treatments to individual needs.

Furthermore, studies have increasingly focused on the long-term safety and efficacy of stem cell therapies. Rigorous clinical trials are now being conducted to assess the outcomes of these therapies over extended periods. This is crucial for healthcare providers and patients alike, as understanding the long-term impacts is vital for making informed decisions about treatment options and managing expectations regarding therapy results.

Ethical considerations also play a pivotal role in the evolution of stem cell research. As advancements continue, discussions surrounding consent, the sourcing of stem cells, and the potential for exploitation are paramount. Healthcare providers must navigate these complex ethical landscapes to ensure that their practices align with both scientific integrity and patient welfare, while also fostering trust in new therapies among the public.

Moreover, interdisciplinary collaboration has become increasingly important in advancing stem cell research. Biomedical engineers, in conjunction with healthcare providers, are developing sophisticated technologies to enhance the delivery and efficacy of stem cell therapies. This collaboration is essential to overcome existing challenges, such as the immune response to transplanted cells and ensuring that stem cells differentiate into the desired cell types for effective treatment.

As the field continues to evolve, ongoing education and communication among healthcare providers, researchers, and patients are crucial. By staying updated on the latest findings and innovations, healthcare professionals can better inform their patients about the potential benefits and risks of stem cell therapies. This collective effort will be instrumental in establishing a future where stem cell treatments are safe, effective, and ethically sound, ultimately improving the quality of life for individuals with chronic health concerns.

Emerging Technologies

Emerging technologies in the realm of stem cell therapies are poised to revolutionise the landscape of chronic health management. Innovations such as CRISPR gene editing and advanced biomaterials are paving the way for more targeted and effective treatments. These technologies not only promise enhanced efficacy but also aim to address long-term safety concerns that have historically plagued stem cell applications. As healthcare providers and biomedical engineers explore these advancements, the potential to improve patient outcomes becomes increasingly tangible.

One notable development is the integration of artificial intelligence (AI) in stem cell research. AI algorithms can analyse vast datasets to identify patterns and predict treatment responses, enabling personalised medicine approaches. This capability could significantly enhance the precision of stem cell therapies, particularly for individuals with complex chronic conditions. By harnessing machine learning, researchers may uncover insights that lead to safer and more effective treatment protocols.

Moreover, the creation of 3D bioprinting technologies is expanding the possibilities for stem cell applications. This technique allows for the fabrication of tissues and organs that closely mimic natural structures, providing a platform for testing therapies before they are administered to patients. The ability to create tailored biological constructs not only boosts the efficacy of treatments but also mitigates risks associated with traditional grafting and transplantation methods.

As these emerging technologies evolve, ethical considerations must also be addressed. The implementation of novel therapies raises questions about consent, accessibility, and the long-term implications for patients. Healthcare providers must remain vigilant in navigating these ethical landscapes to ensure that advancements in stem cell therapies do not compromise patient welfare. A collaborative approach, involving ethicists, scientists, and clinicians, will be essential in guiding responsible innovation.

Ultimately, the future of stem cell therapies is bright, driven by emerging technologies that prioritise safety and efficacy. As we stand on the cusp of these breakthroughs, it is imperative for healthcare providers and researchers to engage actively in discussions about the implications of these innovations. By fostering an environment of collaboration and ethical consideration, we can ensure that the benefits of stem cell advancements are realised while safeguarding patient health and wellbeing.

Global Perspectives and Collaborations

Global perspectives on stem cell therapies are essential to understand the diverse approaches taken across different countries. In regions like Europe, there is a strong emphasis on regulatory frameworks that ensure patient safety while fostering innovation. This balance is crucial as it determines the pace at which new therapies can be developed and made available to those in need. By examining these perspectives, healthcare providers and biomedical engineers can glean insights into best practices and potential pitfalls in the field.

Collaborations between nations and institutions are pivotal for advancing stem cell research. International partnerships allow for sharing of knowledge, resources, and expertise, which can lead to breakthroughs that may not be possible in isolation. Such collaborations can also help in conducting multi-centre clinical trials, enhancing the robustness of data regarding the long-term safety and efficacy of treatments. For patients with chronic health conditions, this global effort could translate into faster access to effective therapies.

Ethical considerations are paramount in the global discourse on stem cell therapies. Different countries have varying ethical standards and regulations, which can impact the development and application of these therapies. It is vital for healthcare providers to be aware of these differences, as they can influence patient care and treatment options. Engaging in international dialogues can foster a better understanding of ethical issues and help establish universally accepted guidelines that prioritise patient welfare.

The role of technology in facilitating global collaborations cannot be overlooked. Advanced communication tools and data-sharing platforms enable researchers and clinicians from various parts of the world to connect and collaborate seamlessly. These technologies not only streamline research processes but also help in disseminating findings more rapidly, thereby accelerating the translation of research into clinical practice. For biomedical engineers, this technological integration is crucial for developing and refining stem cell therapies that are safe and effective.

Finally, the future of stem cell therapies will heavily depend on sustained global collaboration and shared commitment to ethical practices. As the field continues to evolve, ongoing dialogue between healthcare providers, researchers, and patients will be essential. By working together, stakeholders can ensure that advancements in stem cell therapies are both innovative and responsible, ultimately improving outcomes for individuals with chronic health concerns around the globe.

Conclusion

Summary of Key Findings

The exploration of stem cell therapies has yielded significant insights into their long-term safety and efficacy. Research indicates that while these therapies offer promising avenues for treating chronic health concerns, the outcomes can vary widely based on the type of stem cells used and the conditions being treated. Comprehensive studies have shown that some patients experience substantial benefits, while others may encounter adverse effects, highlighting the need for meticulous patient selection and monitoring.

Ethical considerations also play a crucial role in the application of stem cell therapies. The sourcing of stem cells, particularly from embryonic sources, raises moral questions that must be addressed by healthcare providers and researchers alike. Ensuring that these therapies are conducted in an ethically responsible manner is essential for maintaining public trust and advancing scientific progress in this field.

Moreover, the landscape of regulatory frameworks surrounding stem cell therapies is evolving. Various countries have different approaches to the approval and oversight of these treatments, which can impact their availability and application. Healthcare providers must remain informed about the regulations in their respective regions to ensure compliance and to guide patients accurately.

Patient education is another key finding from the research. Many individuals with chronic health concerns may not fully understand the potential risks and benefits associated with stem cell therapies. Therefore, healthcare providers have a pivotal role in communicating these factors effectively, enabling informed decision-making for patients considering these innovative treatments.

In conclusion, the key findings related to stem cell therapies underscore the importance of a multifaceted approach that encompasses safety, efficacy, ethical considerations, and patient education. As the field continues to advance, ongoing research and dialogue among healthcare providers, biomedical engineers, and patients will be essential to navigate the complexities of stem cell therapies and to maximise their potential benefits while minimising risks.

Implications for Healthcare Providers

The implications for healthcare providers concerning stem cell therapies are profound and multifaceted. As these therapies gain traction, it is essential for providers to understand the long-term safety and efficacy of the treatments they recommend. This understanding not only affects patient outcomes but also the overall credibility of the healthcare system. Healthcare providers must remain informed about the latest research and clinical trials to ensure that they are offering evidence-based treatments to their patients.

Moreover, the ethical considerations surrounding stem cell therapies cannot be overlooked. Healthcare providers have a responsibility to discuss the potential benefits and risks associated with these treatments with their patients. This includes being transparent about the limitations of current research and the possibility of adverse effects. By fostering open communication, providers can help patients make informed decisions regarding their treatment options while maintaining an ethical practice.

In addition, healthcare providers must consider the regulatory landscape surrounding stem cell therapies. As regulations evolve, it is crucial for providers to stay updated on legal requirements and guidelines. This knowledge will help ensure compliance and protect both the healthcare provider and the patient from potential legal ramifications. Understanding the regulatory environment also aids in the promotion of safe and effective practices within the field.

The implications extend beyond direct patient care; they also influence interdisciplinary collaboration. Healthcare providers, biomedical engineers, and researchers need to work together to advance the field of stem cell therapies. By sharing expertise and resources, these professionals can enhance the development of innovative treatments that prioritise patient safety and long-term efficacy. Collaborative efforts can lead to breakthroughs that benefit a broader range of patients with chronic health concerns.

Lastly, continuous education and training are paramount for healthcare providers involved in stem cell therapies. As new findings emerge, providers must adapt their practices to incorporate the latest evidence. This commitment to lifelong learning will not only improve patient care but also foster trust within the community. By prioritising education, healthcare providers can confidently navigate the complexities of stem cell therapies and their implications for future healthcare delivery.

Call to Action for Ongoing Research and Development

As we stand on the precipice of a new era in regenerative medicine, the call for ongoing research and development in stem cell therapies has never been more urgent. Health care providers, biomedical engineers, and individuals living with chronic health issues must unite in their efforts to advance understanding and application of these transformative therapies. The long-term safety and efficacy of stem cell treatments remain critical concerns that necessitate rigorous investigation and collaboration across various disciplines.

To ensure that stem cell therapies are both safe and effective, it is essential to establish comprehensive research frameworks that prioritise patient safety. This involves not only evaluating the immediate outcomes of stem cell interventions but also monitoring patients over extended periods. By doing so, we can gather invaluable data that informs clinical practices and regulatory policies, ultimately enhancing the therapeutic landscape for chronic health conditions.

Furthermore, the integration of technology into stem cell research presents a unique opportunity to accelerate advancements. Biomedical engineers are encouraged to innovate and develop new methodologies that can improve the delivery and functionality of stem cell therapies. This includes utilising cutting-edge imaging techniques and data analytics to better understand the biological mechanisms at play, thereby advancing our knowledge and capabilities in this field.

Collaboration among stakeholders is paramount. Health care providers should engage with researchers and patients alike to create a holistic approach to stem cell therapy development. By fostering an environment of open communication and shared knowledge, we can collectively address the ethical considerations surrounding stem cell use, ensuring that patient welfare remains at the forefront of all research efforts.

In conclusion, the path forward in stem cell therapies is paved with both challenges and immense potential. A concerted call to action for ongoing research and development is essential for unlocking the full benefits of these therapies. By committing to long-term studies and embracing innovation, we can pave the way for safe, effective, and ethically sound stem cell treatments that hold the promise of improved health outcomes for countless individuals.

Pause for thought

- In stem cell research, preclinical safety assessments are critical, it is necessary to allow the identification of potential risk so that they can be mitigated before clinical trials commence. This assessment typically involves a series of laboratory studies and animal testing designed to evaluate the biological behaviour of stem cells and their derivatives. By carefully examining the safety profile of these therapies, researchers can provide essential data that supports regulatory approval and patient safety.

- During the preclinical safety assessments, the long-term effects of stem cell transplantation is essential; this involves monitoring for any adverse events such as tumour formation or immune reactions which may may not be apparent until months or years after treatment. Longitudinal studies using animal models are conducted to assess the persistence of stem cells and their input overtime. The findings from these studies inform healthcare providers about the potential risks and benefits associated with stem cell therapies in patients with chronic health conditions.

- The characteristics of the stem cell product is essential. This involves assessing purity, potency and identity of the cells used in therapies. Testing ensures that stem cells are free from contaminants and possess the necessary characteristics to achieve the desired therapeutic outcomes. Quality control measures are essential to maintain consistency across batches as deviation can influence the safety and efficacy of treatment.

- Clinical trials progress through several phases. Phase 1 trial primarily focus on safety involving a small number of participants to assess the treatment tolerability and initial efficiency. In phase 2, the emphasis shifts from merely assessing safety to evaluating the treatment efficacy a larger group of patients. In this phase, there is usually a control group to provide a comparative analysis of the outcomes allowing determination of optimal dosage and treatment protocols. Phase 3 trials are the final stage before a treatment is approved for general use and involve large numbers of participants across multiple centres. This phase aims to confirm the therapy's effectiveness, monitor side effects in a large population and compare the new treatment with standard therapies. The data collected during this phase is critical for regulating approval and must demonstrate that the treatment works and is safe for widespread use.

- Longterm safety profiles of stem cell therapies are becoming increasingly important as these treatments advance and are integrated into clinical practice. Initial outcomes from stem cell therapies can be promising, long term implications require scrutinising a variety of factors, including the source of stem cells, the method of administration and the underlying condition being treated can influence the safety profile.

- Patients with chronic health concerns because of their limited options the allure of stem cell therapy is particularly strong. The onus is, therefore, on the health care provider to ensure patients are fully informed about the uncertainties and potential risks associated with long-term outcomes. Transparent communication and patient education therefore play pivotal roles in managing expectations and fostering trust between patients and providers.

- The long-term implications of stem cell therapies are still being explored, so although studies involving stem cell transplants for conditions like multiple sclerosis and spinal cord injuries have demonstrated significant improvements in patients quality of life, there is still the unknown long-term implication so findings must be interpreted with caution.

- The success rates of stem cell treatment vary significantly depending on the condition being treated. In the case of acute leukaemia, clinical trials have shown that stem cells transplants can result in remission rates exceeding 60%. This high success rate is encouraging when exploring the potential of stem cell therapy in haematological disorders, when compared with spinal cord injuries, the success rate is not as encouraging. Current studies indicate a relatively low success rate of only 20%in its ability to restore significant motor function.

- Studies suggest that stem cell therapies could play a crucial role in altering disease progression rather than merely alleviating symptoms; however long-term efficacy and safety remain subjects of rigorous investigation as the potential for adverse effects must be fully understood before widespread clinical application.

- In studies in which stem cells are used to treat heart disease, the reported success rates range between 20 and 40%. These therapies have promise in improving heart function and reducing the risk of further cardiac events. The heterogeneity of patient responses necessitates a more personalised approach, which considers individual health profiles and specific cardiac conditions.

Take Home Nuggets

- The efficacy of stem cell therapy is influenced by many factors that muse be carefully considered by health care providers and researchers. Among them are the source of stem cells used in treatment, are they adult stem cells, embryonic stem cells or induced pluripotent stem cells. Each of these sources have unique properties and can affect their ability to differentiate into the desired cell types and integrate into the host tissue.

- The method of administration of the stem cell also impact the efficiency of treatment whether they be administered by the intravenous route, whether they be administered by local injection or through other techniques impacts the efficiency of of treatment, each method has its own advantages and challenges, influencing the cells survival, migration, and engraftment rates.

- The microenvironment into which cells are introduced also plays a vital role in their efficacy. Factors such as inflammation, the presence of growth factors, and the overall health of the surrounding tissue can either facilitate or hinder stem cell function. Knowledge of these microenvironments is important in designing therapies and creating biomaterials that support stem cell survival and integration.

- Patient specific factors, including age, genetic background, and pre-existing health conditions can further complicate the effectiveness of stem cell therapies. Individual variations can influence the body's immune response to the transplanted cells and their ability to regenerate damaged tissues. Tailoring treatments to account for these variations are essential for improving long-term outcomes and ensuring the safety of patients undergoing stem cell therapies.

- It is imperative that the research continues to better understand these influencing factors and refine treatment strategies. Continuous evaluation of safety and efficacy through rigorous scientific inquiry will both enhance the reliability of stem cell therapy and foster public trust in these treatments.

- Ethical frameworks within stem cell research is essential for guiding practices that ensure the safety and efficacy of therapies. The landscape of stem cell research is fraught with moral dilemmas. Concerns related to the status of the embryo and the implications of its use in research creates ethical concerns specifically as regards to the status of the embryo and the implications of its use.

- The principle of beneficence, which emphasises the obligation to maximise benefits whilst minimising harm is particularly relevant in stem cell therapies. Researchers and practitioners must critically assess the long-term safety and efficacy of treatments, balancing innovation with the potential risk involved. This involves rigorous clinical trials and post market surveillance to monitor adverse effects and long-term outcomes thereby reinforcing the ethical commitment to patient welfare.

- Equity in access is a vital cog in stem cell therapies. Disparity in health care provision can lead to unequal opportunities for patients with chronic health concerns. Ethical frameworks advocate for polices that promote fair distribution of resources and access to cutting edge therapies ensuring that all patients, regardless of socioeconomic status, can benefit from advancements in stem cell research.

- Regulatory oversight bodies play a crucial role in the development and application of stem cell therapies. It ensures that these innovative treatments adhere to established safety and efficacy standards designed to protect patients. Regulatory bodies such as the food and drug administration in the United States of America and the Medicines and Health Regulatory Agency (MHRA) in the United Kingdom are tasked with evaluating the scientific evidence behind stem cells interventions. By reviewing clinical trial data and manufacturing processes, these organisations help to mitigate risks associated with new therapies before they reach the market.

- The landscape of regulatory oversight is constantly evolving, particularly as advancement in stem cells and the potential for exploitation or harm to vulnerable populations. There is therefore a need for ongoing dialogue between regulatory agencies, researchers and health care providers. Collaborative efforts can lead to the formulation of adaptive regulations that accommodate innovative therapies while still safeguarding patient safety. Such discussions are essential to ensure regulations remain relevant and effective.

Chapter 10
Introduction to Genetic Engineering

Overview of Genetic Engineering

Genetic engineering has emerged as a groundbreaking field, revolutionising various aspects of biomedical research and healthcare. At its core, genetic engineering involves the manipulation of an organism's DNA to achieve desired traits, whether for therapeutic purposes or enhancements. This technology is particularly significant in the context of stem cell research, where the potential to modify embryonic stem cells could lead to advancements in regenerative medicine. However, the rapid evolution of these technologies brings forth a myriad of ethical and moral dilemmas that must be addressed by professionals in the field.

One of the central ethical concerns surrounding genetic engineering is the moral status of human embryos from which stem cells are derived. The debate often centres on the rights of embryos versus the potential benefits of stem cell therapies. The implications of this research extend beyond individual cases, raising questions about human rights and the ethical treatment of all forms of life. As biomedical engineers and healthcare professionals navigate these complex issues, they must consider the societal impacts of their work, particularly in relation to the concept of 'designer babies' and genetic enhancements.

The notion of 'designer babies' encapsulates the potential for genetic engineering to create individuals with specific traits, leading to significant ethical debates. Critics argue that such practices could exacerbate societal inequalities, as access to genetic modifications may be limited to those with financial means. This raises critical questions about fairness and justice in healthcare, and the potential for genetic discrimination in employment and insurance. As these technologies advance, it becomes increasingly important for professionals to advocate for equitable access and the responsible use of genetic engineering.

Religious perspectives also play a crucial role in the discourse on stem cell research and genetic modification. Different faiths offer varied interpretations of the morality of manipulating human life at its earliest stages. Understanding these perspectives is vital for biomedical engineers and healthcare professionals, as they engage with patients and communities that may hold strong beliefs about the sanctity of life. Moreover, considerations of consent, especially regarding the use of genetic material from deceased individuals, add another layer of complexity to the ethical landscape of genetic engineering.

Finally, the role of government regulation in overseeing stem cell research and genetic technologies cannot be overlooked. As advancements continue to unfold, clear guidelines and policies are essential to ensure ethical practices and safeguard public health. The intersection of environmental ethics related to genetic engineering in agriculture further complicates the discussion, as the implications of altering genetic material extend beyond human health to encompass ecological considerations. In summary, the overview of genetic engineering highlights the need for ongoing dialogue among biomedical engineers, researchers, and policymakers to navigate the ethical challenges that lie ahead.

The Concept of Designer Babies

Definition and Origins

The term "designer babies" refers to infants whose genetic characteristics have been artificially selected or modified through advanced genetic engineering techniques. This concept has its roots in the broader field of genetic engineering, which encompasses a range of practices aimed at altering the genetic makeup of organisms. The origins of genetic engineering can be traced back to the early 1970s with the advent of recombinant DNA technology, which allowed scientists to splice genes from one organism into another. As advancements in biotechnology have continued, the conversation around the ethical implications of these practices has gained momentum, particularly in relation to human embryos.

Embryonic stem cell research emerged as a significant area of interest in the late 20th century when scientists discovered that these cells could differentiate into virtually any cell type in the body. This discovery opened new possibilities for regenerative medicine and therapeutic interventions. However, the use of human embryos in such research raises profound ethical questions, particularly concerning the moral status of the embryo. Many argue that the destruction of embryos for research purposes equates to the destruction of potential human life, thus invoking debates around human rights and the ethical treatment of embryos.

The ethics of gene editing in human embryos, particularly with technologies like CRISPR-Cas9, has further complicated the dialogue surrounding designer babies. Proponents assert that gene editing can eliminate genetic disorders and enhance human capabilities, while critics warn of the potential for unforeseen consequences and the slippery slope towards eugenics. This dichotomy poses significant ethical dilemmas, as society grapples with the implications of altering human genetics and the societal inequalities that may arise from such technologies.

Religious perspectives on stem cell research and genetic modification add another layer of complexity to these discussions. Various faith traditions offer differing views on the sanctity of life and the moral implications of manipulating human genetics. For instance, certain religious groups may oppose embryonic stem cell research on the grounds that it undermines the value of human life, while others may advocate for the therapeutic potential of stem cell therapies. This diversity of beliefs underscores the importance of inclusive dialogue among stakeholders in the biomedical field.

Finally, the potential for genetic discrimination in employment and insurance markets raises concerns about privacy and consent in the context of genetic information. As genetic technologies advance, it becomes crucial to establish robust regulatory frameworks that protect individuals from discrimination based on their genetic profiles. Additionally, the environmental ethics related to genetic engineering in agriculture highlight the necessity for a balanced approach that considers both human and ecological welfare. The ongoing evolution of genetic engineering and its implications necessitates a thoughtful examination of the ethical landscape surrounding its applications.

Advances in Genetic Engineering Techniques

Advancements in genetic engineering techniques have revolutionised the field of biomedical research, offering unprecedented opportunities for manipulating genetic material. Techniques such as CRISPR-Cas9 have enabled precise editing of DNA, allowing scientists to target and modify specific genes with remarkable accuracy. This has significant implications for stem cell research, particularly in the development of therapies aimed at treating genetic disorders and other diseases. However, these advancements also raise important ethical questions surrounding the manipulation of human embryos and the potential for creating "designer babies" with selected traits.

The ethical implications of gene editing in human embryos are profound and complex. One of the major concerns is the moral status of embryos derived from human stem cells, which poses a dilemma in balancing scientific progress with respect for human life. Critics argue that altering the genetic makeup of embryos could lead to unforeseen consequences, both for the individual and society at large. The debate intensifies when considering the potential for genetic discrimination, where individuals may be judged or denied opportunities based on their genetic traits.

Moreover, the societal inequalities that may arise from the availability of advanced genetic therapies cannot be overlooked. As stem cell therapies become more accessible, there is a risk that only those who can afford such treatments will benefit, exacerbating existing health disparities. This brings into question the role of government regulation in ensuring equitable access to these technologies and protecting vulnerable populations from exploitation. The intersection of genetic engineering and social justice highlights the need for a comprehensive ethical framework to guide research and application in this rapidly evolving field.

Religious perspectives also play a crucial role in shaping the discourse on stem cell research and genetic modification. Many faith traditions have differing views on the moral implications of manipulating human life at its earliest stages. These perspectives can influence public opinion and policymaking, creating a complex landscape for researchers and healthcare professionals. Engaging with these viewpoints is essential for fostering a dialogue that respects diverse beliefs while advancing scientific understanding.

In conclusion, the advances in genetic engineering techniques present both remarkable opportunities and significant ethical challenges. As biomedical engineers, stem cell researchers, and healthcare professionals navigate this evolving landscape, it is vital to consider the broader implications of their work. The intersection of science, ethics, and society demands a thoughtful approach to ensure that the benefits of genetic engineering are realised without compromising fundamental human rights and ethical principles.

Ethical and Moral Dilemmas of Stem Cell Research

Major Ethical Concerns

The advent of genetic engineering and stem cell research has ushered in a new era of possibilities in biomedical science, yet it brings forth significant ethical concerns that demand rigorous scrutiny. One of the most pressing dilemmas revolves around the moral status of embryos used in research. Many argue that human embryos, especially those derived from in vitro fertilisation, possess a right to life, raising questions about the ethics of their destruction for scientific advancement. This debate often pits scientific progress against deeply held moral beliefs, particularly in religious communities that view life as beginning at conception.

Another critical ethical issue pertains to the implications of gene editing in human embryos. The potential to eradicate genetic disorders and enhance human capabilities raises profound questions about consent and the long-term effects on future generations. The idea of 'designer babies'—children genetically engineered to possess specific traits—further complicates this landscape, as it introduces concerns about eugenics and the societal implications of creating a genetic divide. The question of who gets access to these technologies and whether they may exacerbate existing inequalities in healthcare remains a significant concern.

Moreover, the use of stem cells derived from human embryos presents a unique intersection of ethics and human rights. Advocates for stem cell research often highlight its potential to treat debilitating diseases, yet opponents argue that this research infringes on the rights of the embryos involved. This conflict raises critical questions about the prioritisation of scientific advancement over the rights of potential human life, forcing professionals in the field to navigate a morally complex terrain.

The issue of consent is equally vital, particularly concerning the use of genetic material from deceased individuals. Ethical guidelines must ensure that the wishes of the deceased are respected, and their families adequately informed about how their genetic material may be used. This aspect of bioethics is crucial in maintaining the trust between researchers and the public, as any perceived violation of respect for individual autonomy can lead to significant backlash against genetic research.

Lastly, the role of government regulation in overseeing genetic technologies and stem cell research cannot be overstated. Effective governance is essential to balance the potential benefits of these innovations with the ethical concerns they raise. Policymakers must consider the ethical implications of genetic discrimination in employment and insurance, ensuring that advancements do not result in societal inequalities. The integration of ethical considerations into regulatory frameworks will be pivotal in guiding the responsible development of genetic engineering and stem cell research.

Balancing Scientific Progress and Ethical Standards

The rapid advancements in genetic engineering and stem cell research present a profound challenge in balancing scientific progress with ethical standards. As biomedical engineers and health care professionals delve deeper into the possibilities of creating 'designer babies' through gene editing, they encounter significant ethical dilemmas. These dilemmas often revolve around the moral status of human embryos and the implications of manipulating genetic material. The discourse is further complicated by varying societal beliefs and the potential for genetic discrimination, which raises questions about equity in healthcare access and employment opportunities.

Embryonic stem cell research ignites intense debate regarding human rights and the moral standing of stem cells derived from embryos. Critics argue that the destruction of embryos for research purposes undermines the value of human life, while proponents highlight the potential for groundbreaking therapies that could alleviate suffering for millions. This moral tension necessitates a nuanced understanding of the implications of such research, making it essential for professionals in the field to engage with both scientific and ethical perspectives.

Furthermore, the concept of 'designer babies' introduces additional ethical considerations, particularly around parental consent and the selection of traits. As gene editing technologies become more accessible, the prospect of parents choosing specific genetic attributes for their children raises concerns about societal inequalities. This practice could lead to a divide between those who can afford genetic modifications and those who cannot, exacerbating existing disparities in health and social outcomes.

Religious perspectives also play a crucial role in shaping the ethical landscape of genetic engineering and stem cell research. Various faiths offer differing viewpoints on the sanctity of life and the appropriateness of intervention at the embryonic stage. These beliefs influence public opinion and policymaking, highlighting the need for comprehensive discussions that consider diverse ethical frameworks while navigating the complexities of scientific innovation.

Lastly, government regulation will be pivotal in ensuring that advancements in genetic technologies are pursued responsibly and ethically. Striking the right balance between fostering innovation and protecting human rights will require ongoing dialogue among stakeholders, including scientists, ethicists, policymakers, and the public. As this field continues to evolve, the challenge remains to uphold ethical standards while embracing the potential benefits of scientific progress in genetic engineering and stem cell research.

Implications of Embryonic Stem Cell Research on Human Rights

Human Rights Considerations

The advancement of genetic engineering and stem cell research has ignited a significant debate surrounding human rights considerations. As biomedical engineers and health care professionals delve into the potential of manipulating human genetics, they must grapple with the ethical implications of their work, particularly regarding the moral status of embryos. This raises questions about whether embryos should be afforded the same rights as fully developed individuals, and how these rights may influence research practices and regulatory frameworks.

Embryonic stem cell research poses a profound dilemma regarding human rights. The extraction of stem cells from embryos often leads to the destruction of the embryo, which some argue is tantamount to taking a human life. This perspective is especially prominent among various religious groups that advocate for the sanctity of life from conception. As such, the implications of this research intersect with deeply held beliefs about personhood and the rights of the unborn, necessitating a careful evaluation of ethical boundaries in scientific exploration.

The ethics of gene editing in human embryos further complicates the conversation around human rights. While the potential benefits of eradicating genetic disorders are immense, the prospect of creating 'designer babies' introduces concerns about eugenics and societal inequalities. The ability to select for certain traits could lead to a new form of discrimination based on genetic predispositions, thereby exacerbating existing social disparities. Biomedical engineers must consider how their innovations might contribute to or alleviate these inequalities in access to health care and genetic technologies.

Consent, particularly regarding the use of genetic material from deceased individuals, is another critical aspect of human rights that cannot be overlooked. The ethical implications of using such genetic material without explicit consent pose significant challenges, especially when considering the rights of individuals and their families. This highlights the necessity for robust ethical guidelines and regulatory oversight to ensure that the rights of all parties involved are respected and protected.

In conclusion, as the landscape of genetic engineering and stem cell research continues to evolve, it is imperative for professionals in the field to engage with the moral and ethical challenges that arise. The intersection of human rights, genetic technologies, and societal implications demands ongoing dialogue and reflection. By prioritising ethical considerations, biomedical engineers and health care professionals can contribute to a future where advancements in genetic research align with the protection of human dignity and rights.

The Debate on Personhood

The debate on personhood in the context of genetic engineering and stem cell research is a complex and multifaceted issue that raises significant ethical questions. At its core, the personhood debate revolves around defining when human life begins and what criteria must be met for an entity to be considered a person. This discussion is particularly pertinent to embryonic stem cell research, where the destruction of embryos for scientific purposes raises concerns about the moral status of these entities. Many argue that personhood begins at conception, while others believe it emerges later in development, creating a divide that complicates the regulation of stem cell research and genetic technologies.

One of the key ethical dilemmas related to personhood is the implications for human rights. If embryos are granted personhood status, it could lead to restrictions on research that relies on embryonic stem cells, potentially stifling advancements in regenerative medicine. Conversely, denying personhood may open the door to practices that some deem ethically questionable, such as the creation of 'designer babies' through gene editing. This tension highlights the need for a careful balancing act between advancing scientific research and respecting moral beliefs about the sanctity of life.

Religious perspectives play a significant role in shaping opinions on personhood and stem cell research. Many religious groups advocate for the protection of embryos, viewing them as sacred and deserving of rights. This belief can lead to strong opposition against genetic engineering practices that involve manipulating human embryos. Conversely, some religious traditions may support the use of stem cells for therapeutic purposes, viewing it to alleviate suffering. This array of beliefs adds further complexity to the personhood debate, as differing interpretations of religious doctrine can influence public policy and ethical guidelines in biomedical research.

Additionally, the debate extends to the potential for genetic discrimination in various sectors, including employment and insurance. If personhood is established at the embryonic stage, it raises questions about how genetic information can be used or misused in society. Concerns about discrimination based on genetic predisposition can lead to calls for stringent regulations to protect individuals' rights. The intersection of genetics, ethics, and societal implications necessitates a thorough examination of how personhood impacts not only scientific progress but also the broader social fabric.

Finally, the role of government regulation in stem cell research and genetic technologies cannot be overstated. Policymakers must navigate the murky waters of ethics and science to create frameworks that respect personhood while fostering innovation. This requires an inclusive dialogue among scientists, ethicists, and the public to ensure that the boundaries of research are defined thoughtfully and responsibly. Addressing the personhood debate is crucial for the future of genetic engineering and stem cell research, as it shapes the ethical landscape in which these technologies operate.

The Ethics of Gene Editing in Human Embryos

Current Techniques and Technologies

The field of genetic engineering has witnessed remarkable advancements, particularly in the context of creating designer babies. Techniques such as CRISPR-Cas9 have revolutionised the ability to edit genes with unprecedented precision, allowing for the potential elimination of hereditary diseases. This gene-editing technology provides biomedical engineers and researchers with the tools to modify genetic material, paving the way for significant changes in human development. However, these developments come with profound ethical and moral dilemmas that must be carefully navigated.

Embryonic stem cell research continues to provoke intense debate, particularly concerning human rights and the moral status of embryos. The capacity of these stem cells to differentiate into any cell type offers immense potential for regenerative medicine, yet the process often raises questions about the sanctity of life. Healthcare professionals and students must grapple with the implications of utilising human embryos for research purposes, balancing scientific progress against ethical principles. This dilemma is further complicated by differing religious perspectives on the beginning of life and the acceptability of using embryonic cells.

As genetic engineering progresses, the concept of designer babies raises concerns about societal inequalities. Access to advanced genetic technologies may be limited to wealthier segments of the population, leading to a widening gap in health outcomes. The potential for genetic discrimination in employment and insurance adds another layer of complexity, as individuals with genetically engineered traits may experience biases. Therefore, it is crucial for health care professionals to advocate for equitable access to these technologies, ensuring that advancements benefit all members of society.

Government regulation plays a pivotal role in overseeing stem cell research and genetic technologies. Regulatory frameworks must address the ethical implications of genetic modification while fostering an environment conducive to innovation. Policymakers face the challenge of striking a balance between promoting scientific advancement and protecting individual rights, particularly concerning consent and the use of genetic material from deceased individuals. The development of comprehensive regulations is essential to navigate the complex landscape of genetic engineering and its societal impact.

The environmental ethics surrounding genetic engineering extend beyond human health, influencing agricultural practices as well. The use of genetically modified organisms (GMOs) raises questions about ecological balance and biodiversity. As biomedical engineers explore the potential applications of genetic technologies, they must consider the broader implications for the environment and society. Addressing these ethical concerns will be crucial in shaping a responsible approach to genetic engineering that respects both human and environmental rights.

Ethical Frameworks for Gene Editing

The ethical frameworks surrounding gene editing are complex and multifaceted, particularly as they pertain to the emerging field of genetic engineering. As biomedical engineers and health care professionals grapple with the implications of their work, it is crucial to establish a set of guiding principles that can navigate the moral dilemmas inherent in this technology. These frameworks often draw on various philosophical theories, including utilitarianism, which evaluates the consequences of actions, and deontological ethics, which focuses on the morality of actions themselves. By applying these theories, professionals can better understand the ethical landscape of gene editing and its impact on society.

One major ethical concern is the moral status of stem cells derived from human embryos. Advocates for embryonic stem cell research argue that these cells offer the potential for groundbreaking therapies, while opponents raise questions about the rights of the embryo. This debate is not merely academic; it has real implications for legislation and funding in biomedical research. Understanding the ethical implications of using embryonic stem cells is vital for professionals involved in stem cell research, as it informs their responsibilities towards patients and society at large.

Additionally, the concept of 'designer babies' poses significant ethical challenges. Gene editing technologies like CRISPR raise questions about the desirability and morality of selecting for specific traits, such as intelligence or physical appearance. This manipulation of human genetics can exacerbate existing societal inequalities, as access to such technologies may be limited to affluent individuals or communities. Hence, biomedical engineers and health care professionals must consider the broader societal implications of their work and strive to ensure equitable access to genetic advancements.

Religious perspectives also play a crucial role in the discourse surrounding gene editing and stem cell research. Various faith traditions offer differing views on the sanctity of life and the ethical ramifications of manipulating human genetics. Health care professionals must navigate these diverse beliefs while providing care and making informed decisions that respect the values of their patients. Engaging with these religious perspectives can also help foster a more inclusive dialogue about the ethical considerations of gene editing.

Finally, the regulation of genetic technologies is essential for establishing ethical standards in gene editing and stem cell research. Government oversight can help mitigate risks such as genetic discrimination in employment and insurance, ensuring that individuals are not unfairly treated based on their genetic information. By understanding the role of regulation, biomedical engineers and health care professionals can advocate for policies that prioritise ethical concerns while promoting scientific advancement. Ultimately, a robust ethical framework is necessary to guide the responsible development and application of genetic engineering technologies in a manner that respects human rights and societal values.

The Moral Status of Stem Cells Derived from Human Embryos

Philosophical Perspectives

Philosophical perspectives on genetic engineering and stem cell research delve into the ethical and moral dilemmas that surround these technologies. Central to this discourse is the question of what constitutes human life and the rights associated with it. The implications of using embryonic stem cells raise significant concerns regarding the moral status of embryos. Many argue that the potential for life imbues embryos with rights that must be respected, while others contend that the benefits of research and potential cures justify their use in scientific advancement.

The ethics of gene editing in human embryos further complicates the philosophical landscape. Techniques such as CRISPR allow for precise modifications to DNA, leading to the possibility of 'designer babies' who may be genetically enhanced for specific traits. This power raises profound questions about parental choice, the nature of consent, and the potential for societal inequality. If genetic enhancements become available only to the affluent, a new divide may emerge, exacerbating existing disparities in health and opportunity.

Religious perspectives also play a significant role in the ethical debates surrounding stem cell research and genetic modification. Many faith-based viewpoints advocate for the sanctity of life from conception, objecting to practices that may undermine the dignity of human beings. Conversely, some religious groups may support scientific advancements that alleviate suffering and promote well-being, creating a complex interplay between faith, ethics, and scientific progress.

Consent is another pivotal issue, particularly when considering the use of genetic material from deceased individuals. The ethical implications of obtaining and utilising such material without clear consent from the individual or their family raise questions about autonomy and respect for persons. Furthermore, the potential for genetic discrimination in employment and insurance sectors poses significant challenges, highlighting the need for robust ethical frameworks to protect individuals from misuse of genetic information.

Lastly, the environmental ethics related to genetic engineering in agriculture cannot be overlooked. The manipulation of genetic material for improved crop yields or resistance to pests involves considerations of ecological impacts and sustainability. Balancing the benefits of increased food production against the risks to biodiversity and the environment is a philosophical challenge that reflects broader ethical concerns about the direction of genetic technologies in society.

Legal Perspectives and Legislation

The legal landscape surrounding genetic engineering and stem cell research is complex and multifaceted, reflecting a broad spectrum of ethical, moral, and societal concerns. Governments worldwide are grappling with the implications of advancements in biotechnology, particularly regarding the creation of 'designer babies'. Legislation varies significantly from country to country, with some nations embracing genetic modification technologies while others impose strict prohibitions. This divergence underscores the necessity for a coherent legal framework that addresses not only the scientific possibilities but also the ethical dilemmas inherent in such technologies.

One major concern in this domain is the moral status of embryonic stem cells. The use of human embryos in research raises profound questions about when life begins and the rights of these early-stage entities. As laws evolve, they must balance scientific progress with respect for human rights and dignity. Legislators face the challenging task of ensuring that the rights of individuals, particularly those of potential future persons, are not overlooked in the pursuit of medical and scientific advancement.

In addition to human rights considerations, the ethical implications of gene editing in human embryos have sparked intense debate among bioethicists, scientists, and the public. The potential to eliminate genetic diseases before birth presents a transformative opportunity but also raises fears of genetic discrimination and societal inequality. The question of consent, especially in cases where genetic material from deceased individuals is utilised, adds another layer of complexity to the legal discourse surrounding genetic technologies.

Furthermore, religious perspectives play a significant role in shaping public opinion and legislation on stem cell research and genetic modification. Different faiths offer varying interpretations of the sanctity of life and the ethicality of manipulating human genetics. This diversity of beliefs complicates the establishment of universal legal standards and highlights the need for inclusive dialogue among stakeholders to navigate these sensitive issues.

Lastly, the role of government regulation is crucial in ensuring that stem cell therapies and genetic engineering practices are conducted ethically and responsibly. Policymakers must consider the implications of these technologies on societal inequalities, protecting vulnerable populations from exploitation while fostering innovation. Establishing clear guidelines can help mitigate risks associated with genetic discrimination in employment and insurance, ensuring that advancements in biomedical science contribute positively to society as a whole.

Genetic Engineering and Societal Inequalities

Impact on Health Disparities

The advent of genetic engineering and stem cell research has profound implications for health disparities, particularly in how these technologies might be applied across different socio-economic groups. As biomedical engineers and healthcare professionals explore the potential of designer babies, it is crucial to consider who has access to these advancements. If only affluent families can afford genetic modifications or treatments derived from stem cell research, societal inequalities may be exacerbated, leading to a widening gap in health outcomes between the rich and the poor.

Moreover, the moral status of stem cells, particularly those derived from human embryos, raises significant ethical questions. The debate surrounding the use of embryonic stem cells often centres on the rights of the embryo versus the potential benefits of research. This dilemma is intensified when considering how the benefits of such research are distributed. If the ethical implications are not carefully navigated, we risk creating a system where certain lives are deemed more valuable than others based on economic status or access to advanced medical technologies.

The potential for genetic discrimination is another pressing concern associated with the rise of designer babies. As gene editing becomes more commonplace, there is a risk that individuals could face discrimination in employment or insurance based on their genetic makeup. This possibility underscores the need for robust regulations that protect individuals from such biases while ensuring that the benefits of genetic advancements are shared equitably across society.

Furthermore, the religious perspectives on stem cell research and genetic modification add another layer of complexity to the discussion of health disparities. Various faith groups hold differing views on the sanctity of life and the moral implications of altering human genetics. These beliefs can influence public policy and funding priorities, ultimately affecting who benefits from advancements in genetic engineering and stem cell therapies.

In conclusion, the intersection of genetic engineering, stem cell research, and health disparities presents a challenging landscape for biomedical professionals. The ethical implications of these technologies must be carefully considered to ensure that they do not perpetuate existing inequalities. As we move forward, it will be essential for the healthcare community to advocate for equitable access to these life-changing innovations, fostering a future where all individuals can benefit from advances in genetic science.

Access to Genetic Technologies

Access to genetic technologies has become a pivotal issue in contemporary biomedical discussions, particularly concerning the ethical implications surrounding their use. As advancements in genetic engineering and stem cell research continue to evolve, the access to these technologies raises significant moral dilemmas. Stakeholders, including biomedical engineers and health care professionals, must navigate complex questions about the appropriate use of such powerful tools, particularly in relation to human rights and the moral status of stem cells derived from embryos.

The implications of embryonic stem cell research are profound, as they intersect with various human rights concerns. The debate often centres on the moral status of embryos and whether they should be afforded the same ethical considerations as fully developed humans. This question is particularly pressing for health care professionals who are at the forefront of implementing these technologies in clinical settings. The ongoing discourse on the ethics of gene editing in human embryos further complicates access, as it raises issues about consent, potential misuse, and long-term societal impacts.

Moreover, the concept of 'designer babies' has sparked intense discussions about genetic engineering's role in shaping future generations. While the allure of eradicating genetic diseases is appealing, it also leads to fears of exacerbating societal inequalities. Those with greater access to genetic technologies could potentially create disparities in health outcomes, further entrenching existing inequalities. This aspect of access to genetic technologies is critical for biomedical engineers and researchers who must consider the broader societal implications of their work.

Religious perspectives on stem cell research and genetic modification also play a crucial role in shaping public opinion and policy. Different faiths offer varying viewpoints on the sanctity of life and the moral obligations of science, which influences how access to these technologies is perceived and regulated. As such, understanding these perspectives is essential for health care professionals who must engage with patients and communities that hold diverse beliefs about genetic engineering.

Finally, the potential for genetic discrimination in employment and insurance poses a significant ethical challenge as access to genetic technologies becomes more widespread. As individuals gain access to their genetic information, the risk of misuse by employers or insurance companies grows. These raises pressing questions about privacy, consent, and the responsibilities of those who work with genetic data. With government regulation playing a pivotal role in shaping the landscape of genetic technologies, continued dialogue among stakeholders is essential to ensure ethical practices in this rapidly evolving field.

Religious Perspectives on Stem Cell Research and Genetic Modification

Views from Major Religions

The ethical landscape surrounding genetic engineering and stem cell research is profoundly influenced by the views of major religions. Different faiths have unique perspectives on the sanctity of life, the moral status of embryos, and the implications of altering human genetics. For instance, many Christian denominations view the embryo as a sacred creation, leading to opposition against embryonic stem cell research. In contrast, some more liberal religious groups may accept certain forms of genetic modification if they contribute to healing and alleviating suffering. This divergence highlights the complex interplay between faith, ethics, and scientific advancement.

Islam presents a nuanced view on genetic engineering, where the preservation of life and health is paramount. Scholars within the faith debate the permissibility of genetic modifications, often emphasising the importance of intentions behind such interventions. If genetic engineering serves to prevent disease or enhance quality of life, it may be viewed more favourably. However, concerns about 'playing God' and the potential for genetic discrimination are significant ethical dilemmas that require careful consideration by Muslim bioethicists.

Buddhism introduces another perspective, primarily focusing on the concepts of suffering and compassion. The potential benefits of stem cell research and genetic engineering must be weighed against the possible harms, not only to individuals but also to society. The Buddhist principle of interconnectedness calls for an examination of how genetic modifications could impact social inequalities and the environment. This holistic approach urges biomedical engineers to consider broader societal implications when engaging in genetic research.

Judaism, with its rich ethical tradition, often approaches the subject of stem cell research with a balance of innovation and caution. The preservation of life is a core tenet, leading to support for research that can save lives. However, the moral status of embryos remains a contentious issue, with various interpretations influencing different Jewish communities. This diversity in opinion underscores the importance of dialogue between religious leaders and scientists to navigate the ethical complexities of genetic engineering.

In conclusion, the views of major religions on genetic engineering and stem cell research provide a crucial framework for understanding the ethical implications of these technologies. As biomedical engineers and health care professionals navigate these challenges, recognising the diverse religious perspectives can enhance ethical decision-making and promote a more inclusive approach to genetic advancements. Engaging with faith communities can also foster public trust and dialogue around the moral dilemmas inherent in creating 'designer babies' and utilising stem cell therapies.

The Role of Faith in Ethical Decision-Making

In the realm of biomedical ethics, faith plays a significant role in shaping the perspectives of professionals engaged in genetic engineering and stem cell research. For many, religious beliefs provide a framework for understanding the moral consequences of manipulating human life. This influence can guide decision-making processes when confronted with ethical dilemmas, such as the moral status of embryonic stem cells and the implications of creating 'designer babies'. The intersection between faith and ethics is particularly pronounced in discussions about human rights and the sanctity of life, prompting professionals to consider not just the scientific advancements but also the spiritual ramifications of their work.

The ethical implications of embryonic stem cell research are often debated within the context of various faith traditions. Many religious groups argue that human life begins at conception, thus attributing full moral status to embryos. This belief can lead to significant opposition against practices that involve the destruction of embryos for research purposes. Conversely, some faith perspectives may support the use of stem cells for therapeutic reasons, viewing the alleviation of suffering as a paramount ethical duty. This divergence in beliefs highlights the complex interplay between faith and the ethical frameworks biomedical professionals utilise in their work.

In addition to the moral status of embryos, gene editing in human embryos raises profound ethical questions that intersect with faith-based views. The potential to alter genetic traits invites a variety of responses rooted in religious teachings about creation and the natural order. Some faiths may assert that human beings should not interfere with the genetic blueprint established by a higher power, while others may embrace the technology as a means to enhance human well-being. Such discussions necessitate a careful consideration of how faith influences the ethical boundaries of genetic modification and the responsibilities of those in the biomedical field.

Moreover, the implications of genetic engineering extend beyond individual ethics to encompass societal issues, such as inequality and discrimination. Faith communities often advocate for social justice, urging biomedical professionals to consider how advancements in genetics might exacerbate existing disparities in health care and access to technology. The potential for genetic discrimination in employment and insurance further complicates the ethical landscape, prompting a need for regulations that protect individuals from bias based on their genetic information. Here, faith serves as a guiding principle in advocating for equitable practices in the face of emerging technologies.

Finally, the role of consent, especially concerning the use of genetic material from deceased individuals, raises additional ethical considerations informed by faith. Many religious traditions emphasise the importance of respecting the deceased and their families, which can complicate the ethical landscape surrounding genetic research. As biomedical engineers and health care professionals navigate these multifaceted issues, faith can serve as a vital compass, guiding them towards decisions that honour both scientific progress and the moral values upheld by their beliefs.

Consent and the Use of Genetic Material from Deceased Individuals

Legal and Ethical Issues Surrounding Consent

The issue of consent in the context of genetic engineering and stem cell research is fraught with complexity, as it intersects with legal, ethical, and moral considerations. Informed consent is a fundamental principle in biomedical research, yet the nuances of genetic manipulation raise questions about the nature of consent itself. For instance, how do we navigate consent when dealing with embryos or genetic material derived from deceased individuals? The challenge lies in ensuring that those providing consent fully understand the implications of their decisions, which may not be straightforward given the rapidly evolving nature of genetic technologies.

Furthermore, the ethical implications surrounding consent extend to the concept of 'designer babies', where parents may seek genetic modifications to enhance their offspring's traits. The potential for coercion or undue influence in these decisions is significant, particularly in a society where genetic advantages could translate into social inequalities. The debate over consent in this realm must also consider the moral status of embryos and whether they possess rights that should be respected, thereby complicating the consent process.

The implications of embryonic stem cell research also raise critical legal questions about human rights. As researchers seek to develop therapies that harness the potential of stem cells, the legal frameworks governing consent must evolve to address the rights of the embryos involved. The potential for genetic discrimination in employment and insurance further complicates the landscape, as individuals may be judged based on their genetic makeup, raising urgent ethical concerns about privacy and autonomy.

Religious perspectives on stem cell research and genetic modification add another layer of complexity to the discussion. Different faiths hold varying views on the sanctity of life and the moral implications of altering human genetics. These beliefs can significantly influence public opinion on consent and the acceptability of genetic engineering practices, necessitating respectful dialogue among stakeholders to navigate these diverse perspectives.

Lastly, the role of government regulation in stem cell research and genetic technologies cannot be understated. Effective regulation is essential to ensure that consent processes are transparent and that individuals are protected from exploitation. Policymakers must grapple with balancing innovation in genetic engineering with ethical considerations surrounding consent, aiming to foster a responsible approach that prioritises individual rights while advancing scientific progress.

Case Studies and Precedents

The realm of genetic engineering and stem cell research is rife with case studies that illustrate the profound ethical implications of these technologies. One prominent case involves the use of embryonic stem cells, which has sparked significant debate regarding the moral status of embryos. For instance, the derivation of stem cells from human embryos raises questions about when life begins and the rights of the embryo versus the potential benefits to society. This case highlights the complexities of balancing scientific advancement with ethical considerations, a dilemma that continues to challenge researchers and healthcare professionals alike.

Another significant case is the development of CRISPR technology, which allows for precise gene editing in embryos. The controversy surrounding its use came to the forefront when a Chinese scientist claimed to have created the first genetically edited babies. This event ignited a global conversation about the ethics of gene editing, particularly concerning the long-term implications for humanity. The moral ramifications of editing human embryos extend beyond individual cases, pointing to broader societal concerns, including the potential for genetic discrimination and the exacerbation of social inequalities.

Additionally, the implications of stem cell therapies on societal inequalities cannot be overlooked. Evidence from various studies suggests that access to advanced stem cell treatments is often limited by socioeconomic status, leading to disparities in health outcomes. This raises ethical questions about justice and equity in healthcare, as those with fewer resources may be left behind in the advancements of genetic engineering. Such inequalities highlight the need for careful consideration of how these technologies are implemented and who benefits from them.

Religious perspectives also play a crucial role in shaping the discourse around stem cell research and genetic modification. Different faiths offer varied interpretations of the moral status of embryos and the acceptability of intervening in natural processes. These beliefs influence public opinion and can impact government regulations surrounding stem cell research. Understanding these diverse perspectives is essential for biomedical engineers and health care professionals to navigate the ethical landscape of their work.

Finally, the issue of consent, particularly regarding the use of genetic material from deceased individuals, presents another ethical challenge. The legal and ethical frameworks surrounding consent in genetic research are still evolving, and cases where such material is used without clear consent raise serious ethical concerns. This highlights the need for robust policies and regulations to protect individual rights while promoting scientific progress. As the field of genetic engineering continues to advance, these case studies serve as important precedents that inform the ongoing ethical dialogue in biomedical research.

Genetic Discrimination in Employment and Insurance

Overview of Genetic Discrimination

Genetic discrimination is an emerging concern in the wake of advancements in genetic engineering and biotechnology. As biomedical engineers and researchers delve deeper into the complexities of human genetics, the potential for discrimination based on genetic information becomes increasingly apparent. This phenomenon raises significant ethical and moral dilemmas, particularly regarding the implications of genetic data in various sectors, including employment and insurance. The prospect that individuals may be treated differently due to their genetic predispositions poses a challenge to the principles of equality and justice in society.

The implications of genetic discrimination extend beyond individual rights, affecting societal structures and health care access. With the increasing use of genetic testing, there is a risk that certain groups may face unfair treatment based on their genetic profiles. For example, individuals identified as having a higher risk for specific diseases might encounter barriers when seeking employment or health insurance. This situation highlights the urgent need for robust regulations and ethical guidelines to protect individuals from the misuse of genetic information.

Furthermore, the concept of 'designer babies' introduces another layer of complexity to the discussion of genetic discrimination. As genetic engineering technologies advance, the ability to select for desirable traits in embryos could lead to a societal divide between those who can afford such interventions and those who cannot. This disparity raises profound ethical questions about equity in health care and the moral status of genetically modified individuals. The potential for a new form of inequality based on genetic enhancements is a pressing concern within the biomedical community.

Religious perspectives also play a significant role in the discourse surrounding genetic discrimination and genetic engineering. Various faiths approach the moral status of embryos and the ethics of genetic modification differently, which can influence public opinion and policy decisions. Understanding these diverse viewpoints is essential for health care professionals and researchers as they navigate the ethical landscape of stem cell research and genetic technologies. Engaging with these perspectives can foster a more inclusive dialogue about the implications of genetic advancements.

In conclusion, the overview of genetic discrimination reveals a complex interplay of ethical, social, and legal issues that demand careful consideration. As advancements in genetic engineering continue to progress, it is imperative that biomedical engineers, health care professionals, and researchers advocate for ethical frameworks that safeguard against discrimination. By addressing these challenges head-on, the field can work towards a future where genetic advancements benefit all individuals equitably, rather than exacerbating existing inequalities.

Legal Protections and Gaps

The legal landscape surrounding genetic engineering and stem cell research is a complex tapestry of protections and gaps that reflect societal values and ethical considerations. In many countries, legislation governs the use of human embryos in research, with varying degrees of stringency. While some nations impose strict regulations to safeguard human rights and moral considerations, others adopt a more laissez-faire approach, allowing for greater experimentation. This inconsistency in legal frameworks creates a patchwork of protections that can lead to confusion and ethical dilemmas for biomedical engineers and health care professionals involved in this field.

One significant area of concern is the moral status of embryonic stem cells, which raises profound ethical questions regarding the rights of embryos. In jurisdictions where embryos are afforded legal protection, researchers must navigate the delicate balance between scientific advancement and respect for potential human life. This moral quandary is further complicated by differing religious perspectives, which influence public opinion and, consequently, legislative action. As a result, the ethical implications of using embryonic stem cells can vary dramatically across regions, presenting additional challenges for those working in stem cell research.

Moreover, the potential for genetic discrimination poses another layer of complexity in the legal framework surrounding genetic engineering. As advancements in gene editing technologies become more prevalent, concerns about how genetic information may be used in employment and insurance contexts have emerged. The lack of comprehensive legislation to protect individuals from genetic discrimination raises ethical issues about consent and the use of genetic material, particularly concerning deceased individuals. This gap in legal protections necessitates a critical examination of how society values genetic information and the rights of individuals in the face of rapid technological advancements.

The implications of stem cell therapies on societal inequalities also warrant attention. As these therapies become more accessible, there is a risk that disparities in health care access could widen, disproportionately affecting underprivileged groups. The ethical responsibility of biomedical engineers and health care professionals extends beyond the laboratory; they must advocate for equitable access to innovative therapies to prevent exacerbating existing health inequalities. Government regulation plays a pivotal role in ensuring that advancements in genetic engineering benefit society as a whole, rather than a privileged few.

In conclusion, the intersection of legal protections and ethical considerations in genetic engineering and stem cell research presents a multifaceted challenge. As the field continues to evolve, it is imperative for biomedical engineers, stem cell researchers, and health care professionals to engage in ongoing dialogue about the ethical implications of their work. This dialogue should encompass the moral status of embryos, the potential for discrimination, and the societal impact of emerging therapies, ensuring that the pursuit of scientific knowledge aligns with the protection of human rights and ethical standards.

Environmental Ethics Related to Genetic Engineering in Agriculture

Ethical Considerations in Agricultural Biotechnology

The ethical considerations surrounding agricultural biotechnology are vast and complex, particularly as they intersect with the fields of biomedical engineering and genetic research. One of the primary dilemmas is the moral status of genetically modified organisms (GMOs) and their impact on biodiversity. This raises questions about the long-term consequences of altering natural ecosystems and the potential for unforeseen ecological repercussions. As professionals in stem cell research and health care, it is essential to recognise the implications of these modifications not just on human health but also on environmental integrity.

Another significant ethical concern pertains to the rights of individuals and communities affected by agricultural biotechnology. The introduction of genetically engineered crops can lead to monopolistic practices by large corporations, often at the expense of small farmers and rural communities. This disparity can exacerbate existing societal inequalities and raises the question of consent regarding the use of genetic material sourced from local biodiversity. Such issues highlight the need for a regulatory framework that prioritises both human and environmental rights, ensuring equitable access to biotechnology benefits.

Moreover, the implications of gene editing technologies, such as CRISPR, extend beyond agriculture into the realm of human health, particularly in the context of 'designer babies'. This concept sparks intense debate about the ethical boundaries of genetic enhancement versus genetic modification aimed at disease prevention. Health care professionals must grapple with the moral implications of choosing traits for future generations, considering the potential for genetic discrimination in employment and insurance, which could arise from such technologies.

Religious perspectives also play a crucial role in shaping the ethical landscape of agricultural biotechnology. Different belief systems provide diverse viewpoints on the sanctity of life and the morality of manipulating genetic material. Engaging with these perspectives is vital for biomedical engineers and health care practitioners, as it fosters a more inclusive dialogue about the implications of genetic engineering and stem cell research. Understanding these beliefs can help navigate the ethical complexities and promote a more holistic approach to bioethics.

Finally, the role of government regulation is paramount in overseeing the ethical application of biotechnology in agriculture and health care. Effective governance can mitigate risks associated with genetic engineering by establishing clear guidelines and ethical standards. This regulatory framework is essential to ensure that advancements in biotechnology are pursued responsibly, balancing innovation with ethical considerations. As stakeholders in this field, it is our responsibility to advocate for regulations that safeguard human rights, promote social equity, and protect the environment while embracing the potential benefits of biotechnology.

Impacts on Biodiversity and Ecosystems

The implications of genetic engineering and stem cell research on biodiversity and ecosystems are profound and complex. As biomedical engineers and researchers delve into the manipulation of genetic material, the potential for unintended consequences on natural ecosystems arises. The creation of genetically modified organisms (GMOs), while aimed at improving human health and agricultural productivity, poses risks to existing species and their habitats. The interaction between engineered organisms and wild populations can lead to disruptions in ecological balance, raising significant concerns for the preservation of biodiversity.

One of the critical areas of concern is the alteration of species through genetic modification. The introduction of genetically engineered traits into wild populations can result in the loss of genetic diversity, which is vital for the resilience of ecosystems. For instance, crops engineered for pest resistance may unintentionally harm beneficial insects, leading to a cascade of ecological effects. This interconnection highlights the need for careful consideration of the ethical implications surrounding the release of genetically modified organisms into the environment, as it may infringe upon the rights of non-human species and their habitats.

Furthermore, the impacts on ecosystems extend beyond immediate ecological concerns to long-term sustainability issues. As stem cell therapies and genetic modifications become more prevalent, the potential for creating 'designer babies' raises ethical questions about the prioritisation of certain genetic traits over others.

This not only poses risks to human health but also challenges the natural evolutionary processes that have shaped biodiversity over millennia. The ethical dilemma lies in balancing the pursuit of advancements in healthcare with the responsibility to protect and preserve the intricate web of life on Earth.

The role of government regulation in overseeing genetic engineering practices becomes crucial in addressing these issues. Effective policies must be established to evaluate the ecological impacts of genetic modifications, ensuring that biodiversity is safeguarded. Additionally, regulations should encompass the ethical considerations surrounding consent and the utilisation of genetic material, particularly from deceased individuals. This highlights the intersection of human rights and environmental ethics, further complicating the landscape of genetic engineering.

In conclusion, the impacts of genetic engineering and stem cell research on biodiversity and ecosystems present significant ethical and moral dilemmas. As professionals in the biomedical field, it is imperative to engage in discussions that encompass not only the scientific advancements but also the broader implications for the environment. The future of genetic engineering must be navigated with caution, ensuring that the pursuit of human health does not come at the expense of the planet's ecological integrity.

Government Regulation in Stem Cell Research and Genetic Technologies

Overview of Current Regulations

The landscape of regulations surrounding genetic engineering and stem cell research is intricate and continually evolving. In many countries, legislation aims to balance the potential benefits of these technologies with ethical considerations and societal concerns. Regulatory frameworks vary significantly across jurisdictions, affecting the pace and direction of scientific advancement. For example, some nations have embraced permissive policies that encourage innovation, while others impose strict limitations to prevent perceived ethical transgressions.

Central to these regulations is the moral status of human embryos and the ethical implications of embryonic stem cell research. Debates continue regarding the definition of life and at what point human rights should be conferred. In some regions, laws explicitly prohibit the use of embryonic stem cells, reflecting prevailing religious and cultural beliefs that regard embryos as full human beings. This has led to a significant focus on alternative methods, such as induced pluripotent stem cells, which do not involve the destruction of embryos.

Gene editing technologies, particularly CRISPR, have prompted further regulatory scrutiny. The potential to edit human embryos raises profound ethical questions about 'designer babies' and the implications for future generations. Regulatory bodies are grappling with how to establish guidelines that ensure safety and efficacy while addressing concerns about moral hazards, such as genetic discrimination in employment and insurance. The challenge lies in creating a framework that allows for innovation while safeguarding against misuse.

In addition to domestic regulations, international guidelines play a crucial role in shaping research practices. The World Health Organisation and various ethical committees have sought to establish consensus on the ethical use of genetic technologies. These guidelines often reflect a collective understanding of human rights and ethical obligations, but the divergence in national laws can lead to conflicts, particularly in cross-border research collaborations. Ensuring compliance with both local and international standards remains a significant challenge for biomedical engineers and researchers.

Finally, the role of government regulation extends beyond ethical considerations to encompass societal implications. As advancements in stem cell therapies and genetic engineering continue, there is a growing concern about access and equity. Regulatory frameworks must address the potential for these technologies to exacerbate societal inequalities, ensuring that all individuals, regardless of socioeconomic status, have access to the benefits of scientific progress. This necessitates a comprehensive approach that includes public engagement and dialogue to foster understanding and trust in these emerging technologies.

The Role of Policy in Scientific Advancement

The relationship between policy and scientific advancement is critical in shaping the landscape of biomedical research, particularly in the fields of genetic engineering and stem cell research. Effective policy frameworks can facilitate innovation, ensure ethical compliance, and protect human rights. In contrast, inadequate or poorly designed policies can hinder progress, create confusion, and lead to ethical breaches. Policymakers must navigate complex moral dilemmas, such as the implications of embryonic stem cell research on human rights and the ethical considerations surrounding gene editing in human embryos.

One of the most pressing issues in this domain is the moral status of stem cells derived from human embryos. Policies must address the varying perspectives on when life begins and the rights of these cells versus the potential benefits they may offer for medical advancements. These discussions often intersect with religious beliefs, which can deeply influence public opinion and, consequently, policy decisions. A comprehensive policy approach requires the inclusion of diverse viewpoints to ensure a balanced and just framework that recognises the ethical complexities involved.

Moreover, the role of government regulation in stem cell research and genetic technologies cannot be overstated. Regulations must evolve alongside scientific advancements to ensure that ethical standards are upheld while promoting research that could lead to revolutionary therapies. This includes addressing concerns about genetic discrimination in employment and insurance, as well as the potential societal inequalities that may arise from the availability of advanced stem cell therapies. Policymakers must strive to create an equitable environment where all individuals have access to the benefits of genetic advancements.

Consent remains a critical issue in the use of genetic material, especially concerning deceased individuals. Clear policies must be established to respect the wishes of individuals and their families while allowing for scientific progress. This aspect of policy is vital in building public trust in genetic research and ensuring that ethical standards are maintained. Transparent guidelines can help mitigate misunderstandings and encourage broader acceptance of stem cell research and genetic engineering.

In conclusion, the role of policy in scientific advancement is multifaceted, particularly in the context of genetic engineering and stem cell research. Policymakers must take into account the ethical implications, societal impacts, and diverse perspectives surrounding these technologies. By doing so, they can foster an environment that not only encourages scientific innovation but also protects human rights and promotes social equity. The ongoing dialogue between scientists, ethicists, and policymakers is essential for navigating the complex landscape of biomedical research in a responsible and ethical manner.

Future Directions in Genetic Engineering and Ethical Considerations

Emerging Technologies

Emerging technologies in genetic engineering and stem cell research have the potential to revolutionise healthcare, but they also pose significant ethical and moral dilemmas. The manipulation of human embryos raises questions about the moral status of these entities, leading to heated debates among scientists, ethicists, and policymakers. As biomedical engineers and health professionals explore the possibilities of creating 'designer babies', they must grapple with the implications of such advancements on human rights and societal values, ensuring that scientific progress does not come at the expense of ethical considerations.

The implications of embryonic stem cell research are profound, particularly regarding human rights. The ability to derive pluripotent stem cells from embryos allows for breakthroughs in regenerative medicine, but it also necessitates a careful examination of the rights of the embryos themselves. This intersection of science and ethics demands that healthcare professionals engage in ongoing discussions about the moral status of these cells, as well as the potential for exploitation of vulnerable populations in the pursuit of scientific knowledge.

Gene editing technologies, such as CRISPR, have opened new avenues for correcting genetic disorders but raise ethical concerns regarding their use in human embryos. The prospect of editing the human germline poses questions about consent, particularly when considering the future generations who would inherit these modifications. Furthermore, the potential for genetic discrimination in employment and insurance underscores the need for robust ethical frameworks and regulations to protect individuals from the unintended consequences of genetic enhancements.

Societal inequalities may also be exacerbated by advancements in stem cell therapies and genetic engineering. Access to these cutting-edge treatments is often limited to those with financial means, potentially widening the gap between different socioeconomic groups. As health care professionals, it is critical to advocate for equitable access to these technologies, ensuring that all individuals have the opportunity to benefit from scientific advancements regardless of their background or financial status.

Finally, religious perspectives on stem cell research and genetic modification add another layer of complexity to the ethical landscape. Diverse beliefs about the sanctity of life and the moral considerations surrounding genetic interventions must be acknowledged in any comprehensive debate on these issues. Government regulation will play a vital role in navigating these ethical waters, as policymakers must balance scientific innovation with the moral concerns of society, safeguarding human rights while fostering a responsible approach to genetic research.

Preparing for Ethical Challenges Ahead

As we advance into the realm of genetic engineering and stem cell research, it is imperative that biomedical engineers, stem cell researchers, health care professionals, and students prepare for the ethical challenges that lie ahead. The rapid pace of scientific innovation brings with it not only groundbreaking possibilities but also significant moral dilemmas. Key among these are the implications of embryonic stem cell research on human rights, which necessitate a thoughtful examination of how we define and protect the rights of all human beings, including those not yet born.

The ethics of gene editing in human embryos represents another complex area of concern. With technologies such as CRISPR-Cas9 enabling unprecedented genetic modifications, questions arise about the moral status of the embryos involved. Should we consider the potential benefits of eradicating genetic diseases against the ethical implications of altering human biology? A robust dialogue among all stakeholders is essential to navigate these treacherous waters responsibly.

Moreover, the concept of 'designer babies' poses significant risks that extend beyond individual choice into societal inequalities. Genetic engineering has the potential to exacerbate existing disparities, particularly if access to such technologies is limited to affluent families. This raises urgent questions about fairness and justice in health care, as well as the potential for genetic discrimination in employment and insurance, which could further entrench social divides and marginalise vulnerable populations.

Religious perspectives also play a crucial role in shaping public discourse on stem cell research and genetic modification. Different faiths offer varied interpretations of the moral implications surrounding the creation and manipulation of life. Engaging with these perspectives is vital for creating an inclusive dialogue that respects diverse beliefs while striving for ethical consensus in scientific practices.

Lastly, the role of government regulation cannot be underestimated in addressing these ethical challenges. Effective oversight is essential to ensure that advancements in genetic technologies align with societal values and ethical standards. By fostering a collaborative environment where researchers, ethicists, policymakers, and the public can engage, we can better prepare for the moral complexities that genetic engineering and stem cell research will undoubtedly present in the future.

Conclusion

Summary of Key Findings

The exploration of genetic engineering and stem cell research has unveiled significant findings that underscore the complex interplay between science, ethics, and society. One of the foremost issues identified is the ethical and moral dilemmas that arise from embryonic stem cell research. This research often raises questions about the moral status of embryos and the implications of manipulating human life at its earliest stages. The balance between potential medical breakthroughs and respecting human rights remains a contentious debate among biomedical engineers and health care professionals alike.

Furthermore, the advancements in gene editing technologies, particularly CRISPR, have sparked discussions about the ethics of modifying human embryos. The potential to create 'designer babies' poses unique challenges, as it combines the promise of eradicating genetic disorders with the fear of exacerbating societal inequalities. The implications of such technologies extend beyond individual health, raising concerns about genetic discrimination in employment and insurance, as well as the broader societal impact of creating genetically modified individuals.

Another critical finding pertains to the religious perspectives on stem cell research and genetic modification. Various faiths offer differing views on the acceptability of these practices, often rooted in beliefs about the sanctity of life. This divergence highlights the necessity for inclusive dialogue among stakeholders to navigate the ethical landscape of stem cell research and genetic engineering. Engaging diverse viewpoints can aid in developing frameworks that respect both scientific advancement and moral considerations.

Moreover, consent and the use of genetic material from deceased individuals have emerged as vital topics in the discourse surrounding genetic engineering. The ethical implications of utilising such materials without clear consent raise questions about autonomy and respect for the deceased. It is essential for health care professionals to advocate for stringent regulations that uphold ethical standards in the use of genetic materials, ensuring that practices align with societal values and individual rights.

Lastly, the role of government regulation in overseeing stem cell research and genetic technologies is crucial in shaping the future of biomedical innovation. Striking a balance between encouraging scientific progress and safeguarding ethical standards is imperative. Regulatory frameworks must evolve to address the rapid advancements in genetic engineering while considering the potential environmental impacts and societal inequalities that may arise from these technologies. The findings suggest that a collaborative approach, involving researchers, ethicists, and policymakers, is essential for fostering responsible innovation in the field of genetic engineering and stem cell research.

The Path Forward in Ethical Genetic Engineering

As we navigate the future of ethical genetic engineering, it is crucial to confront the myriad of moral dilemmas that accompany advancements in this field. Biomedical engineers and researchers must grapple with the implications of embryonic stem cell research, particularly regarding the moral status of stem cells derived from human embryos. The discussion surrounding the ethical treatment of these cells raises questions about human rights and the responsibilities of scientists in their pursuit of knowledge and innovation. A thoughtful approach is necessary to ensure that progress does not come at the expense of ethical standards that protect human dignity.

The ethics of gene editing in human embryos has gained significant attention in recent years, especially with the advent of technologies such as CRISPR. These tools present unprecedented opportunities to eradicate genetic disorders, yet they also pose ethical questions about 'designer babies' and the potential for genetic discrimination. Healthcare professionals must engage in dialogue about the long-term societal implications of editing the human genome, particularly in how it may exacerbate existing inequalities in healthcare and access to these technologies. Ensuring equitable access to genetic engineering advancements is essential to prevent a widening gap between different socioeconomic groups.

Religious perspectives also play a vital role in shaping the ethical landscape of stem cell research and genetic modification. Many faith traditions have specific teachings regarding the sanctity of life and the moral implications of manipulating human genetics. Engaging with diverse religious viewpoints can foster a more comprehensive ethical framework that respects the beliefs of various communities. Such dialogue is essential in establishing a consensus that honours both scientific advancement and the moral convictions of different cultures.

Consent is another critical aspect of ethical genetic engineering, particularly regarding the use of genetic material from deceased individuals. The complexities surrounding consent highlight the need for clear guidelines and regulations to protect the rights of individuals and their families. As the field progresses, it is imperative for biomedical engineers and researchers to advocate for ethical practices that prioritise informed consent and respect for the deceased and their legacy.

Finally, the role of government regulation in stem cell research and genetic technologies cannot be overstated. Effective regulation is necessary to ensure that research is conducted ethically and that the interests of society are safeguarded. Policymakers must consider the potential for genetic discrimination in employment and insurance, as well as the environmental implications of genetic engineering in agriculture. A robust regulatory framework can help to mitigate these risks while promoting innovation and responsible scientific exploration.

Pause for Thought

- Genetic engineering is a revolutionary groundbreaking field in biomedical research and healthcare. This involves the manipulation of an organism's DNA to achieve desired traits whether for therapeutic purposes or enhancements.

- This can be applied in stem cell research where the potential to modify embryonic stem cell could lead to advancement in regenerative medicine. However, the rapid evolution of these technologies raises the sceptre of ethical and moral dilemmas.

- Arising from genetic engineering is the notion of designer babies, that is the creation of individuals with specific traits leading to significant ethical debates. The implications for exacerbation of societal inequalities and access limited to those with the financial means has been the focus of much discussion.

- Critical questions about fairness and justice in healthcare were triggered as well as the potential for genetic discrimination in employment and insurance.

- The concept of designer babies arose from infants whose genetic characteristics have been satisfactorily selected or modified through advanced genetic engineering techniques. The origins of genetic engineering can be traced back to the early 1970's with the advent of recombinant DNA technology in which scientist were able to splice genes from one organism into another.

- The ethics of gene editing in human embryo's particularly with technologies as CRISPR-Cas9, further complicated the dialogue surrounding designer babies. Some believe that gene editing can eliminate genetic disorders and enhance human capabilities while others warn of its potential for unforeseen consequences and the slippery slope towards eugenics. Society is therefore left to grapple with the implications of altering human genetics and the societal inequalities that may arise from such technologies.

- Human rights considerations have been part of a significant debate as genetic engineering and stem cell research are advanced. Biomedical engineers and health care professionals continue to grapple with the ethical implications of their work, particularly regarding the moral status of embryos. This raises the questions about whether embryos should be awarded the same rights as fully developed individuals and how these rights may influence research practices and regulatory framework.

- The ability to select for certain traits could lead to a new form of discrimination based on genetic predisposition, thereby exacerbating existing social disparities. Biomedical engineers must be clear on how these innovations might contribute to or alleviate inequalities in access to health care and genetic technologies.

- Consent regarding the use of genetic material from deceased individuals is an aspect of human rights that that cannot be overlooked. The ethical implications of using such genetic material without explicit consent pose significant challenges especially when considering the rights of individuals and their families. This underscores the necessity for robust ethical guidelines and regulatory oversight to ensure that the right of all involved patients is protected and respected.

- As the landscape of genetic engineering and stem cell research continue to evolve, it is imperative for professionals in the field to engage with moral and ethical challenges that arise. The intersection of human rights, genetic technologies, and societal implications demand ongoing dialogue and reflection.

Take Home Nuggets

- By prioritising ethical considerations, biomedical engineers and health care professionals can contribute to a future where advancement in genetic research align with the protection of human dignity and rights.

- The debate on personhood continues, the debate revolves around defining the beginning of human life and the prerequisite criterion to be considered a person. This is particularly important for embryonic stem cell research where the destruction of embryos for scientific purposes raises concerns about the moral status of the embryo.

- An ethical dilemma related to personhood is the implications for human rights. If embryos are granted personhood status, it would lead to restrictions on research that uses embryonic stem cells which could stifle advancement in regenerative medicine.

- Denying personhood to embryos may lead to practices that are ethically questionable maybe even repulsive. This therefore indicates the need for a careful balancing act between advancing scientific research and respecting moral beliefs about the sanctity of life. Thus policy makers face the challenge of promoting scientific advancement and protecting individual rights and t that end government regulations play a pivotal role in overseeing stem cell research and genetic technologies, they must consider the broader implications for the environment and society.

- The ethical frameworks surrounding gene editing are complex and multifaceted, as they relate to the emerging field of genetic engineering. As biomedical engineers and health care professionals grapple with implications of their work, it is necessary to establish a set of guiding principles that can navigate the moral dilemmas inherent in this technology. The frameworks use philosophical pillars for support example, utilitarianism which evaluates the consequences of actions whilst deontological ethics focuses on the morality of actions themselves. This allows for a better understanding of the ethical landscape of gene editing and its societal impact.

- The legal landscape surrounding genetic engineering and stem cell research is complex and multifaceted, reflecting a broad spectrum of ethical, moral and societal concerns. Legislation varies significantly from country to country, with some nations embracing genetic modification technologies while others impose strict prohibitions. This diversity underscores the necessity for a coherent legal framework that addresses the scientific possibilities as well as the ethical dilemmas inherent in such technologies. As laws evolve, they must balance scientific progress with respect for human rights and dignity. Legislatures are tasked in ensuring that the rights of individuals are not overlooked in the pursuit of medical and scientific advancement.

- The implications of embryonic stem cell are profound as they intersect with various human rights concerns. The debate often centres on the moral status of embryos and whether they should be afforded the same ethical considerations as fully developed humans. The ongoing discussion on the ethics of gene editing in human embryo further complicates access, as it raises issues of consent, potential misuse and long-term societal impact.

- Major religions and their belief system impact the ethical landscape associated with stem cell research and genetic modification. Different faiths have unique perspectives on the sanctity of life, moral status of the embryo and the implications of altering human genetics. Many Christian denominations view the embryo as a sacred creation, leading to opposition against embryonic stem research. More liberal religious groups may accept focus of genetic modification if they contribute to healing and alleviate suffering. This reveals the complex interplay between faith, ethics and scientific advancement.

- Islam's view on genetic engineering sees the preservation of life and health as paramount. Here scholars debate the permissibility of genetic modifications, often emphasising the importance of intention behind such interventions. If genetic engineering serves to prevent disease or enhance quality of life, it may be viewed more favourably. Buddhism introduces the concept of suffering and compassion. The potential benefits of stem cells research must be weighed against the possible harms to both individuals and society. Judaism on the other hand approaches the subject of stem cell research with a balance of innovation and caution. Here the preservation of life is a core tenet, leading to support for research that can save lives.

www.ingramcontent.com/pod-product-compliance
Lightning Source LLC
Chambersburg PA
CBHW081207130726
47997CB00009B/2585